CORONARY ANGIOGRAPHY – THE NEED FOR IMPROVEMENT IN MEDICAL AND INTERVENTIONAL THERAPY

Edited by **Branislav Baškot**

Coronary Angiography – The Need for Improvement in Medical and Interventional Therapy
Edited by Branislav Baškot

Published by InTech
Janeza Trdine 9, 51000 Rijeka, Croatia

Publishing Process Manager Iva Simcic

Technical Editor Teodora Smiljanic

Cover Designer InTech Design Team

Additional hard copies can be obtained from orders@intechopen.com

Coronary Angiography – The Need for Improvement in Medical
and Interventional Therapy, Edited by Branislav Baškot
p. cm.
ISBN 978-953-307-641-6

For EU product safety concerns:
IN TECH d.o.o., Prolaz Marije Krucifikse Kozulić 3, 51000 Rijeka, Croatia,
info@intechopen.com or visit our website at intechopen.com.

Meet the editor

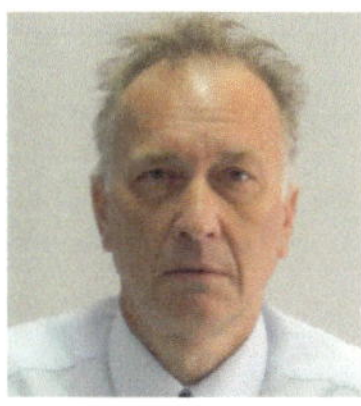

Dr. Branislav Baskot, MD PhD. Assistent Professor; was born 1958. in Ruma, Serbia. He finished Medicine Faculty in Sarajevo, Bosnia and Hercegovina, and specialization of Nuclear Medicine on Military Medical Academy in Belgrade, Serbia in 1994. The main occupation in the field of Nuclear medicine was nuclear cardiology. He obtained his Doctoral degree in 2005.; "Determination of culprit lesion before and after percutaneous coronary intervention by myocardial perfusion imaging" and Master's Degree; "Myocardial perfusion imaging with 99mTc-Tetrofosmin in the diagnosis ischemic heart disease" in 2003. He is an Associate professor of medicine, on Institute of Nuclear Medicine Medical Military Academy Belgrade, Serbia; Associate Professor on US Medical School, the first private medical school in Belgrade, Serbia; Associate Professor on European University Belgrade, Serbia; and Director and owner Department of Nuclear Medicine in Belgrade, Serbia.

Contents

Preface

The mortality from ischemic heart disease has decreased in recent years. The better understanding of risk factors associated with development of coronary artery disease (CAD) has significantly contributed to this decline. Preventive measures such as aggressive therapy of arterial hypertension, diabetes mellitus, and lipid disorders and by campaigning against the smoking are important components of this medical success. Furthermore, improvements in medical and interventional therapy have reduced the complications associated with acute myocardial infarction as well as revascularization.

Interventional cardiology is a branch of cardiology and Andreas Gruentzig is considered the father of interventional cardiology after the development of angioplasty by interventional radiologist Dr Charles Dotter. As we know, interventional procedures have been complicated by restenosis due to the formation of endothelial tissue overgrowth at the lesion site. Restenosis is the body's response to the injury of the vessel wall from angioplasty and to stent as a foreign body. As opposed to bare metal stent, drug eluting stents are covered with a medicine that is slowly dispersed with the goal of suppressing the restenosis reaction. One of the newest innovations in coronary stents is the development of a dissolving stent. Abbott laboratory has used a dissolvable material, polilactic acid that will completely absorb within two years of being implanted. Other key changes happened along the way. Perhaps the most important changes were a modification in mindset so that physicians demonstrated that they could successfully work less invasively within the vascular three. This changes leads to the development of invasive electrophysiologic procedures, such as mapping and ablation, percutaneous application of technology to treat valvular heart disease, and application of percutaneous technologies to treat peripheral arterial disease, and now cerebrovascular disease. Percutaneous methods initially introduced by interventional cardiologists should become the treatment of choice for a multiplicity of cardiovascular conditions.

But we also examined in this book a periprocedural complication of coronary angiography, and coronary intervention. That includes related to cardiac catheterization and diagnostic coronary angiography, and those that occur as a consequence of the specific equipment. However, improvements in devices, the use of stents, and aggressive antiplatelet therapy have significantly reduced the incident of major periprocedural complications, and as an example, the need of emergent coronary artery bypass surgery decreased from 1.5 % in early 90, to 0.14% after 2000 year.

This book should prove to be useful reference for cardiologists, radiologists, nuclear medicine physicians, anesthesiologists, cardiac surgeons, internists and basis scientists, their trainees and medical students who have an interest in this field either from the technical aspects or from clinical viewpoint.

Branislav Baškot MD PhD Ass Prof
Department of Nuclear Medicine Imaging
"Dr Baskot" Belgrade, Serbia

1

Primary Percutaneous Coronary Intervention for ST–Elevation Myocardial Infarction and Door-to-Balloon Time: A Catheterization Laboratory Perspective

Darryl D. Prime and Robert J. Applegate
Wake Forest School of Medicine
United States of America

1. Introduction

Rapid reperfusion improves mortality in patients with acute ST- elevation myocardial infarction (STEMI). Moreover, achieving reperfusion by primary percutaneous coronary intervention (PCI) instead of fibrinolytic therapy is preferred because patients have less strokes, less nonfatal reinfarctions, and a lower mortality rate (Keeley et al., 2003). However, because achieving perfusion with primary PCI sometimes involves transporting patients from the location where the diagnosis was made to a catheterization laboratory, and once in the catheterization laboratory numerous technical and clinical problems must be successfully managed, there is a significant time delay. In some studies, this time delay has been associated with an increased mortality (Boersma, 2006; Nallamothu and Bates, 2003). Furthermore, the advantages of primary PCI over thrombolytic therapy may be negated if the time to reperfusion with primary PCI exceeds that of fibrinolytic therapy by one hour or more (Nallamothu and Bates, 2003). In absolute terms, when patients are selected for the primary PCI strategy, every minute of delay to reperfusion affects the one-year mortality. In one study, the one-year mortality was increased by 7.5% for every 30 minute delay (De Luca et al., 2004). With these factors in mind, the American Heart Association/American College of Cardiology (AHA/ACC) guidelines for STEMI recommend that the interval between arrival at the hospital and treatment of the coronary lesion with a balloon inflation (door-to-balloon time) should be 90 minutes or less (Antman et al., 2004). Conjointly, in the United States the Centers for Medicare and Medicaid Services (CMS) and the Joint Commission on Accreditation of Healthcare Organizations have included this goal as one of their core quality measures. Subsequently, institutions responsible for quality improvement in patients with STEMI were created to focus on factors that increase door-to-balloon times (Singh and Harrington, 2007). Most of the barriers that affect the time interval from patient presentation to the arrival of the patient in the catheterization laboratory have been identified and significant improvements have been made (Bradley et al., 2006; Kraft et al., 2007). Less attention, however, has been directed toward reducing delays after the patient enters the catheterization lab. This chapter will focus on methods clinicians have used to decrease the time between establishment of arterial access and successful coronary reperfusion in patients with STEMI.

2. Electrocardiogram (EKG) - directed PCI in patients with STEMI

In patients with STEMI, an EKG is an essential roadmap if the culprit vessel is visualized and then treated first before performing any other diagnostics. In a retrospective study, Lachance and colleagues used the EKG to determine the culprit vessel in patients undergoing primary PCI for STEMI. In one group, they imaged and then immediately percutaneously treated the culprit vessel before performing a complete coronary and left ventricular evaluation. In another group, they performed complete coronary catheterization and then PCI. Acute myocardial infarction by EKG was defined as chest pain or the equivalent symptoms at rest greater than 30 minutes, with either ST-segment elevation in greater than two contiguous leads (greater than 2 mm in the precordial lead, greater than 1 mm in the limb lead), ST-segment depression greater than 1 mm in the precordial leads, or new or presumed new left bundle branch block (LBBB). In the group where the culprit vessel was treated first, the actual culprit vessel was the presumed culprit vessel by EKG most of the time. Specifically, the EKG correctly diagnosed the culprit vessel in 83 of these 87 patients (95%). In this study, however, patients who had previous coronary artery bypass surgery (CABG) and those with thrombolysis in myocardial infarction (TIMI) 2 to 3 flow in the culprit vessel were excluded from the analysis (LaChance et al., 2008). Similarly, in the retrospective study by Applegate and colleagues, an EKG in the emergency room determined the presumed culprit vessel in the culprit PCI group. The presumed culprit vessel was the actual culprit vessel in 49 of the 50 patients. In one patient, a right coronary guide was chosen but the culprit vessel was a distal dominant left circumflex coronary artery. Left main or severe three-vessel coronary artery disease was found in only 2% of the patients in the culprit vessel group (Applegate et al., 2008).

3. Arterial access

In the catheterization laboratory, several critical but time-consuming steps are performed to help make important decisions not only about revascularization, but also about overall patient management. The first of these involves the location of arterial access. The most common access routes include the femoral, the brachial and the radial artery. In patients undergoing PCI for STEMI, various potent antiplatelet and anticoagulant therapies are required. As a result, bleeding at vascular access sites, particularly the femoral artery, is an important and common cause of morbidity and mortality (Hetherington et al., 2009). Comparatively, the radial artery in this setting, has been associated with minimal or no bleeding complications. Despite this, the femoral artery has been the access site of choice in the United States. Reasons for this include the learning curve associated with performing cardiac catheterizations via the radial artery, and difficulty achieving radial access in certain patients despite having considerable experience. With good reason, operators have been concerned that these difficulties may increase door to balloon times. Several studies have evaluated this concern. Cantor and colleagues in a small multicenter study randomized 50 patients with acute myocardial infarction requiring either primary or rescue PCI to radial or femoral access. Operators in this study had significant experience with the transradial approach. They reported their times from local anesthesia to first balloon inflation at 32 (25th percentile 26, 75th percentile 38) minutes for radial access and 26 minutes (25th percentile 22, 75th percentile 33) for femoral access (P=0.04). Reperfusion success rates were high and comparable with either approach (Cantor et al., 2005). In another randomized study, however, not only were the success rates for perfusion high and similar in both groups, procedure time was less in the transradial group compared to the transfemoral group (44 minutes ± 18, versus 51 minutes ± 21) (Saito et al., 2003). Non-randomized studies investigating these approaches in patients with STEMI, where the location of access is left to the discretion of the interventionalists, have reported lower or similar access to reperfusion times with the transradial approach compared to the femoral approach (Hetherington et al., 2009; Larrazet et al., 2003; Pancholy et al., 2010; Weaver et al., 2010).

These data suggest that the transradial approach may be preferable to the transfemoral approach in patients being treated for STEMI. Furthermore, in patients where femoral access is extremely difficult to obtain, the radial artery provides an attractive alternative. As attractive as the radial approach may seem, there are important points to highlight. There is a significant learning curve associated with radial access. In studies where low failure rates via the radial artery approach were reported, most of the operators already performed more than 1000 radial cardiac catheterizations (Agostoni et al., 2004). In addition, in the non-randomized studies where the choice of access was left to the discretion of the operator, patients with coronary artery bypass grafts of unknown anatomy were more likely to have been performed via the femoral approach. Also, access site crossover is higher when the radial artery access is used. That is, if the initial approach by the radial artery is unsuccessful the procedure has to be performed via the femoral approach. Consistently, a crossover rate of 7% has been observed in most of the studies investigating these approaches. Lastly, the radial approach is often limited by the size of the sheath (not more than 6 French). Placing a 7 or 8 French sheath, which can help provide more support during the procedure, is associated with a higher risk of radial arterial spasm, and thus a lower procedural success rate (Agostoni et al., 2004; Weaver et al., 2010). Despite these obstacles, it seems that a catheterization laboratory team dedicated to the radial approach can achieve comparative door to balloon times with the benefit of decreased morbidity and mortality related to major bleeding in patients with STEMI.

There are little data comparing brachial arteriotomy with other locations of vascular access in patients undergoing PCI for STEMI. In general the brachial approach, like the radial artery approach, is used in patients with severe peripheral vascular disease, or where there is an increased risk of bleeding (due to anticoagulation or recent thrombolytic therapy). Another advantage of this approach, as opposed to the radial artery is the ability to use 7 French or greater catheter sizes. Complications with the brachial artery, however, include median nerve injury from compression by a hematoma, which can potentially lead to irreversible nerve damage. Thus in our laboratory, the radial artery is preferred over the brachial artery for vascular access in selected patients with STEMI.

4. Culprit vessel PCI versus traditional catheterization and PCI for STEMI: Door to balloon times

Comprehensive coronary angiography can identify STEMI patients who may benefit from an urgent surgical approach. Left ventriculography can quantify left ventricular function, left ventricular end-diastolic pressure; exclude mechanical complications including mitral regurgitation, pseudoaneurysms or a ventricular septal defect. This strategy also allows identification of left main and severe three-vessel coronary artery disease upfront. Performing EKG-directed directed PCI, however, after achieving arterial access and prior to routine coronary angiography with or without left ventriculography has been shown to decrease door to balloon times in two small studies (Applegate et al., 2008; LaChance et al., 2008).

In the first study, Applegate and colleagues reviewed 135 consecutive patients who underwent primary PCI for STEMI from July 2005 to June 2007. During the study period, five patients who underwent primary PCI for STEMI were excluded because of incomplete door-to-balloon time data. No other patients were excluded from this analysis. Eighty-five STEMI patients who underwent complete coronary angiography followed by culprit lesion PCI served as the control group. The study group consisted of 50 STEMI patients who first underwent culprit PCI followed by complete coronary angiography. The strategy for achieving reperfusion was at the discretion of the interventionalist performing the procedure. During the study period, six interventionalists performed primary PCI for STEMI. Concern about performing PCI prior to the availability of information from complete coronary angiography, prior coronary artery bypass graft surgery (CABG) and indicators of cardiogenic shock on admission were factors in determining the decision to perform culprit versus traditional PCI by some interventionalists (Applegate et al., 2008).

In the traditional PCI group, vascular access was obtained using the femoral approach. Complete coronary angiography was then performed followed by left ventriculography at the discretion of the interventional cardiologist. Identification of the culprit lesion was based on composite assessment of the ECG, coronary angiogram, and left ventriculogram if available. The choice of equipment for PCI was left to the discretion of the attending physician performing the procedure, including guide catheter shape and size (6 or 7 French). In the culprit PCI group, the location of the presumed infarct lesion was based only on the initial ECG obtained in the emergency department. In these patients, after vascular access was obtained, a guide catheter was advanced and PCI was performed immediately, prior to complete coronary angiography or left ventriculography. Following PCI, coronary angiography was completed, with left ventriculography performed at the discretion of the interventionalist.

The baseline clinical characteristics of the culprit and traditional groups were similar although patients were younger in the culprit vessel group (56 ± 10 years versus 60 ± 13 years) versus the traditional group, p=0.029 (Table 1). The target vessel was more often the right coronary artery (70% versus 49%, p=0.020) in the culprit versus the traditional group. Procedural characteristics were similar, although fewer drug-eluting stents were used in the culprit vessel group (60%) compared to the traditional group (76%, p=0.043). Door-to-balloon times were shorter in the culprit vessel group (66 ± 20 minutes) than in the traditional group (79 ± 28 minutes, p=0.003). This was achieved primarily because of a shorter vascular access-to-balloon time in the culprit group (11 ± 8 minutes) than in the traditional group (18 ± 8 minutes, p<0.001). Door-to-vascular access times were similar for the two groups: 55 ± 18 minutes in the culprit group, versus 61 ± 24 minutes in the traditional group; p=0.10. Ninety- two percent of the culprit group patients achieved a door-to-balloon time <90 minutes, compared to 76% in the traditional group; p=0.023. In 62% of the traditional PCI group, left ventriculography was performed after the PCI. Door-to-balloon times were still significantly lower in the culprit vessel PCI group (17 ± 9 minutes) than in this subgroup of traditional PCI patients (22 ± 7 minutes; p<0.001).

Thirty-day outcomes are shown in Table 2. Planned revascularization procedures after the index PCI were performed in two culprit vessel patients, and in 1 traditional patient; p=0.28.

Characteristic	Traditional PCI {n = 85}	Culprit Vessel PCI {n = 50}	p Value
Male gender, n {%}	70 {82}	39 {78}	0.536
Age, years	60 ± 13	56 ± 10	0.029
Heart failure class III or IV, n {%}	5 {6}	1 {2}	0.412
Current smoker, n {%}	48 {56}	27 {54}	0.780
Diabetes mellitus, n {%}	18 {21}	10 {20}	0.871
Hypertension, n {%}	56 {66}	31 {62}	0.649
Hypercholesterolemia, n {%}	47 {55}	35 {70}	0.091
Vascular disease, n {%}	9 {11}	3 {6}	0.366
History of renal failure, n {%}	3 {4}	1 {2}	0.613
Previous PCI, n {%}	20 {24}	17 {34}	0.188
Previous CABG, n {%}	5 {6}	3 {6}	0.978
Left ventricular ejection fraction, {%}	45 ± 10	45 ± 9	0.921
Vessels disease, n	1.7 ± 0.8	1.6 ± 0.8	0.512
Severe 3-vessel or LMCA disease, n {%}	7 {8}	1{2}	0.138
Cardiogenic shock, n {%}	6 {7}	2 {4}	0.467
IABP inserted, n {%}	6 {7}	2 {4}	0.467
CABG = coronary artery bypass surgery, IABP = intra-aortic balloon pump; LMCA = left main coronary artery disease; PCI = percutaneous coronary intervention			

Table 1. Baseline clinical characteristics by percutaneous coronary intervention method.

Outcome	Traditional PCI {n = 85}	Culprit Vessel PCI {n = 50}	p Value
Planned revascularization, n {%}	1 {1.2}	2 {4.0}	0.283
Death, n {%}	1 {1.4}	1 {2.0}	0.702
Nonfatal MI, n {%}	0 {0}	0 {0}	---
Nonfatal MI or death, n {%}	1 {1.4}	1 {2.0}	0.702
Stent thrombosis, n {%}	0 {0}	0 {0}	---
Target vessel revascularization, n {%}	0 {0}	0 {0}	---
Any major adverse cardiac event, n {%}	1 {1.4}	1 {2.0}	0.702
MI = myocardial infarction; PCI = percutaneous coronary intervention			

Table 2. Major adverse cardiac events out to 1 month by percutaneous coronary intervention method.

There were no stent thromboses or recurrent nonfatal MIs in either group after 30 days of follow up. One patient in each group died during the initial hospitalization (*p*=0.70), and none thereafter.
In this study, door-to-balloon times were reduced when culprit vessel PCI was performed before complete coronary angiography and left ventriculography. The benefit was due to a decrease in the vascular access-to-balloon time of 7 minutes. Importantly, this benefit was achieved when efforts to reduce door-to-balloon times under 90 minutes had already been implemented, with an average door-to- balloon time of 79 minutes in the traditional PCI group. Significant left main or three-vessel coronary artery disease, cardiogenic shock or mechanical complications of MI were infrequently observed and were similar in each group. Specifically, severe three vessel or left main coronary artery disease was seen in 8% of the traditional PCI patients and in 2% of the culprit vessel PCI patients (p=0.138). Cardiogenic shock was seen in 7% of the traditional PCI patients and 4% of the culprit vessel PCI patients (p=0.467). In this study, no mechanical complications were diagnosed by ventriculography. In-hospital and thirty-day outcomes were similar between the two groups.
A similar study performed by Lachance and colleagues compared the door-to-balloon times in a group of STEMI patients assigned to EKG-guided culprit vessel PCI (group 1) and another group assigned to traditional PCI (group 2) retrospectively (Lachance et al., 2008). Two hundred and seventy-nine patients were included in the analysis. These consecutive patients underwent primary PCI at Laval Hospital, Quebec, Canada between May 2006 and August 2007. Eighty-seven patients were in the first group and 192 patients were in the second group. The type of procedural strategy was left to the discretion of the interventionalists. The baseline characteristics, including clinical, procedural and lesion type, were similar between the two groups. Median catheterization lab door-to-balloon times were 21 minutes in group 1 and 25.5 minutes in group 2 (P<0.0001). The median door-to-balloon time was 80 minutes for patients in group 1 and 90 minutes for patients in group 2 (p=0.01). Compared to group 2, more patients in group 1 received reperfusion in less than 90 minutes (63% versus 49%; p=0.04). Three STEMI patients in this cohort were referred for coronary artery bypass surgery. One patient, who had an anterior MI, was in group 2. This patient had a diagnostic right coronary angiogram performed, which revealed moderate stenosis. The left coronary angiogram then revealed severe stenosis of the left main artery and occlusion of the left anterior descending artery. The patient was then referred for urgent coronary artery bypass grafting. The second patient was in group 1 and presented with ST-elevations in the inferior leads. An angiogram of the right coronary artery was performed with a guiding catheter and no significant stenosis was seen. Coronary angiography of the left coronary artery revealed a severe stenosis of the left main. This patient underwent coronary artery bypass grafting two days after coronary angiography. The third patient presented in cardiogenic shock and an echocardiogram was performed before coronary angiography. This revealed a ventricular septal defect and mitral regurgitation. The patient was then referred for urgent cardiac surgery. In the study by Lachance, no mechanical complications were diagnosed by ventriculography. After one year of clinical follow-up, there was no difference between groups in rates of death, reinfarctions, or need for repeat PCI. Because these are small retrospective studies, however, further studies are needed not only to determine if the culprit vessel PCI strategy for STEMI consistently lowers door-to-balloon times, but also, if it improves clinical outcomes.

Observational studies such as ours and that of Lachance may be subject to selection bias. Randomized clinical trials would provide the fairest evaluation of culprit vessel versus traditional PCI for STEMI. The decision to perform culprit versus traditional PCI could have been influenced by important patient and procedural factors that relate to the outcomes of the study, such as age, prior PCI or CABG, and infarct location. While we cannot exclude this possibility, culprit and traditional patient groups had similar baseline clinical and lesion characteristics in both these studies. Moreover, among the interventionalists performing culprit PCI for STEMI, no patient or procedural factors seemed to influence strongly the decision to perform culprit PCI. While there remains a concern that discovery of important clinical information after first performing culprit PCI would surface, in both these studies, this was observed infrequently. These concerns need to be evaluated in larger groups of patients before accepting this strategy as standard clinical practice. Also, the study groups were small and studies in larger groups of patients will need to be performed to determine if the strategy evaluated in this study is both feasible and beneficial in broader clinical practice. Hopefully, longer-term follow-up of cohorts will provide valuable information concerning the relative benefit of culprit vessel versus traditional PCI for STEMI.

5. Culprit vessel PCI versus traditional catheterization and PCI for STEMI: Is there a potential for harm?

Efforts to reduce door-to-balloon times have focused on reducing the time spent prior to getting the patient in the cardiac catheterization laboratory (Bradley et al., 2006; Eagle et al., 2002; Kraft et al., 2007; Kurz et al., 2007). However, there have been few efforts aimed at further reducing door-to-balloon times within the cardiac catheterization laboratory itself (Bradley et al., 2006; Burzotta et al., 2008). Traditionally, patients undergoing urgent percutaneous revascularization initially undergo complete coronary angiography, with or without left ventriculography. This strategy allows identification of life-threatening disease that may require urgent surgery. In the United States, this traditional approach to the patient requiring emergency revascularization, including STEMI patients has been utilized in most laboratories. However, several factors have evolved in the contemporary care of patients with coronary artery disease that are relevant to this approach. First, the actual number of cases undergoing emergency revascularization procedures requiring CABG has dramatically fallen in the past decade (Seshadri et al., 2002; Yang et al., 2005). For example, Yang and colleagues reported a significant decrease in the incidence of emergency CABG from 2.9% to 0.7% to 0.3% across three groups (the "pre-stent" era, 1979 to 1994; the "initial stent era," 1995 to 1999; and the "current stent era," 2000 to 2003 in 23,087 patients undergoing PCI at the Mayo Clinic from 1979 to 2003. This trend was observed despite higher risk features in the more recent patient cohorts. Second, mobilization of the operating room, even under the best of circumstances, generally exceeds a satisfactory time to achieve reperfusion in STEMI patients. Finally, there has been a growing acceptance of hybrid revascularization procedures utilizing both PCI and CABG, either at the same time, or as part of a planned revascularization strategy (Friedrich and Bonatti, 2007). Thus, the identification of left main or three-vessel coronary disease itself is not a contraindication to performing PCI of a culprit vessel in a STEMI patient with a staged CABG as deemed necessary.

6. Traditional catheterization and PCI versus culprit vessel PCI versus a hybrid approach for STEMI

The benefits of performing primary PCI for STEMI, and the need for PCI centers to achieve door-to-balloon times less than 90 minutes, has led to the strategy of performing culprit vessel PCI, even in the setting of left main or significant multivessel disease. Once the decision to perform culprit vessel PCI has been made, the next choice is the stent type, that is, bare metal stent versus drug-eluting stent. The merits of bare metal and drug-eluting stent implantation in STEMI have been the subject of several studies and meta-analyses (De et al., 2009;Hao et al., 2010;Vink et al., 2011;Spaulding et al., 2011). Overall, it appears that drug-eluting stents are as safe as bare metal stents, and reduce rates of target vessel revascularization. Nonetheless, the choice of drug-eluting stents mandates longer term dual antiplatelet therapy than bare metal stents, which is problematic in the patient who may require additional surgical revascularization. While the likelihood of finding significant left main or multivessel disease in STEMI patients is low (Applegate et al., 2008; Lachance et al., 2008), there remains strong concerns that incomplete visualization of the coronary anatomy prior to PCI in STEMI leads to less than optimal decision-making. Traditional complete coronary angiography with multiple orthogonal views followed by left ventriculography is ideal but is time consuming in a situation that demands rapid decisions and treatments. Many operators have adopted a hybrid approach, which allows evaluation of the left main coronary artery with one or two angiograms, and completing a left ventriculogram after the PCI.

We also advocate a hybrid approach as follows (Figure 1) : if the suspected infarct is located in the anterior or lateral left ventricular wall, the first catheter we choose is a left coronary artery guide with the purpose of proceeding with immediate revascularization using a bare metal or drug-eluting stent. The choice of stent in this situation is dependent on both clinical and procedural factors. Our default stent type is a drug-eluting stent unless we are uncertain about compliance with dual-antiplatelet therapy, or we believe that left main or surgical disease is present and will require CABG. In this setting, we believe that an angiogram of the right coronary artery before PCI will not change management. If the suspected infarct-related vessel is the right coronary artery, we perform one or two diagnostic cine angiograms of the left coronary artery to exclude significant left main disease and then perform PCI of the right coronary artery lesion. This identifies left main or three-vessel disease prior to PCI and prevents us from placing drug-eluting stents in patients that will likely need CABG surgery. For STEMI patients with hemodynamic instability, in order to exclude mechanical complications, we also advocate cardiac auscultation, quick look echocardiography and/or left ventriculography before stent implantation.

7. Case presentations

Two cases will be presented to highlight the culprit PCI approach. The first case was a 48-year-old man, with no previous cardiac history, who was admitted with an acute antero-lateral myocardial infarction. The patient was eating dinner at a restaurant when he developed progressive chest pain radiating to the jaw and left arm. He also became diaphoretic. He presented to an outside emergency department and was then transferred to our facility. On physical examination, his vital signs were stable and he had no heart

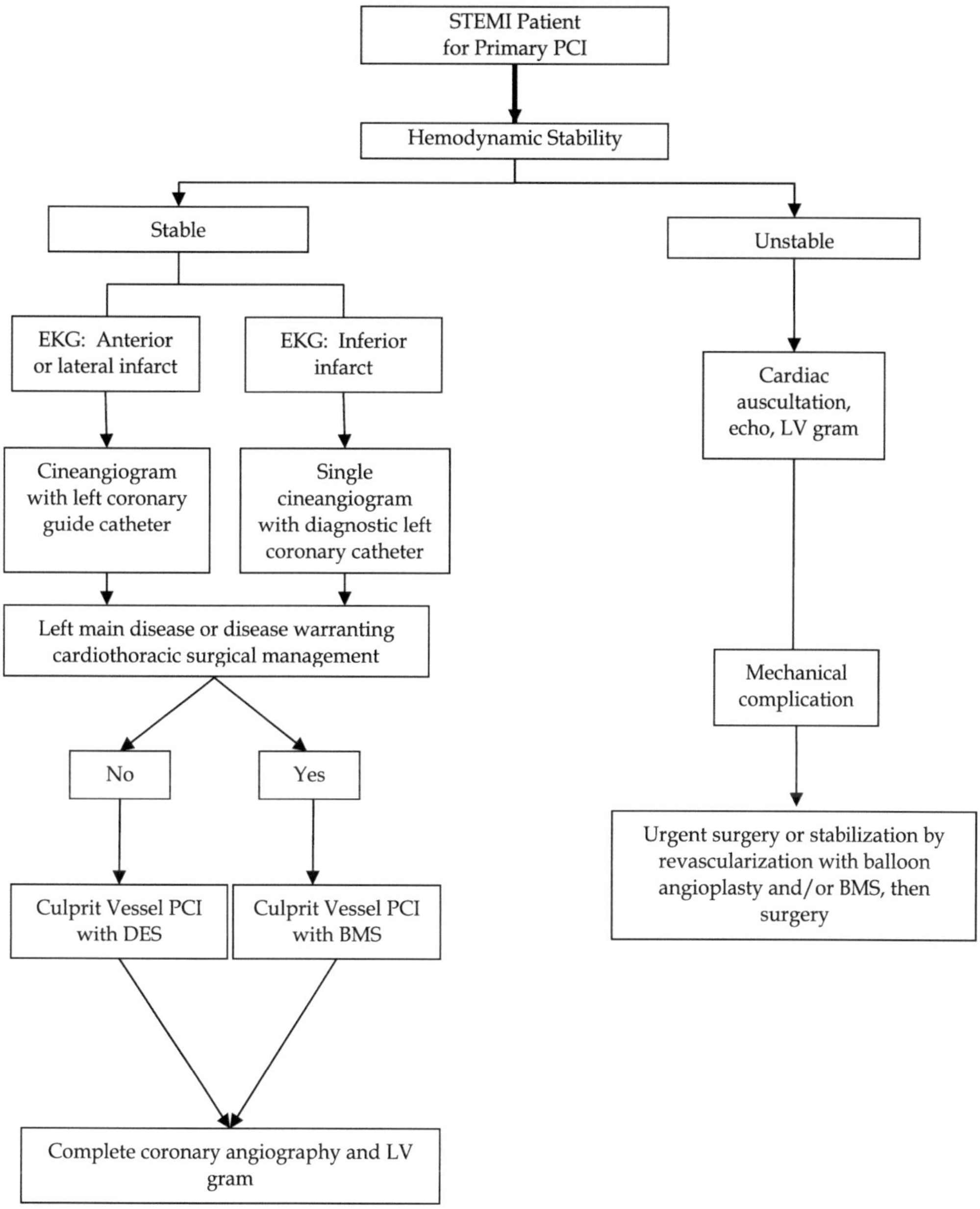

Fig. 1. Algorithm of Hybrid Approach to Primary PCI for STEMI
BMS = bare metal stent, DES = drug-eluting stent, LV gram = left ventriculogram,
echo = echocardiogram

murmur. There were no signs of heart failure. His electrocardiogram demonstrated sinus rhythm with a normal axis and normal intervals. ST elevations and pathological Q waves were present in the anterolateral leads (Figure 2). Laboratory data was not yet available on presentation. Coronary angiography was performed first with a 6 French EBU 3.5 guide catheter (Medtronic Inc., Minneapolis, Minnesota) via the right femoral artery. Complete occlusion of the proximal left anterior descending artery was demonstrated without evidence of collaterals (Figure 3). Percutaneous coronary intervention was then performed with a 2.5 x 12 mm Voyager RX balloon (Abbott Vascular, Chicago, Illinois), followed by a Fetch aspiration thrombectomy catheter (MEDRAD Inc., Warrendale, Pennsylvania). A 3.0 x 18 mm Xience V RX (Abbott Vascular, Chicago, Illinois), drug-eluting stent was then implanted successfully. A 3.5 x 16 mm Voyager NC RX balloon (Abbott Vascular, Chicago, Illinois) was then used to post-dilate the stent. Coronary angiography was then completed. Non-obstructive coronary disease was seen in the right coronary artery. The left ventriculogram demonstrated severe anterolateral hypokinesis and apical dyskinesis. The ejection fraction was 40%. The patient was discharged three days later, free of symptoms.

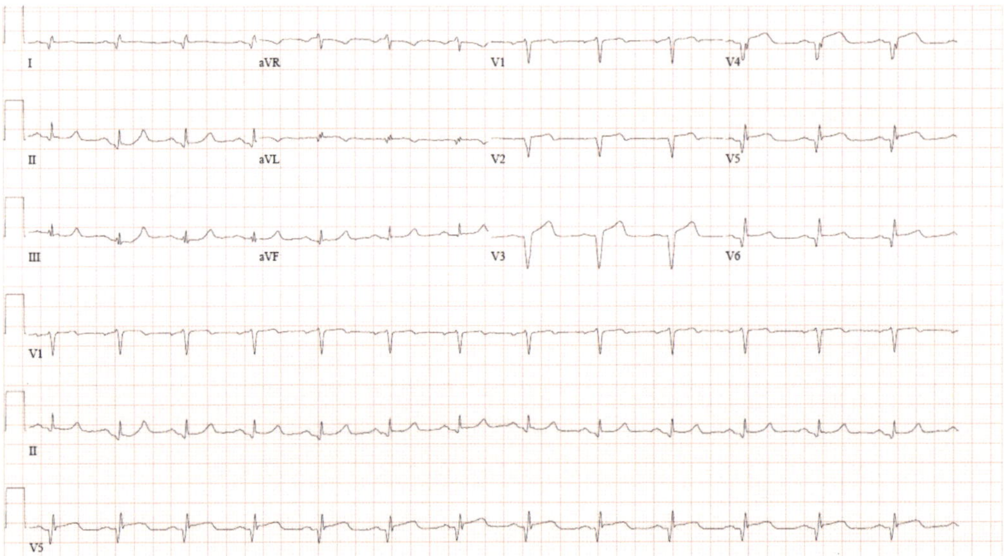

Fig. 2. Case 1, Electrocardiogram

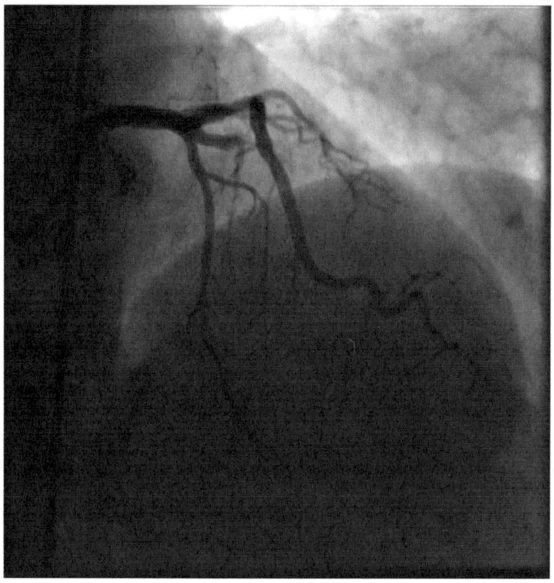

Fig. 3. Case 1, Left Coronary Angiogram

The second case was a 57 year old man with an unknown past medical history who presented with chest pain via the emergency medical services to the emergency room. He was diagnosed with an STEMI in the ambulance. In the emergency room, he developed ventricular fibrillation, requiring cardio-pulmonary resuscitation, multiple cadio - defibrillations, and maximum doses of amiodarone and lidocaine. He was intubated. He eventually developed a stable ventricular tachycardia and was taken to the cardiac catheterization lab. Heart sounds were difficult to appreciate because of the ventilator. His initial EKG in the emergency room demonstrated sinus tachycardia at 123 beats per minute, a left anterior fascicular block, and ST elevations with pathological Q waves in the inferior leads (Figure 4). In the cardiac catheterization lab, the patient required intermittent cardiopulmonary resuscitation, while a 6 French 3.5 ART guide catheter (Boston Scientific/Scimed, Natick, MA) was used to engage the right coronary artery. The right coronary angiogram was the first image acquired. 100% occlusion of the proximal right coronary artery was demonstrated and a 2.5 x 12 mm Voyager RX balloon was used to dilate the coronary artery (Figure 5). After five low-pressure inflations, a VeriFLEX monorail 2.75 x 28 mm bare metal stent (BMS) (Boston Scientific/Scimed, Natick, MA) was implanted successfully across the lesion. The right coronary artery was, at least, co-dominant. Angiography on the left coronary artery was then performed with a diagnostic catheter. This demonstrated a stenosis of 50% in the left main coronary artery and a stenosis of 75% in the left anterior descending artery (Figure 6). The left ventriculogram demonstrated akinesis of the inferior wall and severe hypokinesis of the anterolateral wall. The ejection fraction was 35%. An intra-aortic balloon pump was then placed. The patient did very well, post-procedure. He was extubated two days after admission and was discharged four days after admission. The patient did not undergo CABG surgery during that hospitalization, because he demanded to leave the hospital. Three months after his initial admission the patient underwent CABG. Clopidogrel was discontinued four days prior to the surgery. He

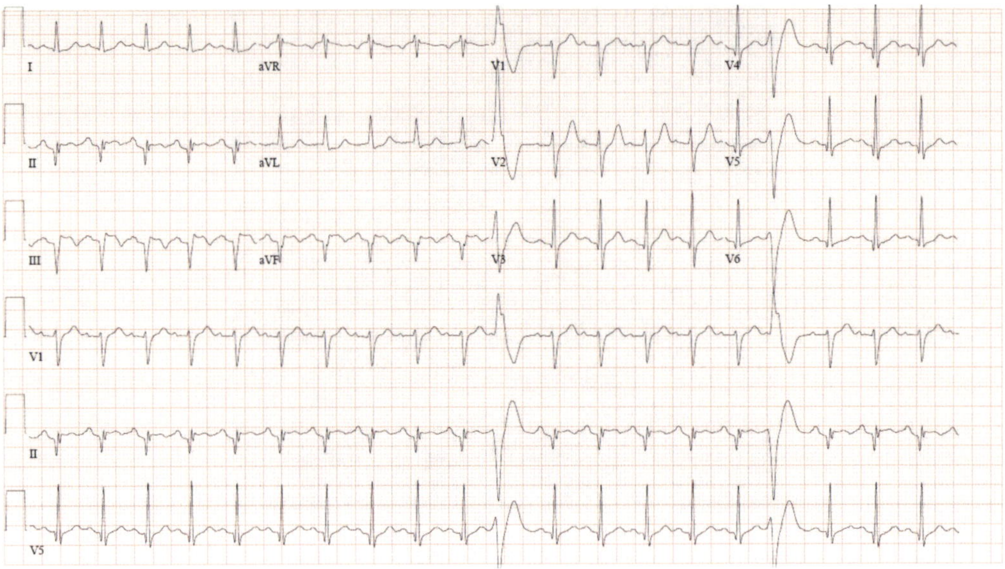

Fig. 4. Case 2, Electrocardiogram

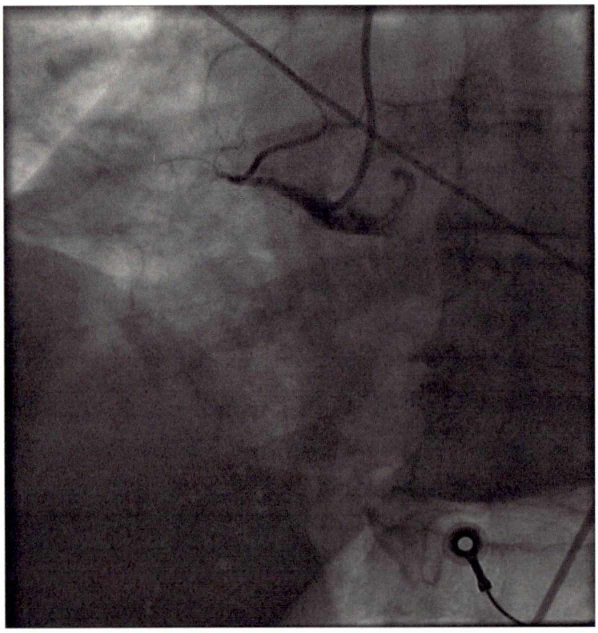

Fig. 5. Case 2, Right Coronary Angiogram

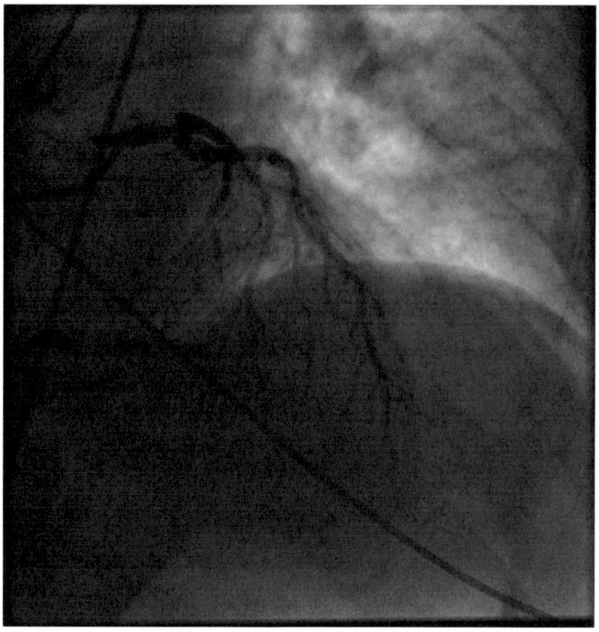

Fig. 6. Case 2, Left Coronary Angiogram

underwent a three vessel bypass with a free skeletonized right internal mammary artery to the first obtuse marginal as a Y graft from the left internal mammary artery, a saphenous vein graft to the posterior descending artery from the aorta, and a skeletonized left internal mammary artery to the left anterior descending as an arterial graft. The patient had no perioperative or postoperative complications.

8. Conclusion

Prior to primary PCI, comprehensive coronary angiography, including left ventricular imaging can provide valuable information for the care of a patient with a STEMI. This approach is time consuming, however, and increased time to reperfusion has been associated with worse outcomes. In the two studies presented, a culprit vessel PCI approach may decrease door-to- balloon times without compromising patient safety. Randomized studies are needed, however, to determine if the incremental decrease in door-to-balloon times using this approach provides clinical benefit. We recommend a hybrid approach, combining certain aspects of comprehensive coronary angiography and the culprit vessel PCI approach. Compared to the femoral approach, the radial arteriotomy is an attractive alternative for vascular access even in the setting of primary PCI for STEMI. Operators experienced with the radial approach report lower or similar access to reperfusion times with the transradial approach compared to the femoral approach.

9. References

Agostoni, P. et al., 2004, Radial versus femoral approach for percutaneous coronary diagnostic and interventional procedures; Systematic overview and meta-analysis of randomized trials: J Am Coll Cardiol, v. 44, no. 2, p. 349-356.

Antman, E. M. et al., 2004, ACC/AHA guidelines for the management of patients with ST-elevation myocardial infarction; A report of the American College of Cardiology/American Heart Association Task Force on Practice Guidelines (Committee to Revise the 1999 Guidelines for the Management of patients with acute myocardial infarction): J Am Coll Cardiol, v. 44, no. 3, p. E1-E211.

Applegate, R. J., S. H. Graham, S. K. Gandhi, M. A. Kutcher, M. T. Sacrinty, R. M. Santos, and W. C. Little, 2008, Culprit vessel PCI versus traditional cath and PCI for STEMI: J Invasive Cardiol., v. 20, no. 5, p. 224-228.

Boersma, E., 2006, Does time matter? A pooled analysis of randomized clinical trials comparing primary percutaneous coronary intervention and in-hospital fibrinolysis in acute myocardial infarction patients: Eur Heart J, v. 27, no. 7, p. 779-788.

Bradley, E. H. et al., 2006, Strategies for reducing the door-to-balloon time in acute myocardial infarction: N Engl J Med, v. 355, no. 22, p. 2308-2320.

Burzotta, F. et al., 2008, Adjunctive devices in primary or rescue PCI: a meta-analysis of randomized trials: Int J Cardiol, v. 123, no. 3, p. 313-321.

Cantor, W. J. et al., 2005, Radial versus femoral access for emergent percutaneous coronary intervention with adjunct glycoprotein IIb/IIIa inhibition in acute myocardial infarction--the RADIAL-AMI pilot randomized trial: Am Heart J, v. 150, no. 3, p. 543-549.

De, L. G. et al., 2009, Efficacy and safety of drug-eluting stents in ST-segment elevation myocardial infarction: a meta-analysis of randomized trials: Int.J.Cardiol., v. 133, no. 2, p. 213-222.

De Luca, G., H. Suryapranata, J. P. Ottervanger, and E. M. Antman, 2004, Time delay to treatment and mortality in primary angioplasty for acute myocardial infarction: every minute of delay counts: Circulation, v. 109, no. 10, p. 1223-1225.

Eagle, K. A., S. G. Goodman, A. Avezum, A. Budaj, C. M. Sullivan, and J. Lopez-Sendon, 2002, Practice variation and missed opportunities for reperfusion in ST-segment-elevation myocardial infarction: findings from the Global Registry of Acute Coronary Events (GRACE): Lancet, v. 359, no. 9304, p. 373-377.

Friedrich, G. J., and J. Bonatti, 2007, Hybrid coronary artery revascularization--review and update 2007: Heart Surg.Forum, v. 10, no. 4, p. E292-E296.

Hao, P. P., Y. G. Chen, X. L. Wang, and Y. Zhang, 2010, Efficacy and safety of drug-eluting stents in patients with acute ST-segment-elevation myocardial infarction: a meta-analysis of randomized controlled trials: Tex.Heart Inst.J., v. 37, no. 5, p. 516-524.

Hetherington, S. L., Z. Adam, R. Morley, M. A. de Belder, J. A. Hall, D. F. Muir, A. G. Sutton, N. Swanson, and R. A. Wright, 2009, Primary percutaneous coronary intervention for acute ST-segment elevation myocardial infarction: changing patterns of vascular access, radial versus femoral artery: Heart, v. 95, no. 19, p. 1612-1618.

Iakovou, I. et al., 2005, Incidence, predictors, and outcome of thrombosis after successful implantation of drug-eluting stents: JAMA, v. 293, no. 17, p. 2126-2130.

Joner, M. et al., 2006, Pathology of drug-eluting stents in humans: delayed healing and late thrombotic risk: J Am Coll Cardiol, v. 48, no. 1, p. 193-202.

Keeley, E. C., J. A. Boura, and C. L. Grines, 2003, Primary angioplasty versus intravenous thrombolytic therapy for acute myocardial infarction: a quantitative review of 23 randomised trials: Lancet, v. 361, no. 9351, p. 13-20.

Kraft, P. L., S. Newman, D. Hanson, W. Anderson, and A. Bastani, 2007, Emergency physician discretion to activate the cardiac catheterization team decreases door-to-balloon time for acute ST-elevation myocardial infarction: Ann Emerg Med, v. 50, no. 5, p. 520-526.

Kurz, M. C., C. Babcock, S. Sinha, J. P. Tupesis, and J. Allegretti, 2007, The impact of emergency physician-initiated primary percutaneous coronary intervention on mean door-to-balloon time in patients with ST-segment-elevation myocardial infarction: Ann Emerg Med, v. 50, no. 5, p. 527-534.

Lachance, P. et al., 2008, ECG-guided immediate intervention at the time of primary PCI to reduce door-to-balloon time in ST-elevation myocardial infarction patients: J Invasive Cardiol, v. 20, no. 11, p. 623-626.

Larrazet, F., F. Philippe, T. Folliguet, M. Slama, T. Meziane, J. Bachet, F. Laborde, and A. Dibie, 2003, [Comparison between radial and femoral approaches in ad hoc coronary angioplasty]: Arch Mal Coeur Vaiss., v. 96, no. 3, p. 175-180.

Nallamothu, B. K., and E. R. Bates, 2003, Percutaneous coronary intervention versus fibrinolytic therapy in acute myocardial infarction: is timing (almost) everything? Am J Cardiol, v. 92, no. 7, p. 824-826.

Pancholy, S., T. Patel, K. Sanghvi, M. Thomas, and T. Patel, 2010, Comparison of door-to-balloon times for primary PCI using transradial versus transfemoral approach: Catheter Cardiovasc Interv, v. 75, no. 7, p. 991-995.

Saito, S., S. Tanaka, Y. Hiroe, Y. Miyashita, S. Takahashi, K. Tanaka, and S. Satake, 2003, Comparative study on transradial approach vs. transfemoral approach in primary stent implantation for patients with acute myocardial infarction: results of the test for myocardial infarction by prospective unicenter randomization for access sites (TEMPURA) trial: Catheter Cardiovasc Interv, v. 59, no. 1, p. 26-33.

Seshadri, N., P. L. Whitlow, N. Acharya, P. Houghtaling, E. H. Blackstone, and S. G. Ellis, 2002, Emergency coronary artery bypass surgery in the contemporary percutaneous coronary intervention era: Circulation, v. 106, no. 18, p. 2346-2350.

Singh, K. P., and R. A. Harrington, 2007, Primary percutaneous coronary intervention in acute myocardial infarction: Med Clin North Am, v. 91, no. 4, p. 639-655.

Spaulding, C. et al., 2011, Four-year follow-up of TYPHOON (trial to assess the use of the CYPHer sirolimus-eluting coronary stent in acute myocardial infarction treated with BallOON angioplasty): JACC.Cardiovasc.Interv., v. 4, no. 1, p. 14-23.

Vink, M. A., M. T. Dirksen, M. J. Suttorp, J. G. Tijssen, E. J. van, M. S. Patterson, T. Slagboom, F. Kiemeneij, and G. J. Laarman, 2011, 5-year follow-up after primary percutaneous coronary intervention with a paclitaxel-eluting stent versus a bare-metal stent in acute ST-segment elevation myocardial infarction: a follow-up study of the PASSION (Paclitaxel-Eluting Versus Conventional Stent in Myocardial Infarction with ST-Segment Elevation) trial: JACC.Cardiovasc.Interv., v. 4, no. 1, p. 24-29.

Weaver, A. N., R. A. Henderson, I. C. Gilchrist, and S. M. Ettinger, 2010, Arterial access and door-to-balloon times for primary percutaneous coronary intervention in patients

presenting with acute ST-elevation myocardial infarction: Catheter Cardiovasc Interv, v. 75, no. 5, p. 695-699.
Yang, E. H., R. J. Gumina, R. J. Lennon, D. R. Holmes, Jr., C. S. Rihal, and M. Singh, 2005, Emergency coronary artery bypass surgery for percutaneous coronary interventions: changes in the incidence, clinical characteristics, and indications from 1979 to 2003: J Am Coll Cardiol, v. 46, no. 11, p. 2004-2009.

2

Risk Stratification and Invasive Strategy in NSTE-ACS

Frantisek Kovar, Milos Knazeje and Marian Mokan
I. Internal Clinic, University Hospital Martin
Slovak republic

1. Introduction

Under the heading of acute coronary syndrome (ACS), we include myocardial infarction with ST segment elevation (STEMI), myocardial infarction without ST segment elevation (NSTEMI) and unstable angina (UA). Given the similar pathophysiological mechanisms, clinical manifestations, diagnostic and therapeutic algorithm UA and NSTEMI are sorted into a common group of ACS without ST segment elevation (NSTE-ACS). ACS is a serious clinical disease, which is associated with higher mortality than stable angina pectoris. High proportion of patients die of sudden death in the early hours of ACS (especially STEMI), before admission to the hospital, therefore it is difficult to assess the real incidence of ACS. The incidence of ACS also depends on the sensitivity of the humoral markers of myocyte necrosis. The annual hospital admissions rate for NSTE-ACS is estimated from the results of registers and surveys about 3 per 1000 inhabitants. The proportion of STEMI represents approximately 20% of NSTE ACS.

1.1 NSTE-ACS

Acute coronary syndromes without ST segment elevation constitute a clinically heterogeneous group. Pathophysiological basis of NSTE-ACS is usually unstable atherosclerotic plaque (with rupture, erosions and inflammatory changes) and the presence of intracoronary thrombosis. Intracoronary thrombus has a high content of platelet and (unlike in STEMI) is non-occlusive or intermittently present. In the USA were hospitalized for ACS 1.57 million patients per 1 year, of which 0.33 million were admitted for STEMI and 1.24 million for NSTE-ACS (0.57 mil. for NSTEMI and 0.67 million for UA). In the same year were performed in the U.S. 1,297,000 coronary angiographies and 658 000 PCIs (Rosamond W et al., 2007). Based on analogous application of these statistics data, it can be expected the annual incidence of 5500 STEMI and 20 600 NSTE-ACS (9500 NSTEMI) in the Slovak Republic.
According to data from the registers of ACS, invasive diagnostics was currently performed in less than half of patients with NSTE-ACS (Fox KA et al., 2003, Bhat DL et al., 2004, Kovar F et al., 2010). Assessment of the benefits of invasive management strategy in NSTE-ACS based on the data from randomized trials is difficult because of number of reasons. High proportion of patients originally enrolled in the conservative arm is then treated invasively and in addition, there were significant differences in the timing of invasive diagnosis in individual studies (less than 2.5 hours to 7 days)) (Cannon CP et al., 2001; Fox KA et al., 2002; Neumann FJ et al., 2003).

The recently published study ICTUS did not present significant difference between groups treated within invasive or conservative arms in terms of mortality, reinfarction or rehospitalization rate for period 1 and 3 year follow-up (22.7% versus 21.2%, p = 0.33). There was observed an increased incidence of early myocardial infarction (15% versus 10%, p = 0.005) among invasive managed patients. During initial hospitalization, however, 76% of patients in the invasive group and 40% of patients scheduled for conservative treatment underwent revascularization procedure (Hirsh A et al., 2007).
Similarly, meta-analysis of more than 4500 patients from randomized trials has suggested that routinely indicated coronary angiography compared with more conservative strategy was associated with increased incidence of early mortality (1.8% vs. 1.1%, p = 0.007) and combined endpoint of death and reinfarction (5.2 % vs. 3.8%, p = 0.002). Long term monitoring however, favored an invasive strategy with a reduction of death and reinfarction (12.2% versus 14.4%, p = 0.001) (Mehta SR et al., 2005).
Some clinical trials were able to document benefit of invasive strategy in NSTE-ACS patients with an increased troponin level in the beginning, but not at its normal levels (Diderholm E et al., 2002, Lagerqvist B et al., 2006).
In a recently published meta-analysis of more than 8300 patients with NSTE-ACS, there has been documented benefits of timely invasive procedure compared with conservative management in order to reduce mortality (4.9% vs. 6.5%, p = 0.001), nonfatal myocardial infarction (7.6 % vs. 9.1%, p = 0.012) over a 2 year follow-up period, without increasing risk of myocardial infarction within 1 month (Bavry AA et al., 2006). Reduction of mortality rate in the early invasive strategy was present during the 5- year follow-up periods in FRISCO II and RITA 3 trials as well (Fox KA et al., 2005; Lagerqvist B et al., 2006).

2. RISC score

As has been pointed out previously, NSTE-ACS is a heterogeneous group of diseases. Coronary angiography can reveal severe stenosis of one or more coronary arteries, narrowing of the left main coronary artery, presence of intracoronary thrombi (FRISC II investigators, 1999; Kovar F et al., 2003, 2004). These facts reflect current recommendations of the European Society of Cardiology (ESC), which emphasize the need for early (and repeated as necessary) risk stratification in patients with NSTE-ACS (Bassand JP et al., 2007).

2.1 GRACE score

The GRACE (Global Registry of acute coronary events) risk score takes into account age, heart rate, systolic blood pressure, serum creatinine level, Killip class on admission, need for resuscitation for cardiac arrest, presence of ST segment depression and increased values of of myocardial necrosis markers (Eagle KA et al., 2004; Fox KA et al., 2006). GRACE score is based on the analysis of a large unselected population from an international registry of all ACS (STEMI and NSTEMI). Evaluated risk factors show independent predictive value for both hospital and 6- month mortality (tab. 1).

2.2 TIMI score

The TIMI (Thrombolysis in myocardial infarction) risk score assesses anamnestic variables (age ≥ 65 years, ≥ 3 risk factors of ischemic heart disease, known coronary artery stenosis >

Risk score (Tertils)	GRACE risk score	Hospital mortality (%)	Mortality within 6 months (%)
low	< 108	<1	<3
mean	109-140	1-3	3-8
high	> 140	> 3	> 8

Table 1. Hospital and six month mortality rate depending on the GRACE risk score

TIMI RISK SCORE	
VARIABLE	POINT
age ≥ 65 years	1
≥ 3 risk factors for vascular disease	1
known coronary artery stenosis > 50%	1
use of aspirin in the last 7 days	1
severe angina within 24 hours	1
ST segment deviations > 0.5 mm	1
positive markers of necrosis	1
Risk score	**0-7**

Table 2. TIMI (Thrombolysis in myocardial infarction) risk score parameters

50%, aspirin therapy in the last 7 days and the actual presence of severe angina within 24 hours, ST segment deviations > 0.5 mm and increased laboratory markers of necrosis (Antman EM et al., 2000). TIMI score is then the sum of individual items (value 0-7) (tab. 2). Its advantage is simplicity, but has not so high predictive accuracy as a comprehensive GRACE score (Figure 1).

2.3 Correlation between coronary angiography findings and the TIMI risk score level

In a retrospective study, we investigated contribution of early risk stratification to the invasive management timing. Population consisted from 424 consecutive NSTE-ACS patients (264 men and 160 women), age 26-87 years (mean age 65,75 years, median 67 years), referred for coronary angiography to the Ist Department of Internal medicine University hospital Martin during the period from December 2009 to October 2010. Patients with NSTE-ACS were stratified according to the TIMI risk score and based on achieved risk score level subsequently divided into three risk groups (Figure 2 and 3):

1. low risk (0-2 points)
2. intermediate risk (3-4 points)
3. high risk (5-7 points)

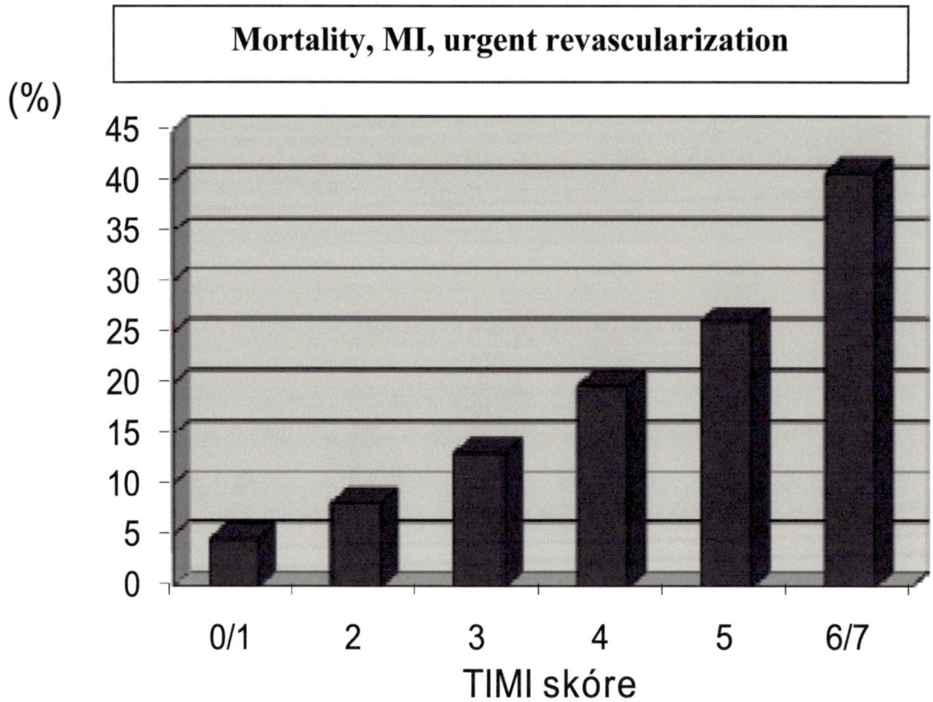

Fig. 1. Incidence of major cardiovascular events based on TIMI risk score level

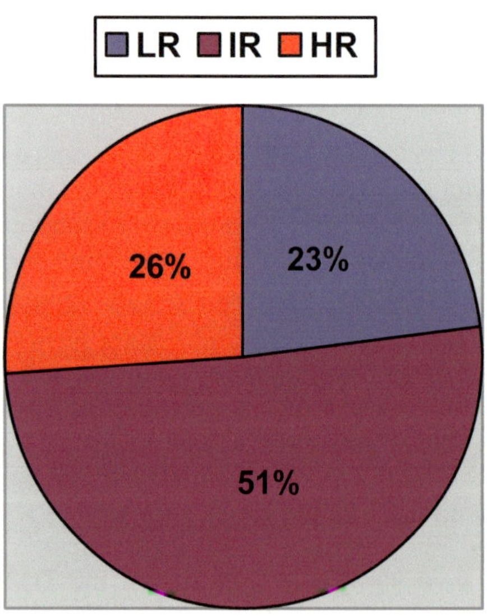

Fig. 2. Risk stratification according TIMI risk score
LR - low risk, IR - intermediate risk, HR - high risk

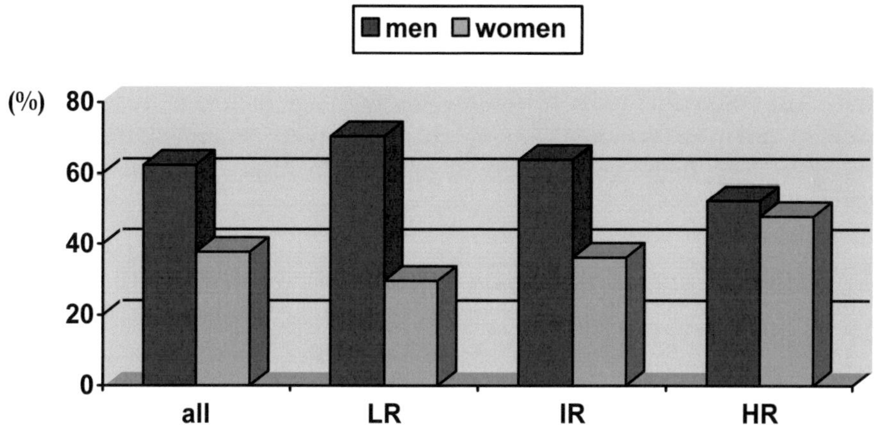

Fig. 3. Proportion of men and women in different risk groups
LR - low risk, IR - intermediate risk, HR - high risk

There were more men than women in the age range bellow 65 years in all risk groups, but this difference was no longer present in the age ≥ 65 years (Figure 4 and 5).

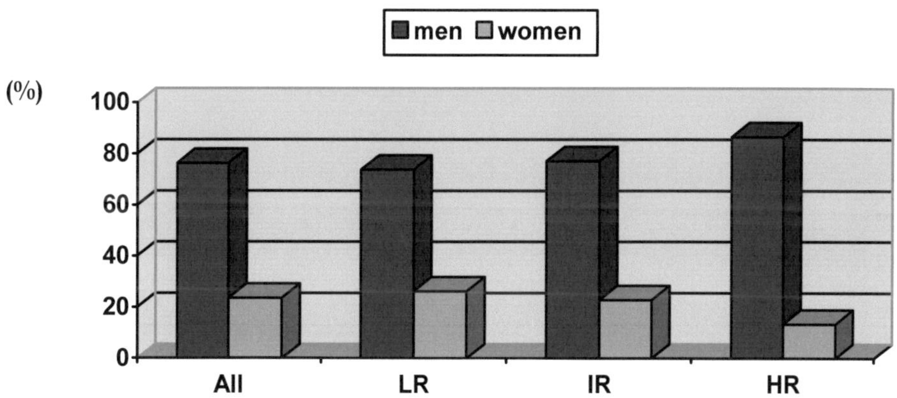

Fig. 4. Proportion of men and women in different risk groups in age below 65 year
LR - low risk, IR - intermediate risk, HR - high risk

Elevated cardiac troponin was identified as most frequent parameter of the TIMI risk score (in 81,8% of patients). Second often parameter occurred presence of ≥ 3 risk factors for coronary artery disease in 60,1% patients (Figure 6).
Frequency of risk factors for coronary artery disease rose with increasing TIMI risk score, so in high-risk group almost 90% of patients had ≥ 3 risk factors (Figure 7).
On coronary angiography was assessed stenosis of:

- main stem of left coronary artery – LMA > 50%
- ramus interventricular anterior - RIA > 75%
- ramus circumflexus – RCX > 75%

- arteria coronaria dextra - RCA > 75%
- multivessel coronary artery disease - stenosis ≥ 3 - coronary arteries

There were more coronary arteries stenoses identified with increasing TIMI risk score (Figure 8). In age range ≥ 65 years in comparison with age bellow 65 year, there were more coronary arteries stenoses among patients with intermediate risk. This relationship was even more pronounced in patients in high TIMI risk score group (Figure 9 and 10).

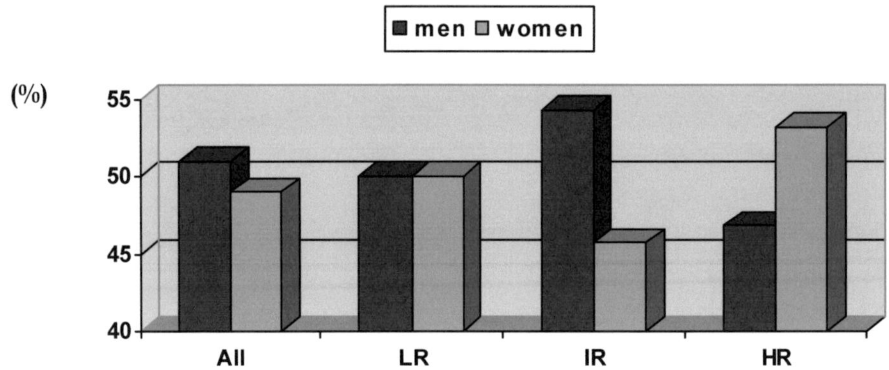

Fig. 5. Proportion of men and women in different risk groups in age ≥ 65 year
LR - low risk, IR - intermediate risk, HR - high risk

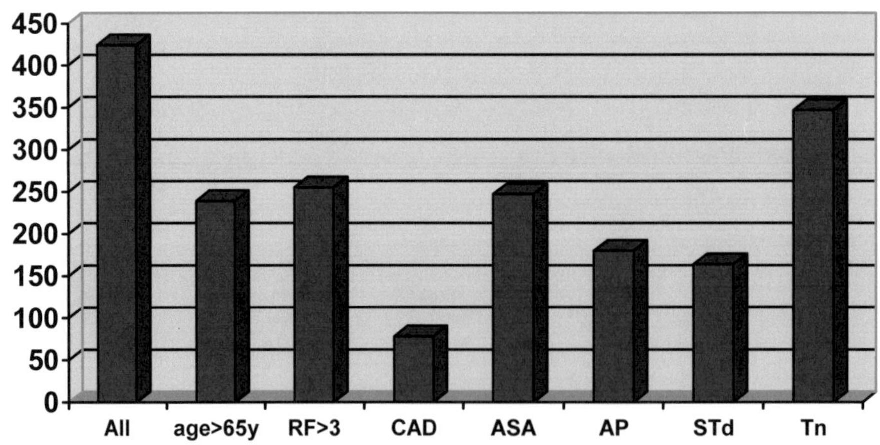

Fig. 6. Incidence of anamnestic, clinical and laboratory parameters of TIMI risk score
RF - risk factor for atherosclerosis, CAD - known coronary artery narrowing > 50%, ASA - acetylsalicylic acid, AP - angina pectoris, STd - ST segment depression ≥ 0.5 mm, Tn - troponin

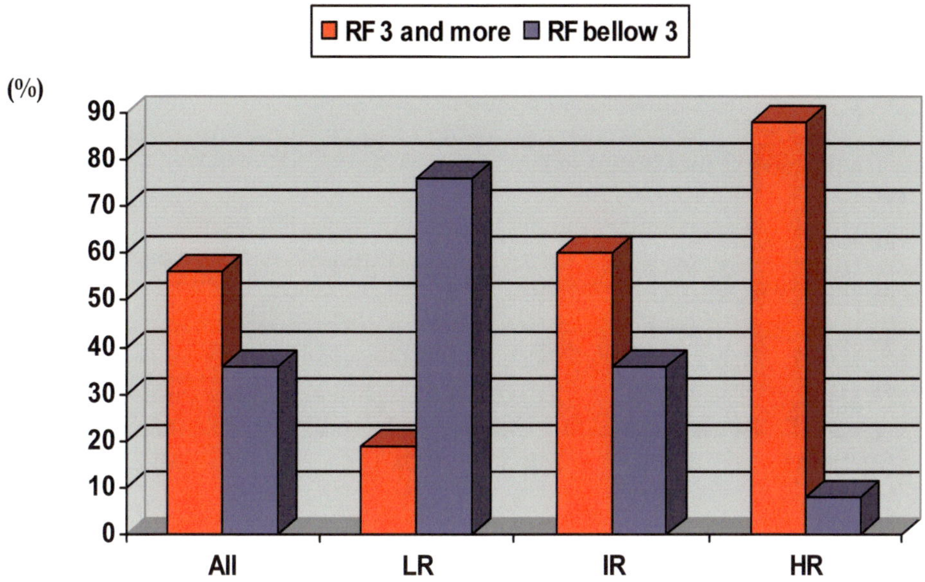

Fig. 7. Proportion of patients with ≥ 3 risk factors for coronary artery disease in different risk groups
LR - low risk, IR - intermediate risk, HR - high risk

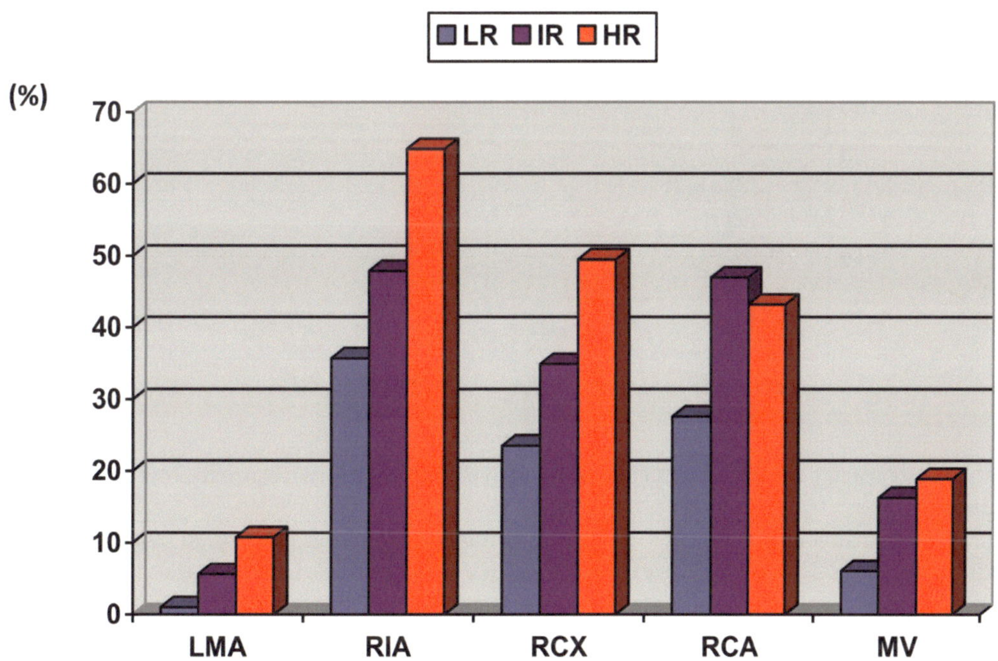

Fig. 8. Coronary arteries stenoses in different risk groups
LMA - left main coronary artery, RIA - ramus interventricularis anterior, RCX - ramus circumflexus, RCA - arteria coronaria dextra, MV - multivessel coronary artery disease

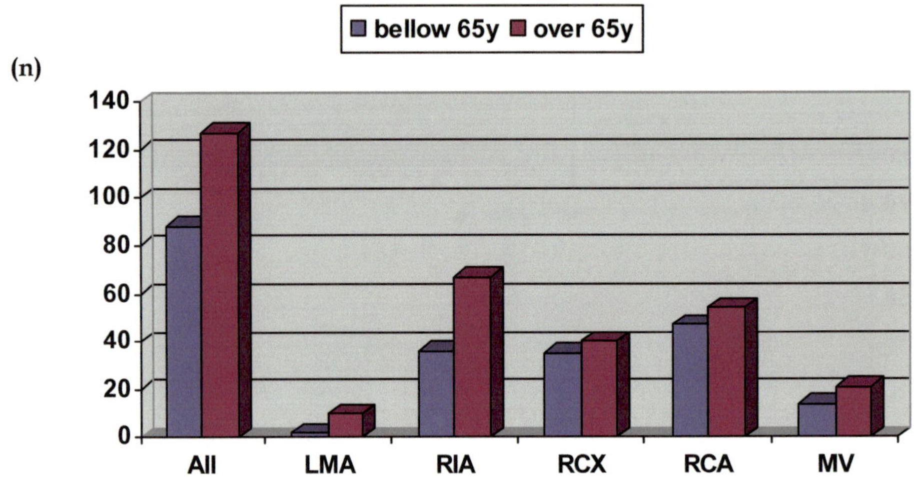

Fig. 9. Coronary arteries stenoses in patients with intermediate TIMI risk score in different age groups
LMA - left main coronary artery, RIA - ramus interventricularis anterior, RCX - ramus circumflexus, RCA - arteria coronaria dextra, MV - multivessel coronary artery disease

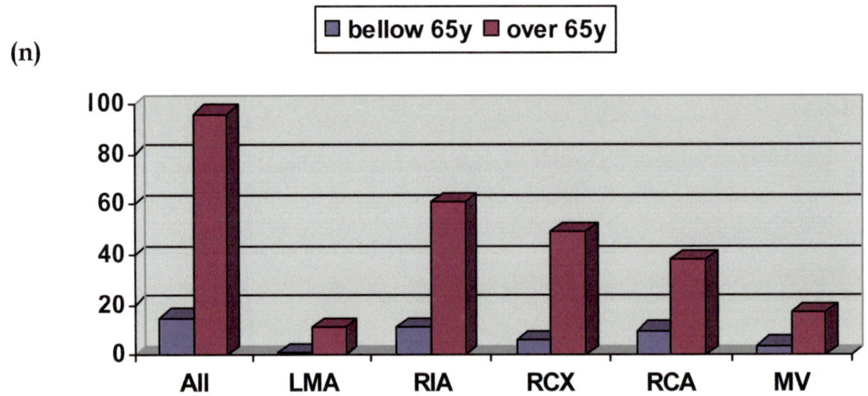

Fig. 10. Coronary arteries stenoses in patients with high TIMI risk score in different age groups
LMA - left main coronary artery, RIA - ramus interventricularis anterior, RCX - ramus circumflexus, RCA - arteria coronaria dextra, MV - multivessel coronary artery disease

Coronary angiography findings were negative in 25,7% of patients. While in the group with low risk, coronary angiography was without significant stenosis in 42,8% of patients, there was so in 25,5% in the intermediate risk group and in only 10,8% of patients in high risk group (Figure 11). Extensive involvement of coronary arteries was assessed by coronary angiography in intermediate and high risk groups.

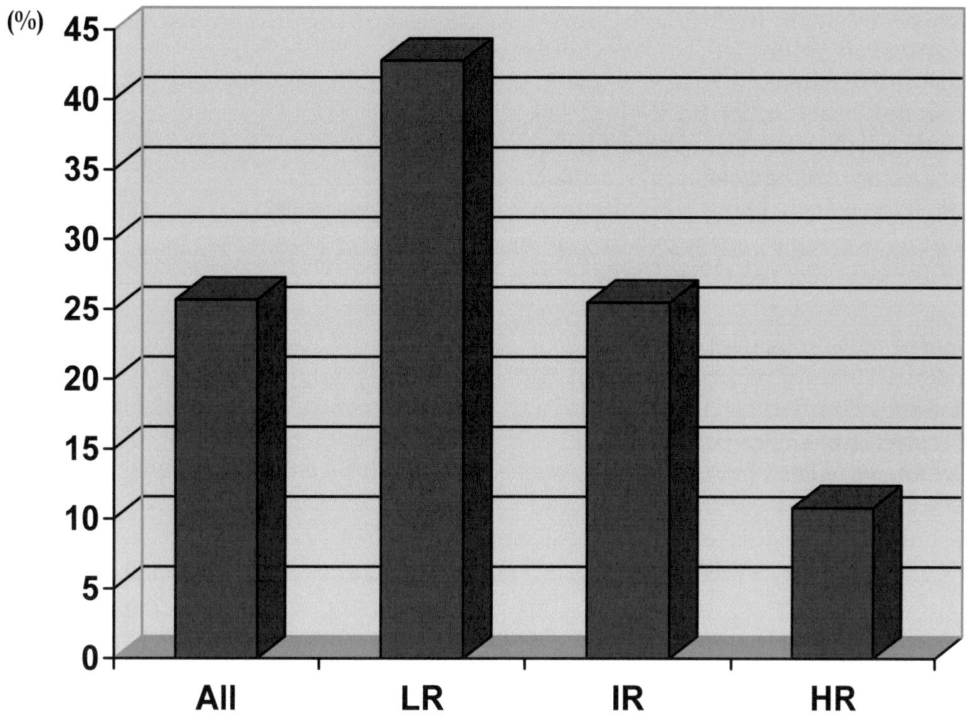

Fig. 11. Proportion of patients without significant coronary artery stenosis in different TIMI risk group
LR - low risk, IR - intermediate risk, HR - high risk

3. Indication and timing of invasive diagnostics

Depending on the risk score level, we can make decisions for the indication of invasive diagnostic and its timing in patients with NSTE-ACS in three modes (urgent, early invasively and elective) (Bassand JP et al., 2007):

3.1 Urgent invasive strategy

It is indicated within 2 hours in patients with high risk score. This strategy is taken in to account particularly in patients with:

a. Refractory angina
b. Recurrent angina despite intensive pharmacologic treatment with presence of deep (≥ 2 mm) ST segment depression or deep negatives T waves on ECG
c. Symptoms of heart failure or hemodynamic instability (incipient signs of shock)
d. Serious arrhythmias (ventricular fibrillation or ventricular tachycardia)

3.2 Early invasive strategy

This strategy is considered in NSTE-ACS patients with high risk of serious ischemic events. Coronary angiography should be performed within 72 hours in this group.

These are patients presenting with:
a. elevated troponin levels
b. dynamic ST segment or T waves changes (≥ 0.5 mm)
c. diabetes mellitus
d. reduced renal function (GFR <1 ml / s)
e. reduced left ventricular ejection fraction <40%
f. angina pectoris early after myocardial infarction
g. angina pectoris within 6 months after coronary intervention (PCI)
h. history of coronary artery bypass grafting (CABG)
i. medium or high risk GRACE score

3.3 Conservative (elective) strategy

It is indicated in those patients who meet all the following criteria:
Are free of:
a. Recurrence of angina pectoris
b. Symptoms of heart failure
c. Major arrhythmias
d. Changes in both initial and second ECG (after 6-12 hours)
e. Elevated troponin levels (at entrance examinations and even after 6-12 hours)

Low risk, as assessed by GRACE or TIMI scores, supports the decision making for a conservative treatment. These patients should undergo an exercise test before hospital discharge and coronary angiography in case of inducible ischemia.

Risk stratification of ACS patients (as recommended by the ESC) is now clearly recommended to identify patients with moderate to high risk of serious cardiovascular complications, who benefit most from both early invasive diagnosis and subsequent coronary arteries revascularization. In so selected risky ACS group coronary angiography has to be performed during index hospitalization.

4. Effect of early treatment strategy on long-term outcomes in NSTE-ACS

Because invasive diagnosis plays an important role in the management of NSTE-ACS, we decided to analyze the clinical course of patients who have been made coronary angiography at the beginning and by finding subsequently revascularization, and also in those patients who refused invasive testing (Kovar F et al., 2007).

4.1 Patients and methods

Prospective analysis of consecutive patients admitted to our clinic with a diagnosis of unstable angina or myocardial infarction without ST segment elevation. All patients received comprehensive standard (according to current recommendations) pharmacologic therapy. Within 48 hours was performed coronary angiography and further revascularization therapy if appropriate. Invasive diagnosis was not performed in patients who refused this procedure.

Initial coronary angiography record was analyzed according to location and type of coronary stenosis (A, B, C), closure of coronary artery was evaluated separately.

Lesion type A: a short concentric stenosis, easily accessible, less calcified, without thrombus, without side branch involving (success rate of intervention> 85%, low risk)

Lesion type B: tubular 10 to 20 mm long, eccentric, with the presence of calcifications, involving ostium of coronary artery, bifurcation stenosis, presence of thrombus (intervention success rate 60-85%, moderately high risk)
Lesion type C: diffuse stenosis> 20 mm, extremely coiled proximal segments, bifurcation lesions with the impossibility to access a lateral branches (success rate of intervention <60%, high risk) (Figure 12 a,b,c).
During the one-year follow-up period there were assessed mortality rate, need for repeated hospitalization for ACS or revascularization and left ventricular ejection fraction (LVEF). These endpoint variables were evaluated in four groups of patiens who: 1) underwent percutaneous coronary intervention (PCI) or 2) surgical revascularization (CABG), 3) after angiography were treated conservatively or 4) refused invasive diagnostics in the beginning.

4.2 Statistical analysis

Any analysis of the effectiveness of the treatment was made in four groups of patients: PCI, CABG, conservative treatment and conservative treatment without initial invasive diagnosis. Two-sided Fisher's exact test in the modification of 2 x 4 was used to test hypotheses about the same effect of therapies. χ^2 test were used for *a posteriori* analysis of categorical variables. As statistically significant we considered differences at significance level of $P < 0,05$.

4.3 Results

During the reporting period were for UA and NSTEMI admitted 183 patients, of which 109 were men aged 35-84 (mean ± SD: 55,9 ± 11,6) years and 74 women aged 44-86 (mean ± SD: 66; 5 ± 12.0) years. History and clinical variables are shown in table 3.

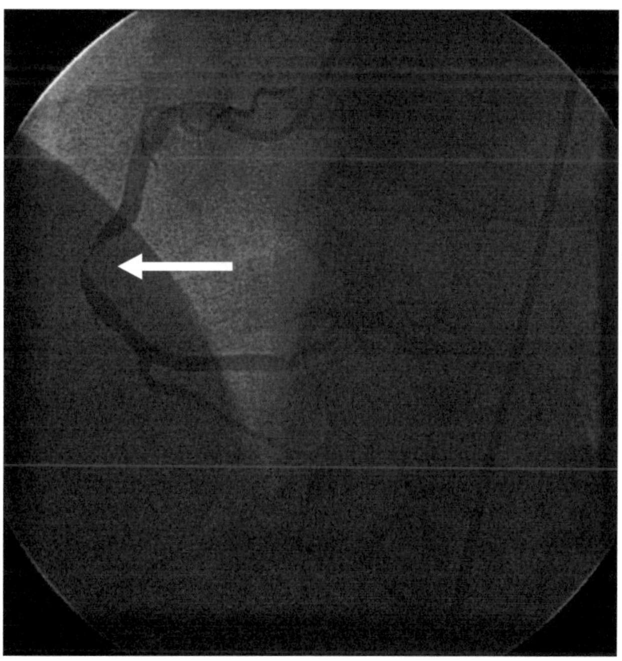

Fig. 12a. Lesion type A

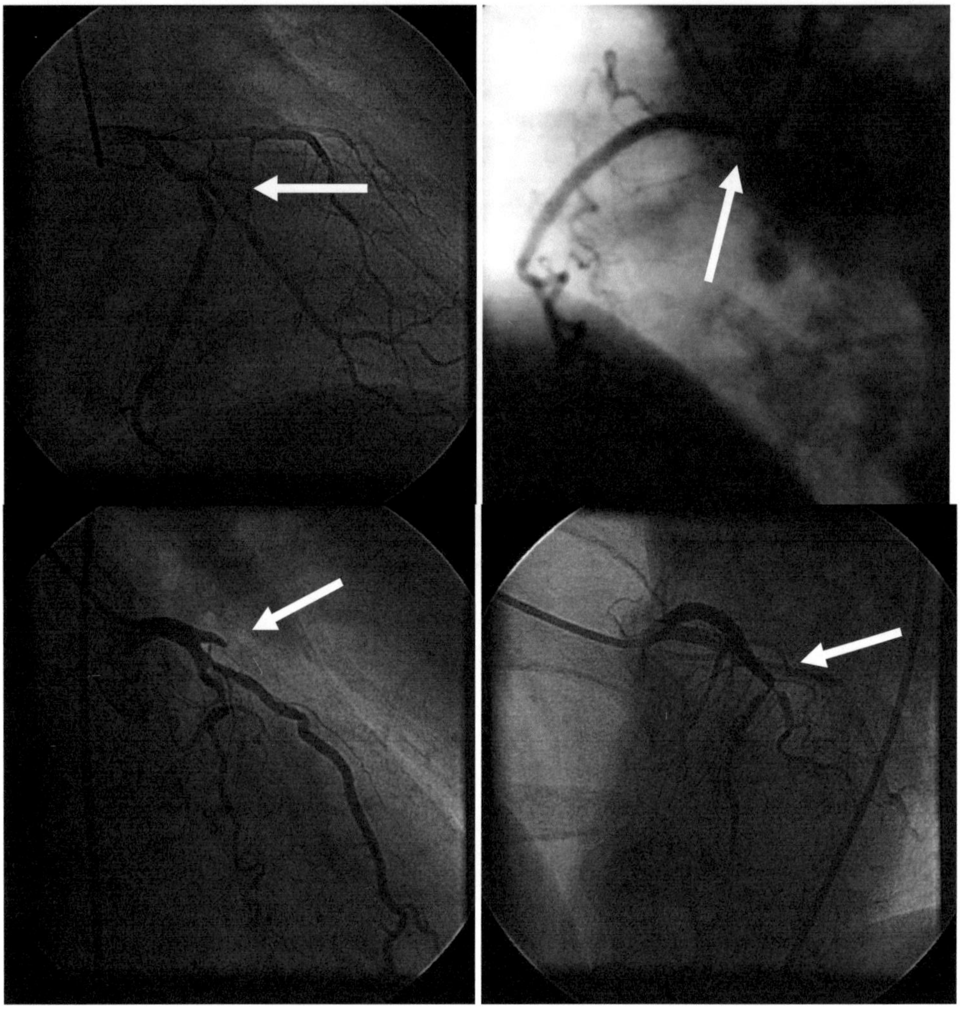

Fig. 12b. Lesions type B

Evaluated population of patients has been at high risk for the presence of cardiovascular risk factors and history of cardiovascular disease: more than 65% patients had hypertension, 37.7% had a myocardial infarction, in nearly 20% was already performed a revascularization of coronary arteries in the past, 9.8% had stroke, hypercholesterolemia was present in 77% and diabetes mellitus in 25.7% of all patients.

Early after hospital admission, 171 patients (93.4%) underwent coronary angiography and 12 (6.6%) patients refused invasive diagnostics (they were also treated conservatively).

There was found in 7.6% of patients closure of coronary arteries, advanced atherosclerotic coronary artery stenosis (stenosis B and C) were evaluated in 67.8% patients on the initial angiography. Frequency of significant coronary arteries stenosis (ramus interventricularis anterior, ramus circumflexus, right coronary artery) was similar (37.4%, 32.8%, respectively 22 %), significant impairment of left main coronary artery was present in 7% of patients.

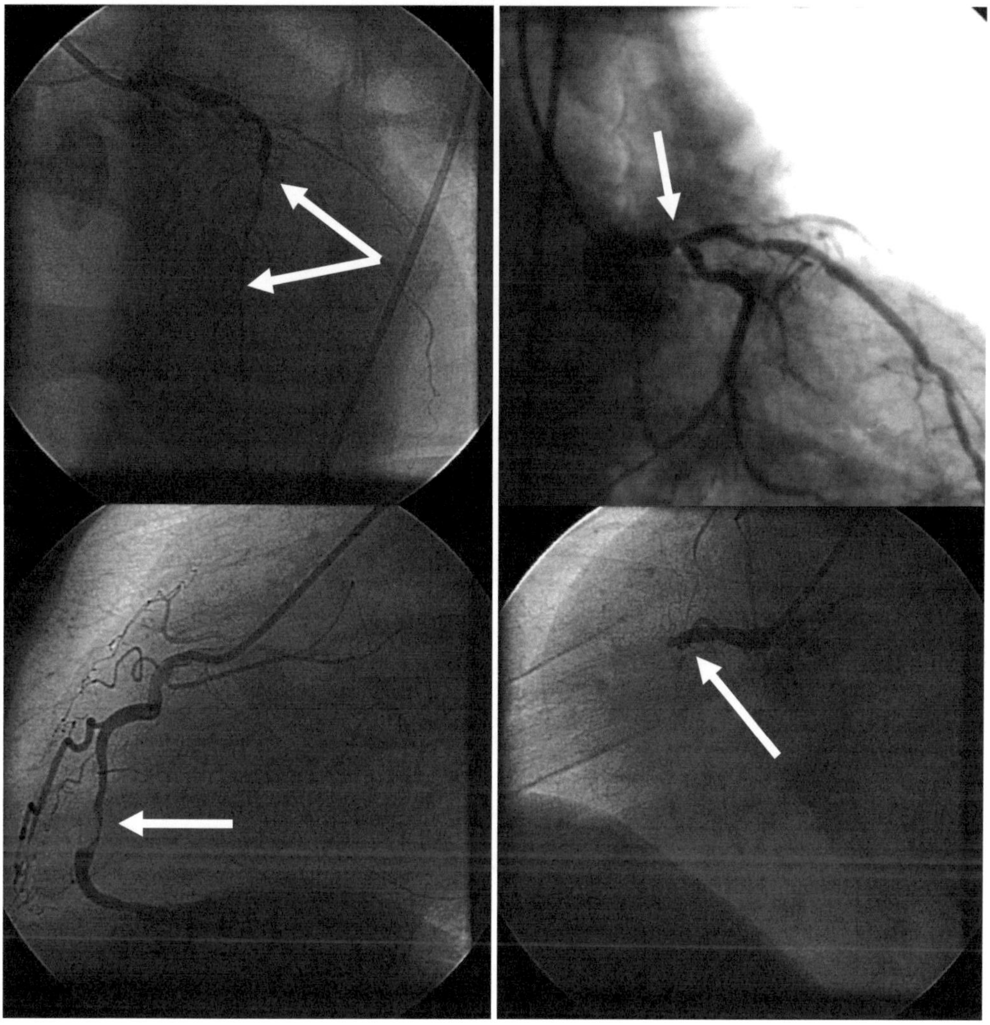

Fig. 12c. Lesions type C

Subsequent coronary revascularization underwent 72.1% of patients (mostly PCI was performed), 21.3% were treated conservatively after angiography and in 6.6% patients was not coronary angiography performed in the beginning.

Table 4. shows the presence of analyzed clinical parameters in different groups during a one-year follow-up, their comparison is in table 5.

There was a trend to higher mortality rate and more frequent need for both repeat hospitalization or revascularization for ACS among patients treated conservatively without angiography at the beginning in comparison with invasive strategy group. LVEF> 50% occurred significantly more in patients treated according angiographic findings compared with patients without initial coronary angiography. The different incidence reached the highest statistical significance when compared group of patients without coronary angiography with patients treated with PCI (a posteriori analysis).

	n	%
No. of patients	183	100,0
men	109	56,3
hypertension	120	65,6
hypercholesterolemia	141	77,0
History of MI	69	37,7
History of PCI	23	12,6
History of CABG	13	7,1
LV insufficiency	39	21,3
history of CVD +	56	30,6
DM	47	25,7
History of ictus	18	9,8
Cigarette smoking	41	22,4
Obesity (BMI ≥ 30)	63	34,4

Table 3. History and clinical variables
MI – myocardial infarction, PCI – percutaneous coronary intervention, CABG – bypass grafting, LV – left ventricle, DM – diabetes mellitus, CVD – cardiovascular disease

1 – year follow up								
	PCI (n = 84)		CABG (n =48)		Without revascularization (n = 39)		Without angiography (n = 12)	
Parameter	n	%	n	%	n	%	n	%
Mortality rate	4	4,8	2	4,2	4	10,3	3	25,0
Rehospitalization for UA / PCI / MI	11	13,1	5	10,4	6	15,4	5	41,7
LVEF ≥ 50%	71	84,5	31	64,6	22	56,4	4	33,3
LVEF <50%	13	15,5	17	35,4	17	43,6	8	66,7

Table 4. 1-year follow up
UA – unstable angina, PCI – percutaneous coronary intervention, MI – myocardial infarction, LVEF – left ventricle ejection fraction

	PCI (N = 84)	CABG (N = 48)	Without Revasc. (N = 39)	Without angiography (N = 12)	P value
mortality rate	4 (4,8)	2 (4,2)	4 (10,3)	2 (16,7)	0,2047
repeat hospitalization	11 (13,1)	5 (10,4)	6 (15,4)	5 (41,7)	0,0811
LVEF ≥ 50%	71 (84,5)	31 (64,6)	22 (56,4)	4 (33,3)	0,0001

Table 5. Comparison of applied therapeutic strategies during 1 year follow up
PCI - percutaneous coronary intervention, LVEF - left ventricle ejection fraction, CABG - bypass grafting

5. SLOVACS registry of acute coronary syndromes

Slovak registry of acute coronary syndromes (SLOVACS) deals with data collection and evaluation of patients hospitalized for ACS since 2007 year. Sheets with information about of ACS patients hospitalization are sent by physicians from various hospital departments (coronary units, intensive care units, cardiology or internal departments).

5.1 Objective

The aim of this analysis is to provide an assessment of management of patients with NSTE-ACS in Slovakia in 2008 year and to assess compliance of fair practice and official recommended guidelines for diagnosis and treatment of ACS without ST segment elevations. The source data for analysis were drawn from the registry of acute coronary syndromes SLOVACS (Kovar F et al., 2010).

5.2 Methods

SLOVACS registry is dedicated to both systematic data collection and subsequent analysis of ACS in Slovakia since 2007 year. This registry is organizationally arranged by Slovak Society of Cardiology (SKS) and National Health Information Centre (NHIC) (Studencan M et al., 2008).
Data on patients with acute coronary syndrome are recruited from sheets of ACS, which are completed and electronically transmitted to the NHIC by physicians from different departments (internal, cardiology, intensive care units, coronary units), where is the patient hospitalized with a diagnosis of ACS. This activity is supervised by the special regional coordinators.
In this particular analysis we evaluated data results in patients with NSTE-ACS and non-specified ACS. If the detailed and clear ECG diagnosis and accurate categorization of ACS at admission was not possible, this ACS was marked like non-specified ACS (presence of left bundle branch block, after repeated myocardial infarction, repolarization changes in left ventricular hypertrophy).
In NSTE-ACS population were assessed selected history variables, age and gender of patients. There was made an analysis of given therapy, with special attention to invasive diagnosis of ACS and revascularization therapy (PCI or surgical). It was also evaluated hospital mortality and subsequent analysis of the causes of death.

5.3 Statistical analysis

Descriptive statistics were calculated for patient groups of men and women in the categories of UA / NSTEMI-ACS and non-specified ACS. Averages and standard deviations (SD) were calculated for continuous variables and for categorical variables were calculated frequency distribution or percentage was used respectively. To estimate the statistical significance of differences, Student's *t-test* for continuous variables and Fisher's exact test for categorical variables were used. For statistically significant differences the significance level of $P < 0{,}05$ was determined. Statistical analysis was performed in SPSS, Windows version 13.0 (SPSS Inc., Chicago, IL, USA).

5.4 Results

There were reported to NHIC 3047 hospitalization for NSTE-ACS and 799 hospitalizations for non-specified ACS during period 1.1.2008 - 31.12.2008. For all subtypes of ACS, women were on average older than men and men diagnosed with NSTE-ACS were significantly older compared with a group of men in the STEMI-ACS (66 ± 12 vs. 61 ± 12, P < 0,001). Tab. 6 shows the proportion of patients in different types of ACS, taking into account age and sex.

	Number of cases			Mean age (years± SD)		
	Total	Men	Women	Total	Men	Women
ACS	6 241	3816 (61.1%)	2425 (38.9%)	67 ± 12	64 ± 12	71 ± 11 a
STEMI	2415 (38.7%)	1593 (66.0%)	822 (34.0%)	64 ± 13	61 ± 12 b	71 ± 12 a
UP / NSTEMI	3047 (48.8%)	1799 (59.0%)	1268 (41.0%)	68 ± 12	66 ± 12	71 ± 11 a
Non-spec. ACS	799 (12.5%)	444 (55.6%)	355 (44.4%)	68 ± 12	65 ± 13	71 ± 11 a

Table 6. Distribution of ACS by type, age and sex
[a] P < 0,001 men vs women, [b] P < 0,001 men with STEMI vs men with NAP/NSTEMI, ACS - acute coronary syndrome, STEMI - acute coronary syndrome with ST segment elevation, UA / NSTEMI - Unstable angina pectoris / myocardial infarction without ST segment elevations

5.5 Anamnestic data

Each patient was systematically assessed with respect to the evidence of hypertension, diabetes mellitus type I or II, history of stroke. As is apparent from the graphs 12 and 13, in both types of ACS was significantly often present arterial hypertension (80.1% respectively 78.3%) and diabetes mellitus type II (30.3% respectively 27.1%) and 12.1% of patients has history of stroke (Figures 13 and 14).

Occurence of concominat diseases in patinens with non-STE-ACS was similar in both SLOVACS registries 2007 and 2008 years (Figure 15).

5.6 Revascularization therapy

Among 3047 patients with NSTE-ACS coronary angiography was performed in 943 patients (30.9%) during index hospitalization, 799 patients (26.2%) were sent to catheterization laboratory from other institutions. Of the 799 patients with non-specified ACS was performed coronary angiography in 284 patients (35.5%). To invasive diagnosis were referred 187 patients (23.4%) from other hospitals (without catheterization facilities).

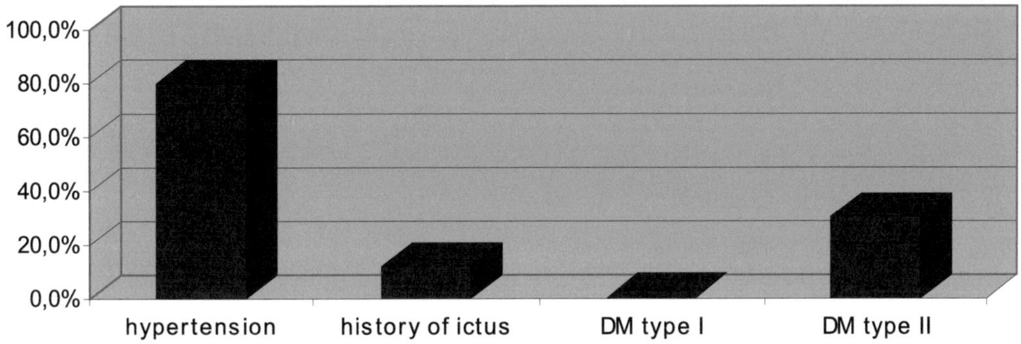

Fig. 13. Occurrence of major diseases observed in patients with UA / NSTEMI
DM - diabetes mellitus, UA / NSTEMI - Unstable angina pectoris / myocardial infarction without ST segment elevations

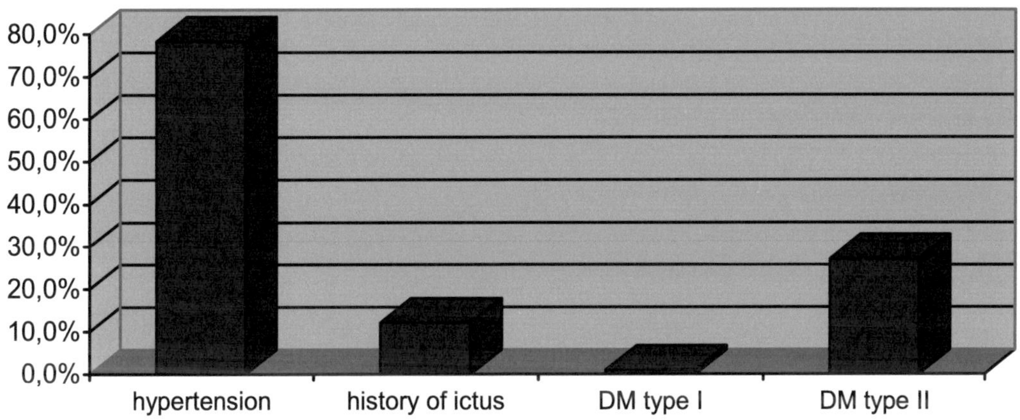

Fig. 14. Occurrence of major diseases observed in patients with non-specified ACS
DM - diabetes mellitus, ACS - acute coronary syndrome

Percutaneous coronary intervention (PCI) was performed in 409 patients (13.4%) with NSTE-ACS and 50 patients (6.3%) with non-specified ACS. During PCI was in NSTE-ACS implanted 370 intracoronary bar metal stents and 76 (20.5%) drug eluting stents. In non-specific ACS patients were during intervention procedures implanted 111 stents, including 17 (15.3%) drug eluting stents.

Surgical revascularization (CABG) was performed during hospitalization for NSTE-ACS in 165 patients (5.4%) or was scheduled electively for additional 128 patients (4.2%). Together was cardiac therapy planned for 293 patients (9.6%). In case of non-specific ACS were performed CABG immediately in 27 patients (3.5%), and planned later in 30 pts. (3.8%), together was cardiac revascularization indicated in 57 patients (7.3%).

5.7 Pharmacological treatment

SLOVACS registry systematically monitor the use of antiplatelet therapy (aspirin, clopidogrel), platelet glycoprotein IIb / IIIa receptor blockers, unfractionated and low molecular weight heparin, beta blockers, angiotensin converting enzyme inhibitors and statins. Use of individual drug groups shows table 7 and 8.

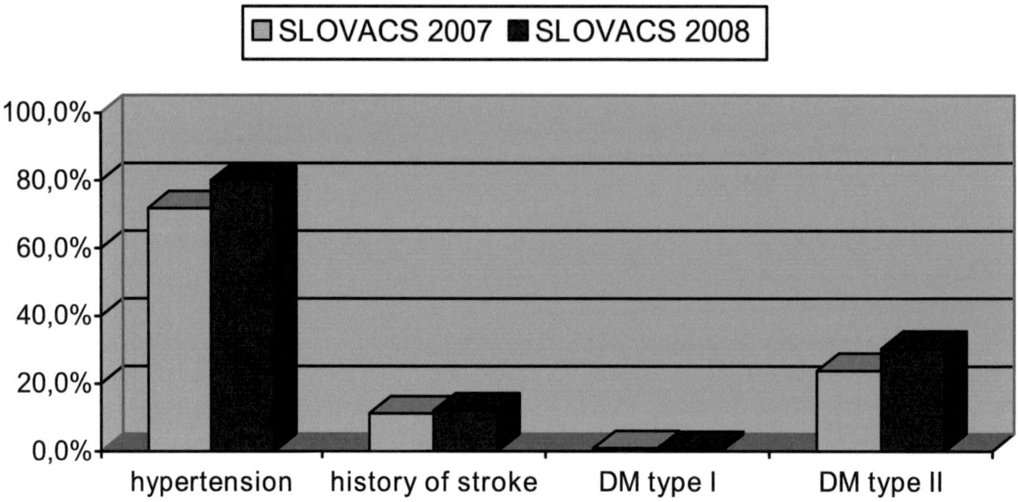

Fig. 15. Comparison of incidence of major diseases in patients with NSTE-ACS in both SLOVACS registry 2007 and 2008 year

Pharmacological treatment	N (%)
Aspirin	2753 (90.4%)
GP IIb / IIIa	70 (2.3%)
Clopidogrel	2636 (86.5%)
Beta-blocker	2471 (81.1%)
Heparin (UFH)	729 (23.9%)
Heparin (LMWH)	2267 (74.4%)
ACE inhibitor	2410 (79.1%)
Statin	2403 (78.9%)

Table 7. Concomitant treatment studied in patients with UA / NSTEMI
GP - platelet glycoprotein IIb / IIIa receptor blockers, UFH - unfractionated heparin, LMWH - low molecular weight heparin, ACE - angiotensin converting enzyme, UA / NSTEMI - Unstable angina pectoris / myocardial infarction without ST segment elevation

5.8 Hospital mortality analysis and causes of death

In group of patients hospitalized with a diagnosis of NSTE-ACS, 109 patients died (3.6%). Analysis of causes of death during hospitalization for men and women in the group with NSTE-ACS is shown in table 9 and 10.

Pharmacological treatment	N (%)
Aspirin	690 (88.6%)
GP IIb / IIIa	19 (2.4%)
Clopidogrel	625 (80.2%)
Beta-blocker	615(79.2%)
Heparin (UFH)	207 (26.6%)
Heparin (LMWH)	507 (65.1%)
ACE inhibitor	619 (79.5%)
Statin	598 (76.9%)

Table 8. Concomitant treatment studied in patients with non-specified ACS
GP - platelet glycoprotein IIb / IIIa receptor blockers, UFH - unfractionated heparin, LMWH - low molecular weight heparin, ACE - angiotensin converting enzyme, UA / NSTEMI - Unstable angina pectoris / myocardial infarction without ST segment elevation

Immediate cause of death	men	women	P
	N (%)	N (%)	
Proportion of all deaths	47 (2.6%)	62 (4.9%)	<0.001
Rupture of interventricular septum	0 (0%)	1 (1.6%)	0,413
Higher degree AV block	0 (0%)	1 (1.6%)	0,413
Cardiogenic shock	15 (31.9%)	22 (35.5%)	0,011
Pulmonary edema	5 (10.6%)	8 (12.9%)	0,076
Ventricular fibrillation	3 (6.4%)	4 (6.5%)	0,206
Other cardiac events	19 (40.4%)	18 (29.0%)	0,087
Stroke	2 (4.3%)	1 (1.6%)	0,426
Other non-cardiac cause	3 (6.4%)	7 (11.3%)	0,049

Table 9. The immediate cause of death in patients with UA / NSTEMI during the hospitalization phase
UA / NSTEMI - Unstable angina pectoris / myocardial infarction without ST segment elevation, AV - atrioventricular

Immediate cause of death	men	women	P
	N (%)	N (%)	
Proportion of all deaths	20 (4.5%)	28 (8.4%)	0.017
Rupture of interventricular septum	0 (0%)	0 (0%)	-
Higher degree AV block	1 (5.0%)	1 (3.4%)	0,494
Cardiogenic shock	7 (35.0%)	14 (50.0%)	0,021
Pulmonary edema	4 (20.0%)	2 (7.1%)	0,283
Ventricular fibrillation	2 (10.0%)	3 (10.7%)	0,271
Other cardiac events	4 (20.0%)	4 (14.3%)	0,261
Stroke	1 (5.0%)	1 (3.4%)	0,494
Other non-cardiac cause	1 (5.0%)	3 (10.7%)	0,195

Table 10. The immediate cause of death in patients non-specified ACS during the hospitalization phase
UA / NSTEMI - Unstable angina pectoris / myocardial infarction without ST segment elevation, AV - atrioventricular

Comparison of hospital mortality data from the register SLOVACS per year 2007 and 2008 and the Euro Heart Survey II provides figure 16.

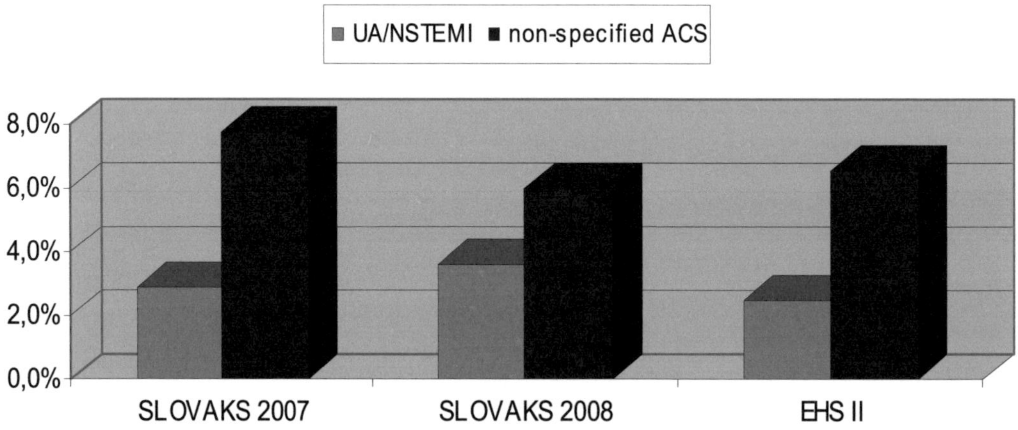

Fig. 16. Hospital mortality rate in patients with UA / NSTEMI ACS and non-specified ACS in SLOVACS registry per year 2007 and 2008 and EHS II
UA / NSTEMI - Unstable angina pectoris / myocardial infarction without ST elevation, ACS - acute coronary syndrome, EHS - Euro Herat survey

As apparent, pharmacologic treatment is administered sufficiently according guidelines. Few, however, were indicated glycoprotein IIb / IIIa platelet receptors blockers, which are applied mainly in patients during coronary intervention. Comparison with data from the register SLOVACS in 2007 and 2008 and Euro Heart Survey I and II is given in figure 17.

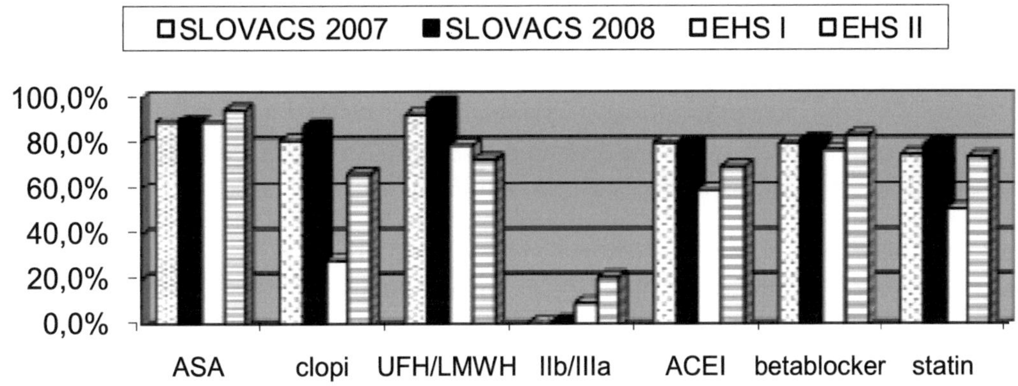

Fig. 17. Comparison of applied concomitant therapy for patients with UA / NSTEMI in the register SLOVACS 2007 and 2008 and EHS I and II
ASA - acetylsalicylic acid, clopi – clopidogrel, IIb/IIIa - platelet glycoprotein receptor blocker, UFH - unfractionated heparin, LMWH - low molecular weight heparin, ACEI - angiotensin converting enzyme inhibitor, EHC - Euro Herat survey

However, disappointing is the low proportion of patients with NSTE-ACS who are indicated for invasive diagnosis and possible subsequent coronary vessels revascularization. Comparison of data from the SLOVAKS registry 2007 and Euro Heart Survey II in terms of indications of coronary angiography and percutaneous coronary intervention in patients with NSTE-ACS shows figure 18.

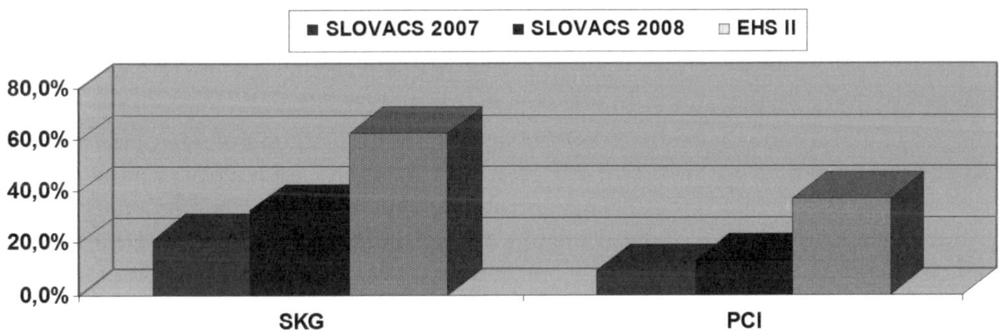

Fig. 18. Consumption of coronary angiography and PCI in patients with UA / NSTEMI according to the data from SLOVACS registry 2007 and 2008 and the EHS II
SKG - selective coronary angiography, PCI - percutaneous coronary intervention, EHS - Euro Heart Survey

Of patients who were not admitted to departments with the option for invasive diagnosis, were transferred to catheterization only 799 of 2405 patients (33.2%). Of the total number of admissions for NSTE-ACS, diagnostic catheterization underwent 943 (30.9%) patients, interventional treatment was performed in 409 patients (13.4%). These data are similar to data from other registries ACS (Polonski L et al., 2007).
There is even more serious situation in the indication of patients for invasive diagnosis among non-specified ACS group, which has highest hospital lethality (6%) in comparison

with various types of ACS. These patients are often elderly, with more significant co morbidity, renal insufficiency (Lev EI et al., 2003). From invasive diagnostic benefit most patients with high risk of cardiovascular complications.

Patients with UA / NSTEMI represent a heterogeneous group of diseases with potentially serious both in-hospital course and long-term prognosis. As was found by the results of SLOVACS registry 2008, there is frequent co morbidity with high presence of hypertension and diabetes mellitus type II in patients with NSTE-ACS. Hospital mortality was 3.6%, in patients with NSTE-ACS and 6% in non-specified ACS, respectively. SLOVACS registry data confirm excellent acceptance of recommendations, relating to the combined pharmacological treatment of NSTE-ACS with a high administeration rate of dual antiplatelet therapy, beta blockers, angiotensin converting enzyme inhibitors, anticoagulant therapy (UFH and LMWH) and statins. In the management of NSTE-ACS would be desirable more frequent application of platelet glycoprotein IIb / IIIa inhibitors, especially in high-risk patients. Unsatisfactory low is the indication rate for invasive diagnostic procedures and revascularization treatment. Only 30.9% of patients with UA / NSTEMI and 23.4% with non-specified ACS have performed selective angiography during the initial hospitalization. PCI was performed in 13.4% patients with NSTE-ACS and only 6.3% patients with non-specified ACS. SLOVACS registry results suggest the need for increased concentration of attention on a consistent risk stratification of patients with NSTE-ACS. In the case of medium or high risk of cardiovascular complications and unfavorable course, patients should be indicated for selective angiography and depend on finding, further coronary artery revascularization. Invasive diagnosis in these patients has to be conducted during the index hospitalization for NSTE-ACS.

6. Impact of bleeding complications on the prognosis of NSTE-ACS

In most cases a vulnerable plaque (with rupture or erosion) in the coronary artery with the presence of intracoronary platelets rich thrombus represents pathophysiologic basis of ACS. The key basic treatment regimen for NSTE-ACS is, therefore, antiplatelet therapy (mostly dual) and application anticoagulants agents (unfractionated heparin, low molecular weight heparin, fondaparinux, and direct thrombin inhibitors). In patients treated with PCI are often administered platelet IIb / IIIa receptor blocker. These combined and effective antithrombotic approaches significantly reduce the incidence of thrombotic complications in NSTE-ACS, but are often associated with an increased risk of bleeding. Recently, systematic attention is paid to the impact of bleeding on prognosis in patients with NSTE-ACS.

6.1 Occurrence

Bleeding complications can achieve varying degrees of severity. The most frequently used assessment is according to the TIMI (Thrombolysis in myocardial infarction) and GUSTO (Global utilization of streptokinase and t-PA for occluded coronary arteries) criteria (Table 11) (Antman EM et al., 2005; GUSTO investigators, 1993).

The incidence of major bleeding complications in the treatment of NSTE-ACS is in the range 2-15% (OASIS-2 investigators, 1999; Ferguso JJ et al., 2004; Bhat DL et al., 2004). Frequency of bleeding is influenced by excessive dose antithrombotic medications, antithrombotic agents alternation (switching), presence of renal dysfunction, higher age of the patient and female gender (Alexander KP et al., 2005; Collet JP et al., 2005). European register GRACE (Global registry of acute coronary events) has identified additional independent predictors of major bleeding complications in NSTE-ACS patients (Table 12) (Moscucci M et al., 2003).

Hemorrhage	Characteristics of bleeding
TIMI classification	
Large	intracranial, decreased Hb ≥ 50 g / l
Small	decrease in Hb 30-50 g / l
Minimum	decrease in Hb <30 g / l
GUSTO classification	
Severe / life -threatening	intracranial or hemodynamically significant or requiring intervention
Medium	requiring transfusion but without hemodynamic disability
Slightly	does not meets the criteria for severe or moderate major bleeding

Table 11. Assessment of severity of bleeding in acute coronary syndrome
TIMI = Thrombolysis in myocardial infarction, GUSTO = Global utilization of streptokinase and t-PA for occluded coronary arteries

Parameter	Adjusted OR	95% CI	P
age (increase per 10year)	1,22	1,10-1,35	0,0002
female sex	1,36	1,07-1,73	0,0116
renal insufficiency	1,53	1,13-2,08	0,0062
history of bleeding	2,18	1,14-4,08	0,014
mean BP (per 20mmHg decrease)	1,14	1,02-1,27	0,019
diuretic therapy	1,91	1,46-2,49	<0.0001
IIb / IIIa receptor blocker therapy	1,86	1,43-2,43	<0.0001
fibrinolysis receptor blocker + IIb / IIIa	4,19	1,68-10,4	0,002
administration of inotropic agents	1,88	1,35-2,62	0,0002
right-sided catheterization	2,01	1,38-2,91	0,0003

Table 12. Independent predictors of major bleeding in NSTE-ACS
NSTE ACS = acute coronary syndrome without ST segment elevation, BP = mean blood pressure

6.2 The prognosis in patients with severe bleeding

Significant increase of hospital mortality rate in patients with ACS and bleeding (OR 1.64, p <0.0001) highlighted the results from the GRACE registry, which collects data of patients with NSTE ACS already since 1999 year (Moscucci M et al., 2003) (Figure 19).

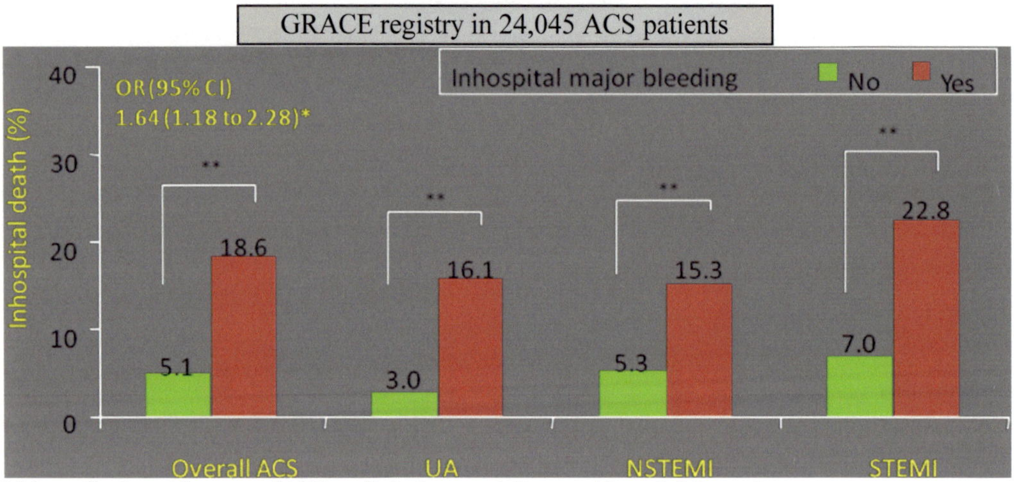

*After adjustment for comorbidities, clinical presentation, and hospital therapies

**p<0.001 for differences in unadjusted death rates

Fig. 19. Association of major bleeding and an increased risk of hospital death in ACS patients

In REPLACE (Randomized Evaluation of PCI linking angiomax to reduced clinical events) - 2 study, patients with major bleeding had 30 times higher risk of death during the 30-day monitoring in comparison with patients without such bleeding complications (5.2% vs. 0.2%; p <0.001). Moreover, the multivariate analysis identified a major bleeding as the third strongest predictor (with renal dysfunction and heart failure) of 1-year mortality (OR 3.53, 95% CI 1.91 to 6.53, p <0.0001) (Stone GW, 2004).

Analysis of more than 26 000 patients from ACS studies GUSTO (Global utilization of streptokinase and t-PA for occluded coronary arteries) IIb, PURSUIT (Platelet glycoprotein IIb / IIIa in unstable angina: receptor suppression using INTEGRILIN therapy) and PARAGON (Platelet IIb / IIIa antagonist for the reduction of acute coronary syndrome events in a global organization network) shows a link between 30-day mortality and severity of bleeding, irrespectively of invasive procedures (Figure 20) (Rao SW et al., 2005).

Another meta-analysis (34 000 patients) from OASIS (Organization to ASSESS strategies in acute ischemic syndromes) registry, OASIS-2 study and CURE (Clopidogrel in unstable angina to Prevent Recurrent Events) study confirmed that serious bleeding is a strong independent predictor of mortality, myocardial infarction and stroke (Table 13) (Eikelboom JE et al., 2006).

Interesting results were shown by a 10-year retrospective analysis of 11 000 patients treated with PCI (Kinnaird TO et al., 2003). Major bleeding was confirmed as an independent risk factor for hospital mortality (OR 3.5, 95% CI 1.9 to 6.7, p = 0.001). Patients with bleeding complications had significantly higher incidence of Q-wave myocardial infarction (1.2% vs. 0.2%, p <0.001), non Q-wave myocardial infarction (30.7% vs. 11.8%, p <0.001) and needs for repeat revascularization (1.9% vs. 0.3%, p <0.001) compared with the group without bleeding. Significantly increased risk of death was associate with bleeding by TIMI criteria rated as small as well (1.8% vs. 0.6%, p <0.001) (Figure 21).

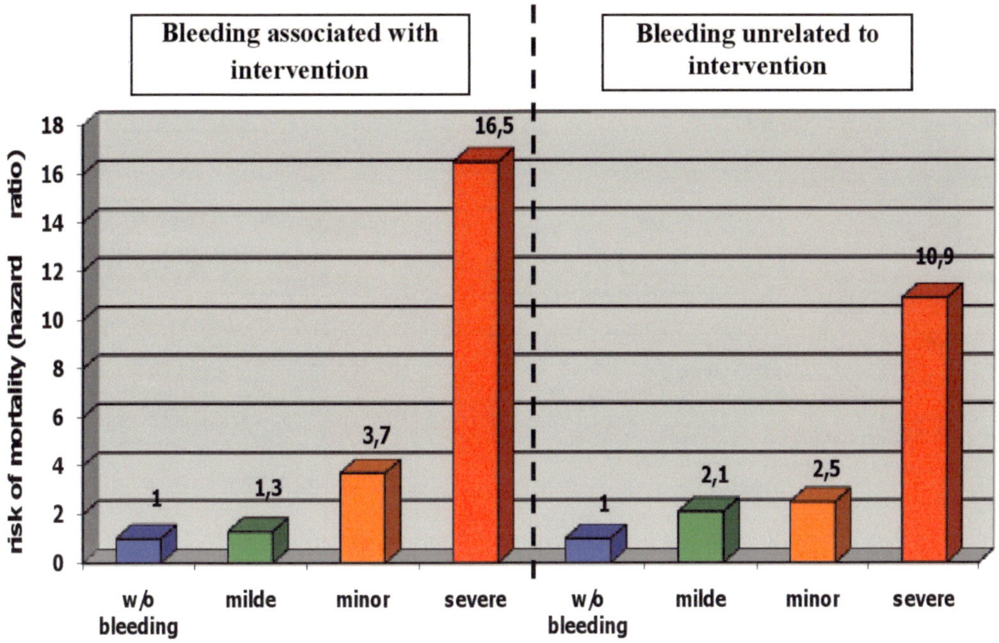

Fig. 20. Effect of bleeding severity by GUSTO criteria on 30-day mortality in patients with NSTE-ACS
GUSTO = Global utilization of streptokinase and t-PA for occluded coronary arteries, NSTE-ACS = acute coronary syndrome without ST segment elevation

OASIS registry, OASIS-2 and CURE (N = 34 126)				
Parameter	**Severe bleeding**	**No major bleeding**	**Adjusted HR (95% CI)**	**P**
Mortality	12.8%	2.5%	5.37 (3,97-7,26)	<0.0001
Myocardial infarction	10.6%	4.1%	4.44 (3,16-6,24)	<0.0001
Stroke	2.6%	0.6%	6.46 (3,54-11,79)	<0.0001

Table 13. Effect of bleeding on the clinical course
OASIS = Organization to assess strategies in acute ischemic syndromes, CURE = Clopidogrel in unstable angina to prevent recurrent events

Unambiguous confirmation of the negative impact of bleeding on the both early and long-term prognosis of patients with NSTE-ACS was brought by randomized trial OASIS-5 (Yusuf S et al., 2006). This clinical study compared the effect of fondaparinux and enoxaparin in the treatment of more than 20 000 patients with NSTE-ACS. Although the primary efficacy endpoint (incidence of death, myocardial infarction or refractory ischemia to day 9) was similar in both groups (5.8% vs. 5.7%, p = ns), treatment with fondaparinux was associated with significantly lower incidence of bleeding complications (2.2% vs. 4.1%, p <0.001). Net clinical benefit, expressed the occurrence of death, myocardial infarction,

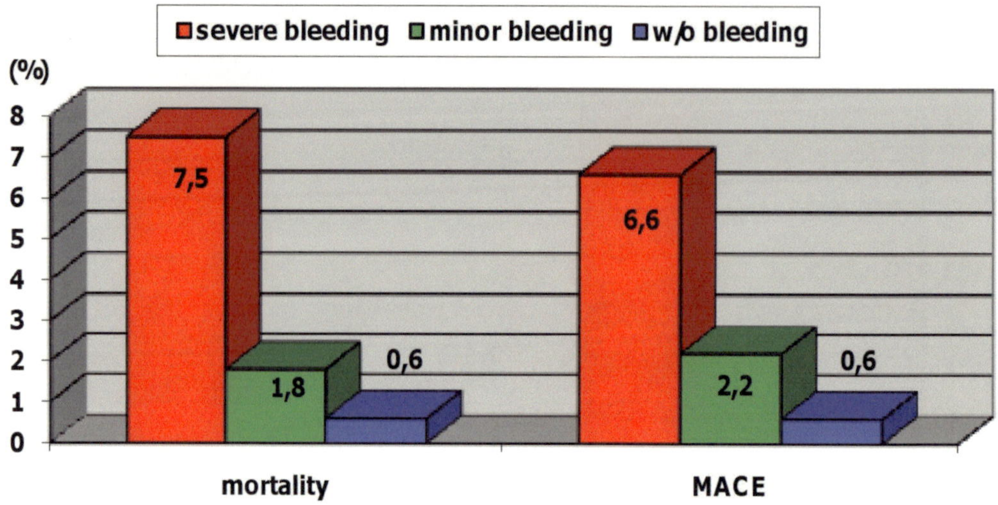

Fig. 21. Effect of bleeding on the hospital course in patients treated with PCI
PCI = percutaneous coronary intervention, MACE = major cardiac events

OASIS-5 (n = 20,078)		
	30 days	180 days
Major bleeding	HR (95% CI)	HR (95% CI)
Death	5.06 (4,59-5,62)	3.16 (2,92-3,44)
Myocardial infarction	5.01 (4,56-5,57)	2.99 (2,75-3,28)
CMP	4.77 (3,95-6,00)	3,30 (2,82-3,97)
Minor bleeding	HR (95% CI)	HR (95% CI)
Death	2.42 (2,03-2,97)	1.76 (1,31-2,37)
Myocardial infarction	1.48 (1,28-1,78)	1,29 (1,15-1,48)
CMP	1.54 (1,06-2,67)	1.48 (0,76-2,89)

Table 14. Effect of bleeding to day 9 at 30 and 180-day course of patients with NSTE-ACS
OASIS = Organization to ASSESS strategies in acute ischemic syndromes, stroke = stroke, NSTE-ACS = acute coronary syndrome without ST segment elevation

refractory ischemia or major bleeding was more favorable in fondaparinux group (7.3% vs. 9.0%, p <0.001). Patients with significant bleeding to 9 day, had during a long-term (30 and 180 days) follow-up in the OASIS-5 study higher cumulative risk of mortality, myocardial infarction and stroke. This increased cumulative risk was present even in group of patients with a small bleeding (Table 14, Figure 22, 23, 24) (Budaj A et al., 2006).

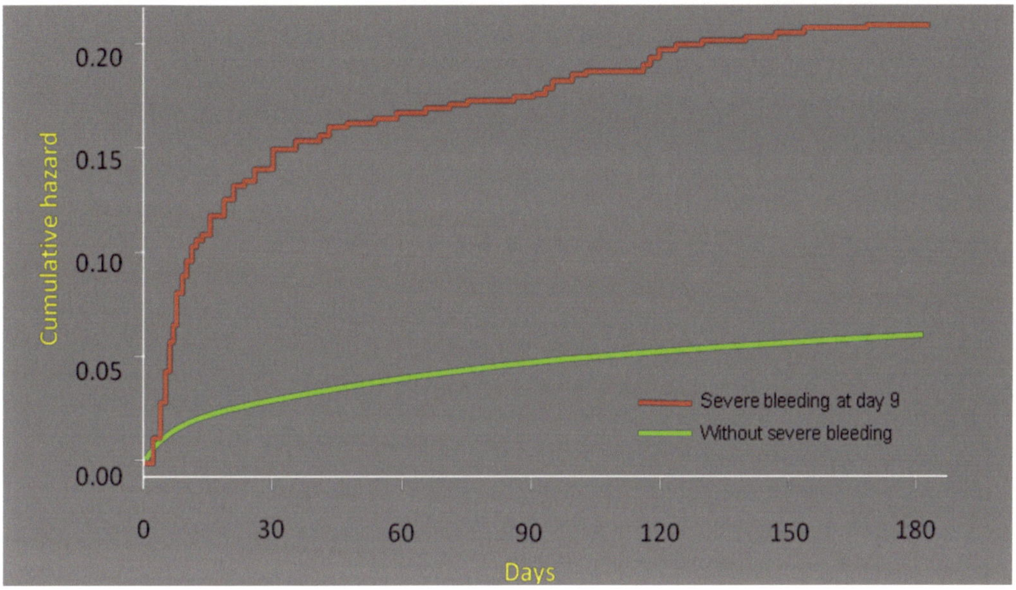

Adjusted HR (95% CI) at day 30: 5.06 (4.59-5.62); at day 180: 3.16 (2.92-3.44)

Fig. 22. Increase mortality rate in patients with severe bleeding at day 9 (all pts at day 30 resp. day 180)

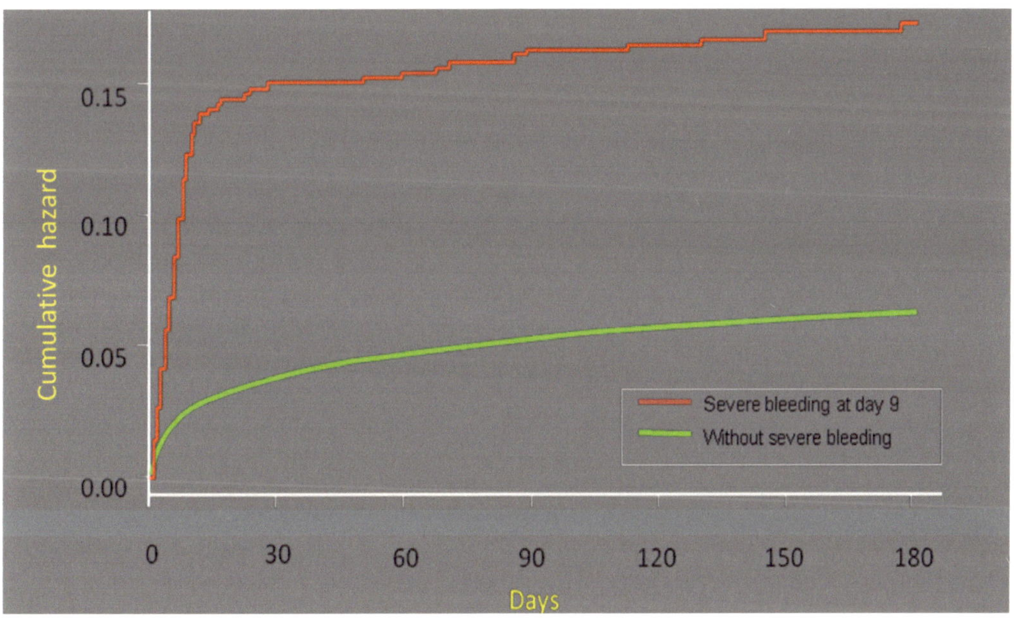

Adjusted HR (95% CI) at day 30: 5.01 (4.56-5.57); at day 180: 2.99 (2.75-3.28)

Fig. 23. Increase risk of myocardial infarction in patients with severe bleeding at day 9 (all pts at day 30 resp. day 180)

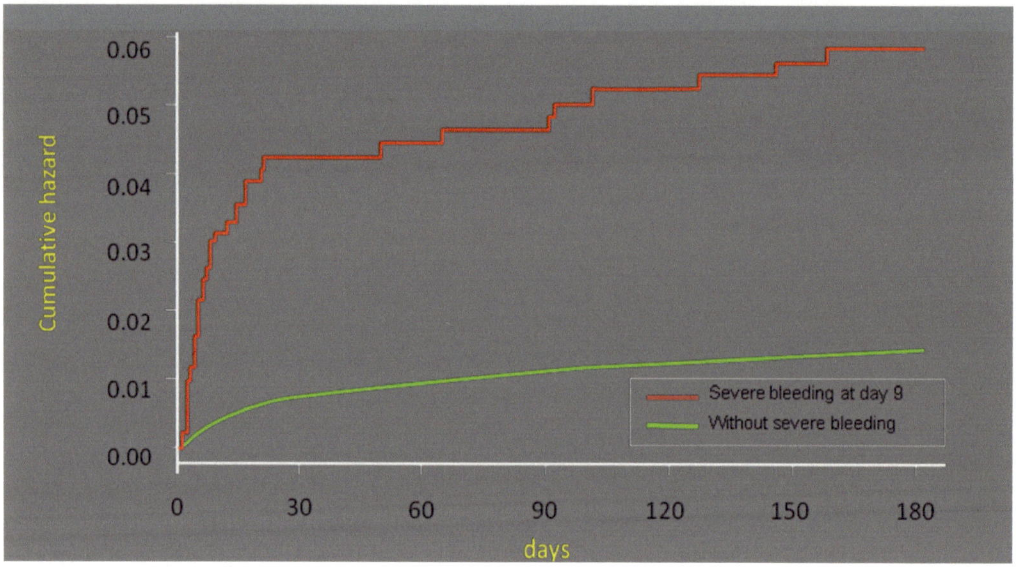

Adjusted HR (95% CI) at day 30: 4.77 (3.95-6.00); at day 180: 3.30 (2.82-3.97)

Fig. 24. Increase risk of stroke in patients with severe bleeding at day 9
(all pts at day 30 resp. day 180)

6.3 The mechanisms for worsening clinical course

There are postulated several mechanisms in connection with bleeding that could worse clinical course in NSTE-ACS (Table 15).

hemodynamic consequences
renal failure
effect of transfusion
prothrombotic and proinflammatory state triggered by bleeding
need to discontinue antiplatelet and anticoagulant therapy

Table 15. Postulated mechanisms of worse course during bleeding

Serious consequence of bleeding is interruption of antithrombotic therapy. Clinically significant bleeding actually required discontinuation of anticoagulant and antiplatelet therapy until resolution. In the case of small transition bleeding is often possible to continue this therapy (Bassand JP et al., 2007).

Application of blood transfusion improves the prognosis of elderly patients with acute myocardial infarction and hematocrit <30% (Wu WC et al., 2001). However, in the hematocrit values > 33% there was not demonstrated the usefulness of a blood transfusion.

By contrast, in several clinical trials and meta-analysis, the administration of blood transfusion was associated with increased mortality, higher incidence of myocardial infarction and refractory ischemia (Sabatine MS et al., 2005; Rao SW et al., 2004) (Figure 25).

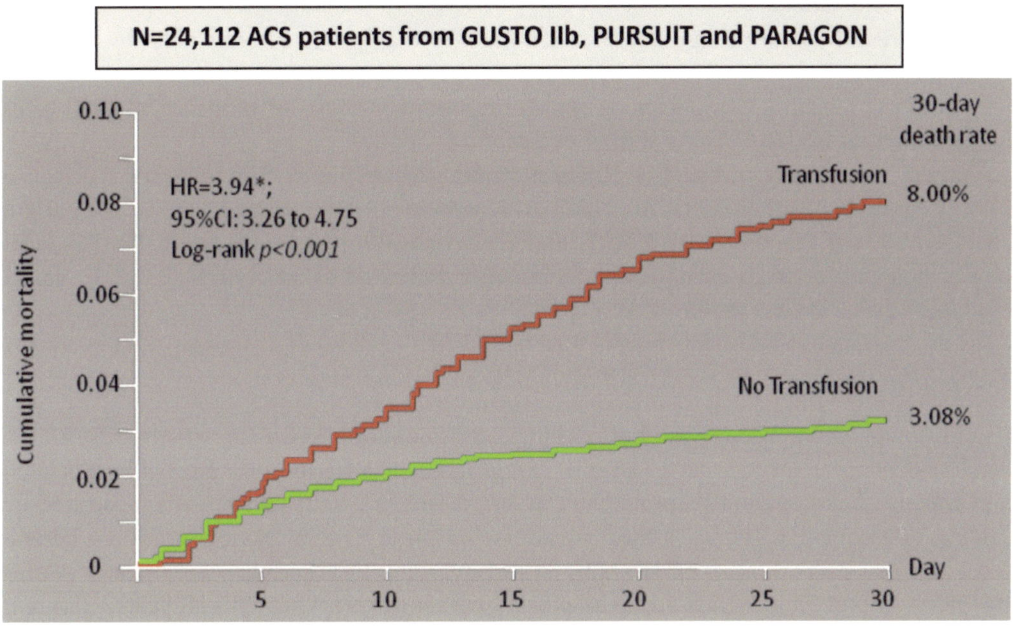

Adjusted for baseline characteristics, bleeding and transfusion propensity and nadir hematocrit

Fig. 25. Association of blood transfusion with an increased 30-day mortality in UA/NSTEMI patients

On the worsening clinical course in patients with NSTE-ACS after transfusion administration may participate:

a. erythrocyte damage
b. influence the metabolism of NO in blood storage
c. impaired release of oxygen from hemoglobin in the reduction content of 2,3 - difosfoglycerate in erythrocytes
d. increase inflammatory mediators (Fransen SV et al., 2008)

Accurate cut-off level of hemoglobin and hematocrit for indication of blood transfusion in patients with NSTE-ACS are not provided. According to current recommendations of the European Society of Cardiology transfusion is not indicated for hemoglobin> 80g / l or hematocrit> 25%, provided that anemia is a hemodynamically well tolerated (Bassand JP et al., 2007).

6.4 Prevention of bleeding complications

Given the demonstrated risk of severe clinical events associated with bleeding and administration of blood transfusions, it is extremely important to use in patients with NSTE-ACS all available measures in bleeding prevention. It is necessary to focus particularly on:

- choice of safe drug (fondaparinux in OASIS-5 study)
- appropriate dosage (taking into account age, gender, creatinine clearance)
- duration of antithrombotic therapy
- timing of early invasive treatment
- choice of arterial access
- combination of anticoagulant and antiplatelet therapy to choose only by certified indications

Prevention of bleeding complications is also important in terms of reducing hospital costs for treatment of NSTE-ACS. As shown by economic analysis of the GUSTO IIb study, with an increase in severity of bleeding, there is prolonged hospitalization and rising financial costs. Length of hospitalization for NSTE-ACS without bleeding was 5.4 days, with slight bleeding 6.9, with moderate 15.0 days, and severe bleeding 16.4 days ($p < 0.01$). Financial cost of hospitalization in each group significantly increased as follows: 14 282 USD vs. 21 674 USD vs. 45 798 USD vs. 66 564 USD ($p < 0.01$) (Rao SV et al., 2008).

7. Conclusion

In addition to a comprehensive pharmacologic treatment of NSTE-ACS, which includes the combined antiplatelet regimens (aspirin, clopidogrel, platelet receptor IIb / IIIa blockers) and effective anticoagulant therapy, plays an important role early invasive diagnosis and by finding subsequent coronary artery revascularization. From invasive procedures benefit most high risk patients with NSTE-ACS, who undergoing PCI. Early invasive strategy is for this risk group of patients safe and is associated with long-term favorable clinical course and substantially influence prognosis.

There is very important in NSTE-ACS patients risk stratification at the beginning and according to the assessed risk scores subsequent decision for urgent or early invasive strategy. In low-risk NSTE-ACS is indicated stress test and in case of inducible ischemia is than followed by coronary angiography before hospital discharge.

Patients with NSTE-ACS represent a risk population with an increased incidence of ischemic and bleeding complications. Bleeding events significantly affect both short and long-term prognosis of patients with NSTE-ACS. This is why it is necessary in the global risk stratification of NSTE-ACS a careful assessment of the risk of bleeding. Balanced assessment of the risk for both thrombotic and bleeding complications allows then to select optimal diagnostic and therapeutic management of patients with NSTE-ACS.

8. References

Alexander KP, Chen AY, Roe MT et al.: Excess dosing of antiplatelet and antithrombin agents in the treatment of non ST segment elevation acute coronary syndromes. JAMA 2005; 294: 3108-3116

Antman EM, Cohen M, Bernink PJ et al.: The TIMI risk score for unstable angina/non ST elevation MI: a method for prognostication and therapeutic decision making. JAMA 2000; 284: 835-842

Antman EM, Morrow DA, McCabe CH et al.: Enoxaparin versus unfractionated heparin as antithrombin therapy in patients receiving fibrinolysis for ST elevation myocardial infarction. Design and rationale for the Enoxaparin and thrombolysis reperfusion for acute myocardial infarction treatment-Thrombolysis in myocardial infarction study 25 (ExTRACT-TIMI 25). Am Heart J 2005; 149: 217-226

Bassand JP, Hamm CW, Ardissino D et al.: Guidelines for the diagnosis and treatment of non ST elevation acute coronary syndromes. The Task force for the diagnosis and treatment of non ST elevation acute coronary syndromes of the European society of cardiology. Eur Heart J 2007; 28:1598-1660

Bavry AA, Kumbhani DJ, Rassi AN et al.: Benefit of early invasive therapy in acute coronary syndromes: a meta-analysis of contemporary randomized clinical trials. J Am Coll Cardiol 2006; 48: 1319-1325

Bhatt DL, Roe MT, Peterson ED et al.: Utilization of early invasive management strategies for high risk patients with non ST elevation acute coronary syndromes: results from the CRUSADE quality improvement initiative. JAMA 2004; 292: 2096-2104

Budaj A, Eikelboom J, Wallentin L et al.: Bleeding complications predict major cardiovascular outcomes in non ST elevation acute coronary syndromes: results from the OASIS-5 trial. J Amer Coll Cardiol 2006; 47: 195A

Cannon CP, Weintraub WS, Demopoulos LA et al.: Comparison of early invasive and conservative strategies in patients with unstable coronary syndromes treated with the glycoprotein IIb/IIIa inhibitor tirofiban. N Engl J Med 2001; 344: 1879-1887

Collet JP, Montalescot G, Angelli G et al.: Non ST segment elevation acute coronary syndrome in patients with renal dysfunction: benefit of low molecular weight heparin alone or with glycoprotein IIb/IIIa inhibitors on outcomes. The Global registry of acute coronary events. Eur Heart J 2005; 26: 2285-2293

Diderholm E, Andren B, Frostfeldt G et al.: The prognostic and therapeutic implications of troponin T levels and ST depression in unstable coronary artery disease: the FRISC II invasive troponin T electrocardiogram substudy. Am Heart J 2002; 143: 760-767

Eagle KA, Lim MJ, Dabbous OH et al.: A validated prediction model for all forms of acute coronary syndrome: estimating the risk of 6-month postdischarge death in an intervational registry. JAMA 2004; 291: 2727-2733

Eikelboom JW, Mehta RS, Anand SS et al.: Adverse impact of bleeding on prognosis in patients with acute coronary syndromes. Circulation 2006; 114: 774-782

Ferguso JJ, Califf RM, Antman et al.: Enoxaparin vs unfractionated heparin in high risk patients with non ST elevation acute coronary syndromes managed with an intended early invasive strategy: primary results of the SYNERGY randomized trial. JAMA 2004; 292: 45-54

Fox KA, Poole Wilson PA, Henderson RA et al.: Interventional versus conservative treatment for patients with unstable angina or non ST elevation myocardial infarction: the British heart foundation RITA 3 randomised trial. Randomised intervention trial of unstable angina. Lancet 2002; 360: 743-751

Fox KA, Goldman SG, Anderson SA et al.: From guidelines to clinical practice: the impact of hospital and geographical characteristics on temporal trends in the management of acute coronary syndromes. The Global registry of acute coronary events (GRACE). Eur Heart J 2003; 24: 1414-1424

Fox KA, Poole Wilson PA, Clayton TC et al.: 5-year outcome of an interventional strategy in non ST elevation acute coronary syndrome: the British heart foundation RITA 3 randomised trial. Lancet 2005; 366: 914-920

Fox KA, Dabbous OH, Goldberg RJ et al.: Prediction of risk of death and myocardial infarction in the six months after presentation with acute coronary syndrome: prospective multinational observational study (GRACE). BMJ 2006; 333: 1091-1094

Fransen E, Maessen J, Dentener M et al.: Impact of blood transfusion on inflammatory mediator release in patients undergoing cardiac surgery. Chest 1999; 116: 1233-1292

FRISC II investigators. Invasive compared with non-invasive treatment in unstable coronary artery disease: FRISC II prospective randomised multicentre study. Lancet 1999; 354: 708-715

The GUSTO investigators. An international randomized trial comparing four thrombolytic strategies for acute myocardial infarction. E Engl J Med 1993; 329: 673-682

Hirsh A, Windhausen F, Tijsen JG et al.: Long term outcome after an early invasive versus selective invasive treatment strategy in patients with non ST elevation coronary syndrome and elevated cardiac troponin T (the ICTUS trial): a follow up study. Lancet 2007; 369: 827-835

Kinnaird TD, Stabile E, Mintz GS et al.: Incidence, predictors and prognostic implications of bleeding and blood transfusion following percutaneous coronary interventions. Am J Cardiol 2003; 92: 930-935

Kovar F, Krajči P, Mečiar P et al.: Invazívna diagnostika a intervenčná liečba akútnych koronárnych syndrómov - vlastné skúsenosti. Kardiol prax. 2003; 1: 109-113

Kovar F, Krajči P, Mečiar P et al.: Klinický a angiografický profil pacientov s akútnym koronárnym syndrómom. Interná med., 2004; 4: 609-613

Kovář F, Krajči P, Margóczy R et al.: Má výber úvodnej liečby u pacientov s akútnym koronárnym syndrómom bez elevácií segmentov ST vplyv na dlhodobý priebeh? Cardiol 2007; 16 (6): 259-264

Kovář F: Možnosti invazívneho manažmentu u pacientov s akútnym koronárnym syndrómom: Je potrebná stratifikácia rizika? Interná med 2008; 1: 31-35

Kovář F, Studenčan M, Hricák V et al.: Manažment pacientov s akútnym koronárnym syndrómom bez elevácií segmentov ST. Analýza údajov registra SLOVAKS z roku 2008. Cardiol, 2010, 19(3), 181-191

Lagerqvist B, Husted S, Kontny F et al.: 5-year outcomes in the FRISC II randomized trial of an invasive versus conservative strategy in non ST elevation acute coronary syndromes: a follow-up study. Lancet 2006; 368: 998-1004

Lev EI, Battler A, Behar S et al.: Frequency, characteristics and outcome of patients hospitalized with acute coronary syndromes with undetermined electrocardiographic patterns. Am J Cardiol 2003; 91: 224-227

Mehta SR, Cannon CP, Fox KA et al.: Routine vs selective invasive strategies in patiens with acute coronary syndromes: a collaborative metaanalysis of randomized trials. JAMA 2005; 293: 2908-2917

Moscucci M, Fox KA, Cannon CP et al.: Predictors of major bleeding in acute coronary syndromes: the Global registry of acute coronary events (GRACE). Eur Heart J 2003; 24: 1815-1823

Neumann FJ, Castrati A, Pogatsa Murray G et al.: Evaluation of prolonged antithrombotic pretreatment („cooling off strategy") before intervention in patients with unstable coronary syndromes: a randomized controlled trial. JAMA 2003; 290: 1593-1599

Organisation to assess strategies for ischemic syndromes (OASIS-2) investigators. Effect of recombinant hirudin (lepirudin) compared with heparin on death, myocardial infarction, refractory angina and revascularization procedures in patients with acute myocardial ischaemia without ST elevation: a randomized trial. Lancet 1999; 353: 429-438

Polonski L, Gasior M, Gierlotka M et al.: Polish registry f acute coronary syndromes (PL-ACS). Characteristics, treatments and outcomes of patients with acute coronary syndromes in Poland. Kardiol Pol 2007; 65: 861-872

Rao SV, Jollis JG, Harrington RA et al.: Relationship of blood transfusion and clinical outcomes in patients with acute coronary syndromes. JAMA 2004;292: 1555–1562

Rao SV, Jolis LG, Harrington RA et al.: Relationship of blood transfusion and clinical outcomes in patients with acute coronary syndromes. JAMA 2004; 292: 1555-1562

Rao SV, O´Grady K, Pieper RS et al.: Impact of Bleeding Severity on Clinical Outcomes Among Patients With Acute Coronary Syndromes. Am J Cardiol 2005; 96: 1200-1206

Rao SV, Kaul PR, Liao L et al.: Association bertween bleeding, blood transfusion and costs among patients with non ST segment elevation acute coronary syndromes. Amer Heart J 2008; 155: 369-374

Rosamond W, Flegal K, Friday G et al.: Heart Disease and Stroke Statistics-2007 Update: A Report From the American Heart Association Statistics Committee and Stroke Statistics Subcommittee. Circulation 2007; 115: e69-e171

Sabatine MS, Morrow DA, Giugliano RP et al.: Association of hemoglobin levels with clinical outcomes in acute coronary syndromes. Circulation 2005; 111: 2042-2049

Stone GW: Advantages of direct thrombin inhibition in high- and low-risk patients. J Invasive Cardiol 2004;16(Suppl G):12-17

Studenčan M, Baráková A, Hlava P et al.: Slovenský register akútnych koronárnych syndrómov (SLOVAKS)-analýza údajov z roku 2007. Cardiol 2008; 17: 179-190

Wu WC, Rathore SS, Wang Y et al.: Blood transfusion in elderly patients with acute myocardial infarction. N Engl J Med 2001; 5: 310-317

Yusuf S, Mehta SR, Chrolavicius S et al.: Efficacy and safety of fondaparinux compared to enoxaparin in 20 078 patients with acute coronary syndromes without ST segment elevation. The OASIS (Organization to assess strategies in acute ischemic syndromes)-5 investigators. N Engl J Med 2006; 354: 1464-1476

3

Trans Radial Access for Diagnostic Coronary Angiography and Percutaneous Coronary Interventions: Current Concepts and Future Challenges

Deepak Natarajan
Moolchand MedCity
New Delhi
India

1. Introduction

Transradial approach (TRA) for diagnostic coronary angiography was first used as early as 1948(1) but was soon abandoned for larger access vessels such as femoral and brachial arteries because catheters then used were too large and cumbersome to be routinely used for radial artery cut down. The radial access technique was re-introduced 2 decades ago and has since then been employed both for diagnostic coronary angiography and percutaneous coronary intervention (PCI). It is however still not as popular as the femoral artery approach (FA) in most parts of the world. The femoral artery has conventionally been the most popular approach despite some limitations, such as presence of peripheral artery disease, anticoagulated patients, obese patients or those who have orthopedic problems of the spine or hip. The patient, with FA, has to lie down for several hours post procedure and this can be arduous in the presence of congestive heart failure or lung disease. The duration of recumbency with the femoral approach albeit shortened by closure devices but controlled trials have yet to demonstrate significantly reduced access site complications, and also such devices are not employed all over the world.

Professor Lucien Campeau, a French Canadian physician described coronary angiography by TRA in 1989 (2-3) and Professor Ferdinand Kiemeneij in Amsterdam performed successful PCI for the first time using the radial approach in 1993(4). Keimeneij also conducted a randomized study involving 900 patients comparing trans femoral, trans brachial and trans radial approaches in patients undergoing percutaneous coronary angioplasty (PTCA). All 3 approaches had equivalent clinical outcomes but local access site complications were substantially less in the TRA subgroup (5).

The TRA has certain advantages over the conventional FA. The radial artery is close to the skin surface and can therefore be more easily palpated and punctured. The radial artery can be easily compressed post procedure and the patient is almost immediately mobile. Moreover the patient can be discharged in a couple of hours after diagnostic coronary angiography and the next day if he has undergone PCI.

2. Allen test

Traditionally cardiologists confirm dual supply to the hand by radial and ulnar arteries by performing the Allen's test (6-7). The hand is supplied by both radial and ulnar arteries. The radial artery is hence not an end artery like the femoral or brachial arteries .In the event of radial artery block, albeit quite uncommon, the hand continues to get blood supply via the ulnar artery.

Many, but not all, interventional cardiologists therefore check for ulnar collateral supply before a procedure by the Allen's test. Both arteries are compressed firmly till the palm of the hand blanches. The ulnar artery is suddenly released and if the palm regains color quickly (within 8-10 seconds) the ulnar artery is patent. Another method, probably more objective is to check waveforms and oxygen saturation by a pulse oximetry/plethysmography. Rapid re-appearance, on release of ulnar artery compression, of arterial pulse waveform documented by an oxygen saturation probe placed on the index finger confirms patency of the ulnar artery (Figures 1-5). Some operators in recent times however have done away with assessing dual hand circulation and almost 30% no longer bother with the Allen test (8).

3. Radial puncture

The first step is the preparation and draping of the wrist (usually right) and the radial artery is punctured with a needle with or without the use of local anesthesia. The needle varies in length form 2-4 cms and 19-21 gauge. Some operators prefer the shorter needles because it is easier to pick the flash of blood observed on puncturing the radial artery. Operators in Asia prefer a hydrophilic sheath covered needle. Patient discomfort is minimal and radial artery spasm non-existent. An introducer wire is threaded through the needle into the radial artery and minute quantity of local anesthesia (1-2 ml) is administered (if not given earlier) at the base of the needle with the introducer wire. Next a tiny superficial incision is made on the skin ensuring the radial artery is not damaged. The puncture by the needle is usually made 2-3 cms above the radial styloid. A dedicated 5 Fr or 6 Fr sheath is introduced into the radial artery, 1,000 -2,000 units of heparin and 50-100 mcg of nitroglycerine administered intra - arterially to prevent thrombus and spasm .The arterial sheath, 5 Fr or 6 Fr, is connected to the pressure transducer to confirm radial artery entry pulse waveform (Figures 6-9).

4. Coronary angiography

We use the Tiger II (Terumo) catheter to hook both left and right coronary arteries during diagnostic coronary angiography, while PCI is performed by standard 6 Fr left and right guiding catheters (Judkins, XB, Amplatz left, EBU and Kimny). Once radial access has been successfully achieved it is easy to navigate diagnostic and guide catheters through the brachial, axillary and subclavian arteries into the ascending arch of aorta. It is important to visualize the negotiation of the catheter right from the wrist to the aorta under fluoroscopy Direct visualization ensures the correct route is adopted preventing vascular complications (Figures 10-15). The right radial artery is preferred by most operators while the left artery is avoided in patients with compromised kidney function as it may be needed for a future arterio-venous shunt. Similarly the left renal artery is not employed in a prospective coronary bypass surgery patient who may need a radial graft. The left radial approach however is particularly helpful for left internal mammary artery PCI, and with traditional diagnostic and guide catheters(Judkins,EBU,XBU etc) are used.

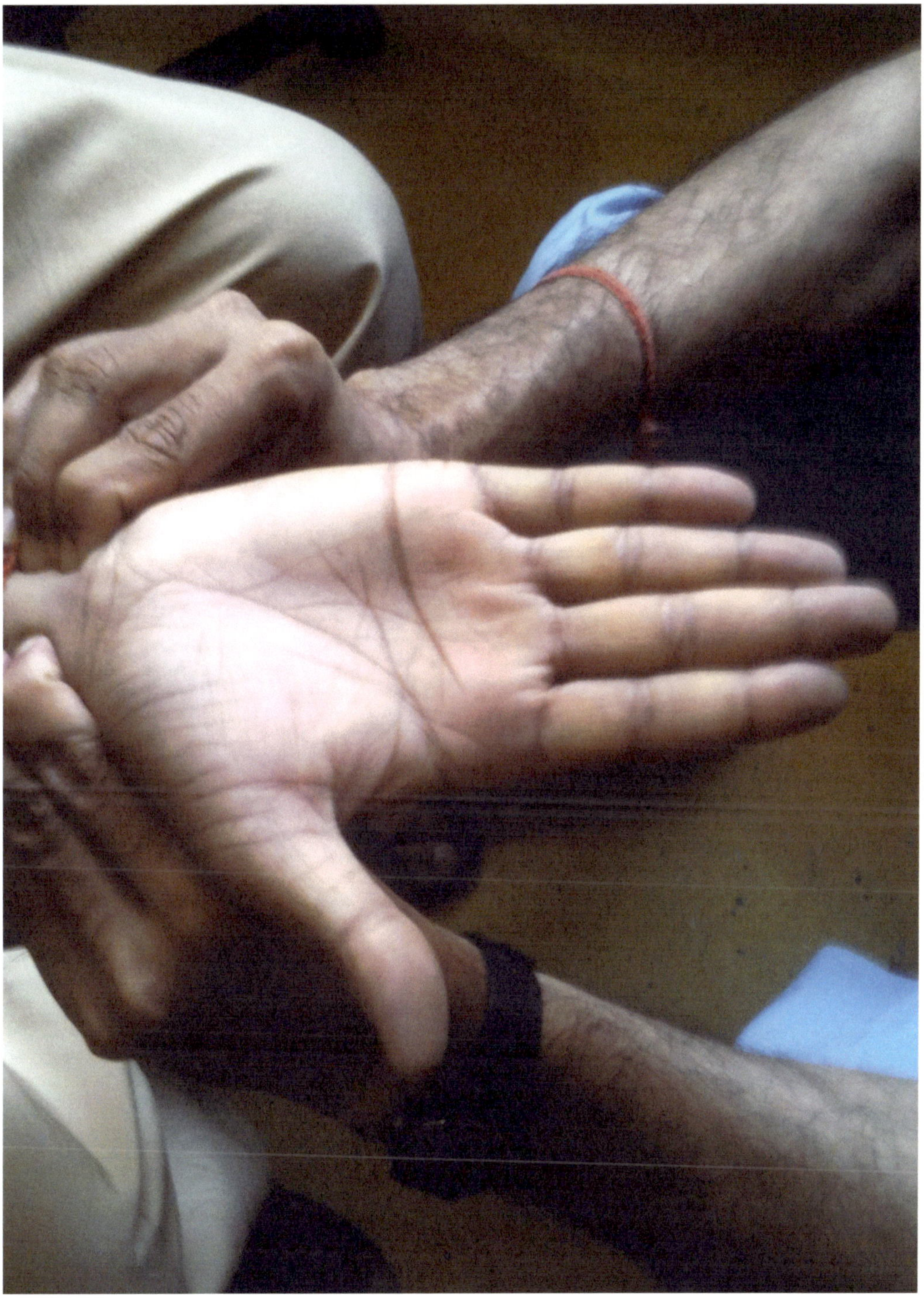

Fig. 1. Blanching of palm with simultaneous compression of radial and ulnar arteries in the right wrist

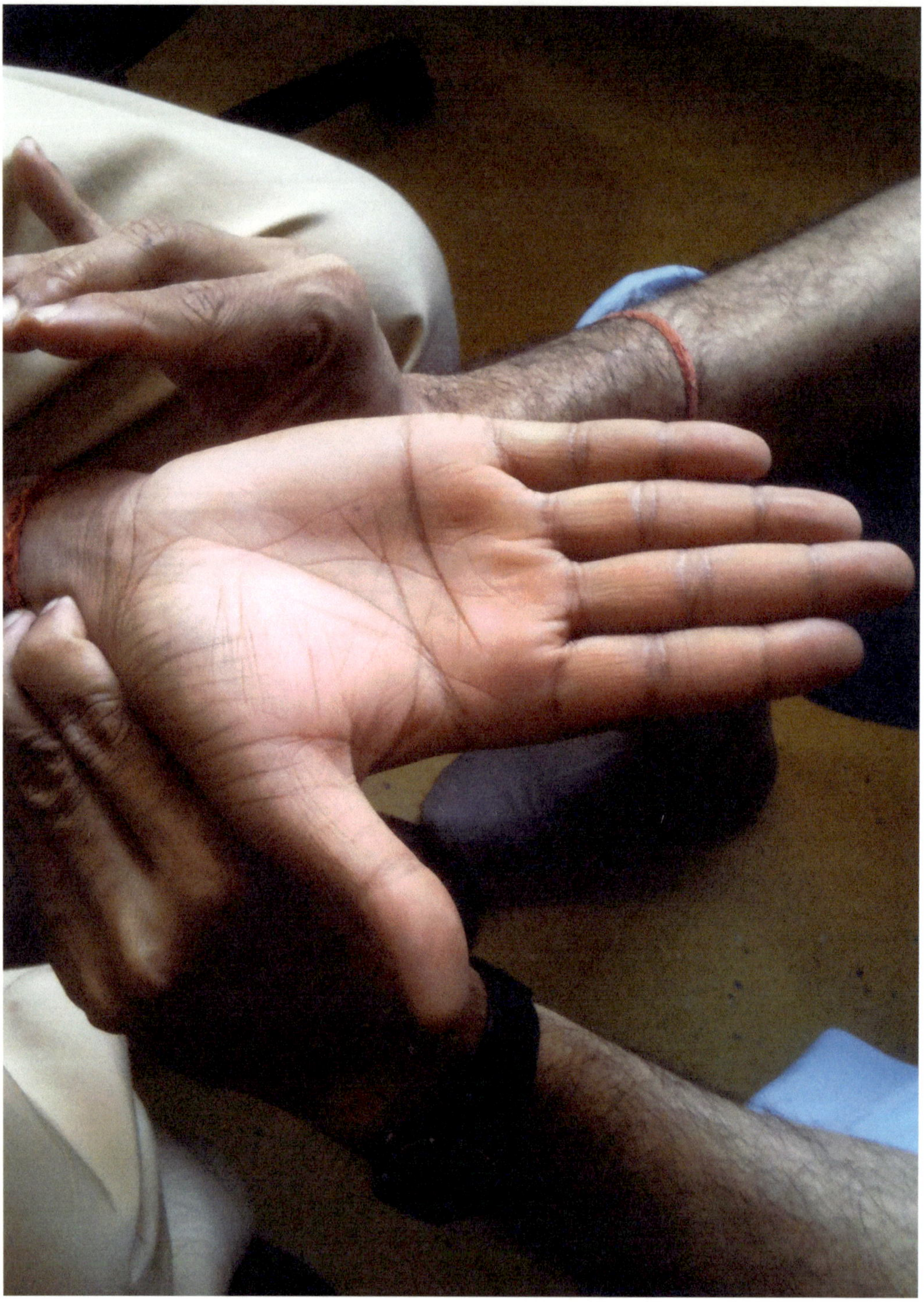

Fig. 2. Recovery of color of the palm on release of ulnar artery suggesting normal ulnar collateral flow

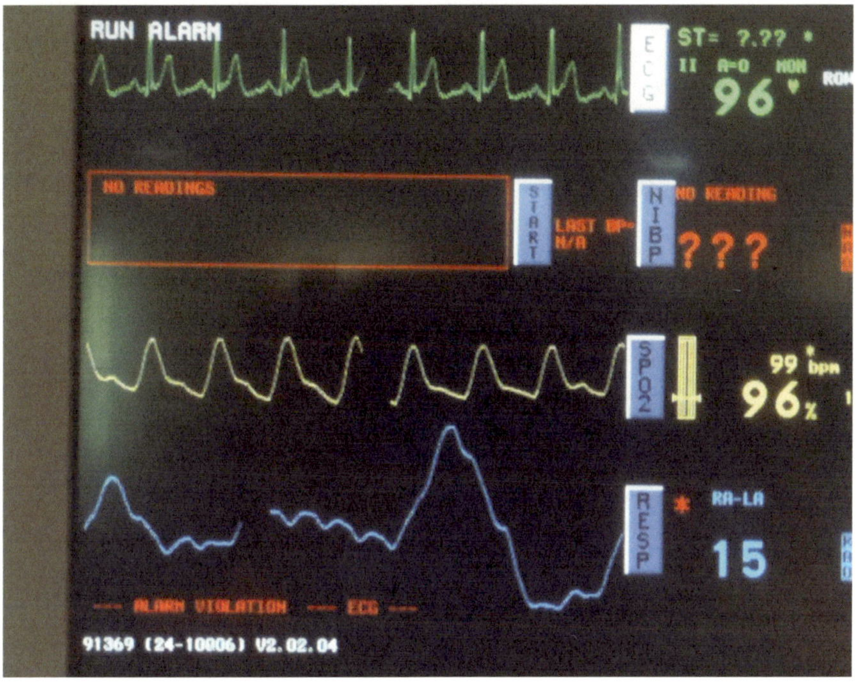

Fig. 3. Normal pulse waveform and oxygen saturation before Allen test

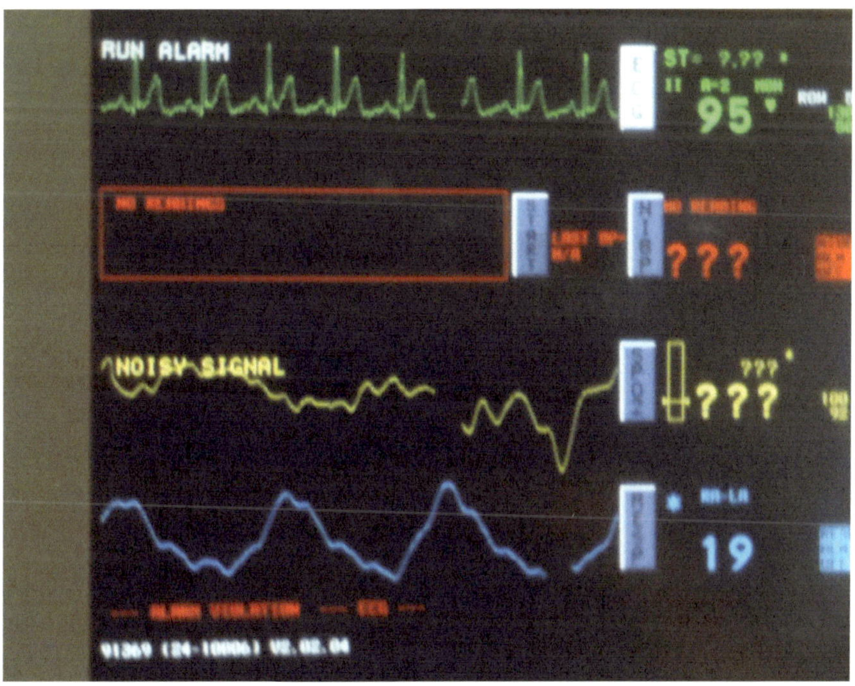

Fig. 4. Disappearance of pulse waveform and inability to read oxygen saturation on compressing radial and ulnar arteries

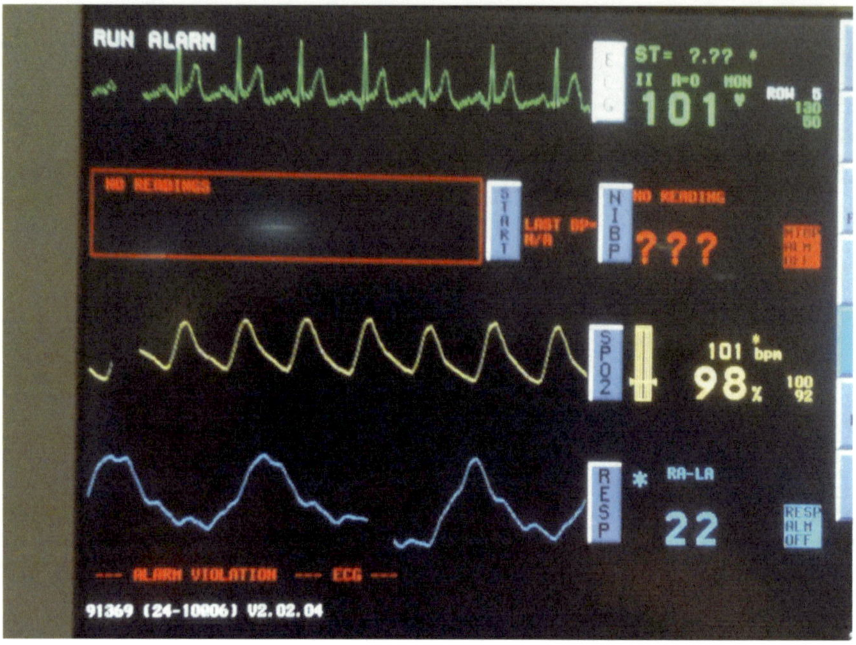

Fig. 5. Prompt recovery of pulse waveform and oxygen saturation on release of ulnar artery

5. Hemostasis

Ensuring complete hemostasis requires simple manual compression because the radial artery is both small and superficial. The earlier practice of administering nitroglycerin and verapamil just prior to sheath removal has also been largely abandoned. In the rare case where vessel spasm is encountered during the procedure nitroglycerin can be useful. Radial artery block subsequent to coronary angiography or PCI is also extremely uncommon. Temporary radial artery block occurs in 5% of patients and can be reduced with pre procedural usage of heparin. In fact more than 50% of TRA operators do not ascertain the incidence of radial artery obstruction subsequent to a procedure or prior to hospital discharge.

Almost 90% of operators use the right radial artery initially and 31% cross over to the contra lateral radial artery if unsuccessful. Fifty four percent of operators opt for the femoral artery in case of initial radial access failure.

6. Discharge

Same day discharge is quite common especially post diagnostic coronary angiography and a substantial number of patients undergoing PCI can also be discharged the same or the following day. Randomized studies have established the safety of same day discharge in patients of acute coronary syndrome (ACS) after uncomplicated PCI (22).

7. Reduction in bleeding complications with RTA as compared to femoral route

Recently it has been recognized that major bleeding results in an odds ratio of 3.5 for in-hospital and 1 year mortality. Surprisingly the hazard at 1 year was greater than that

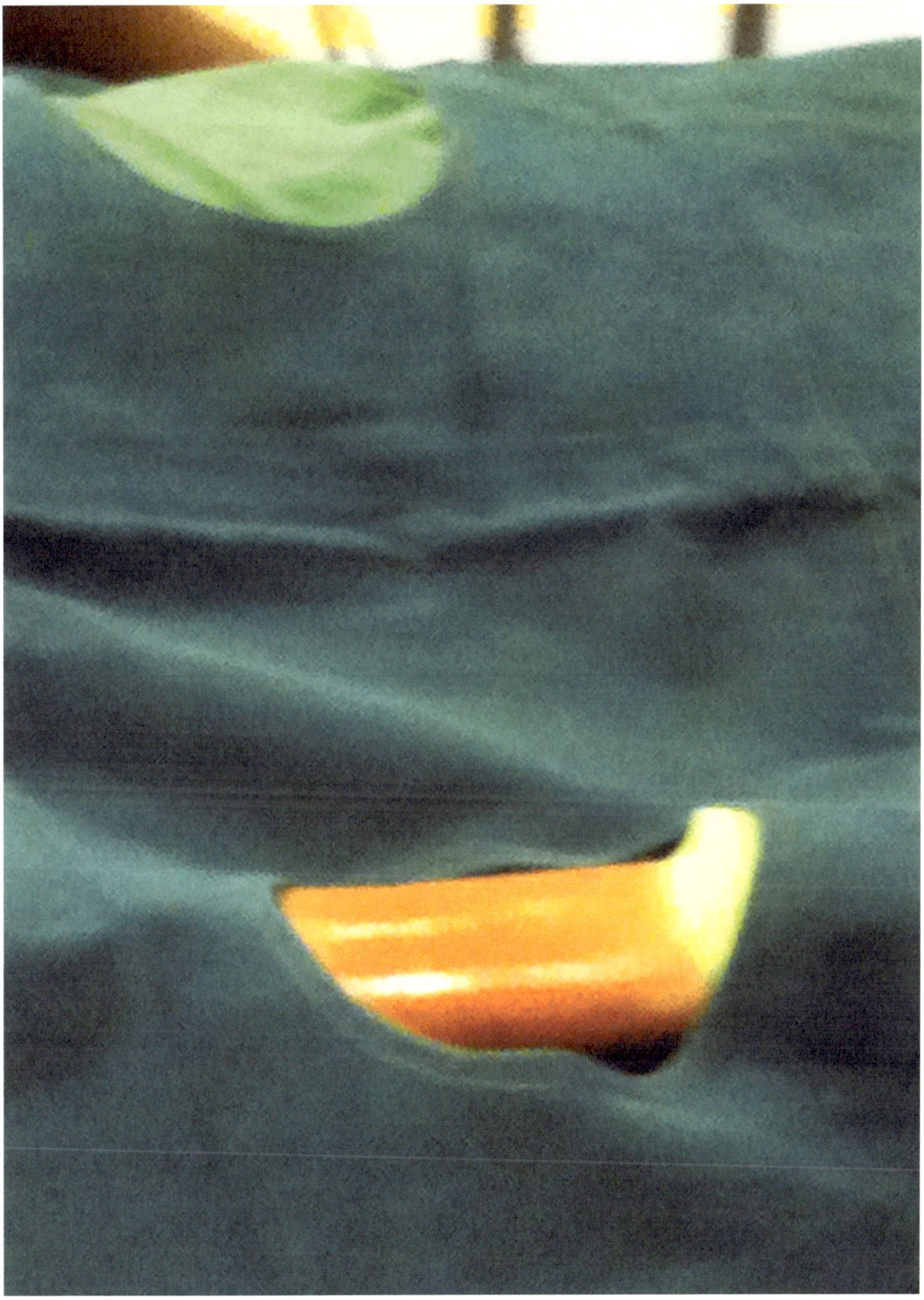

Fig. 6. The right wrist sterilized and draped before radial puncture

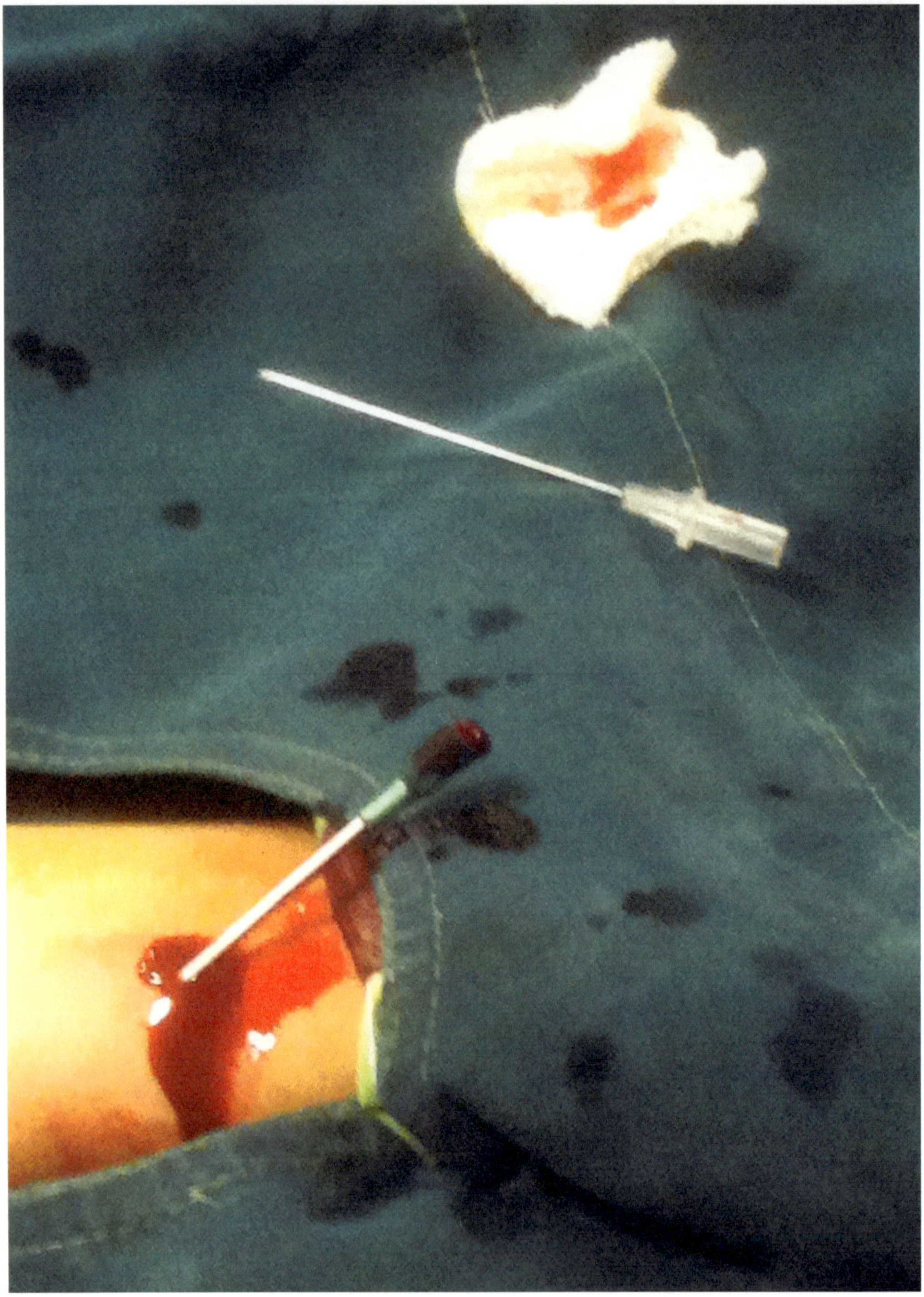

Fig. 7. Radial artery successfully punctured by needle/sheath and the needle removed with sheath in artery lumen displaying back flow of arterial blood

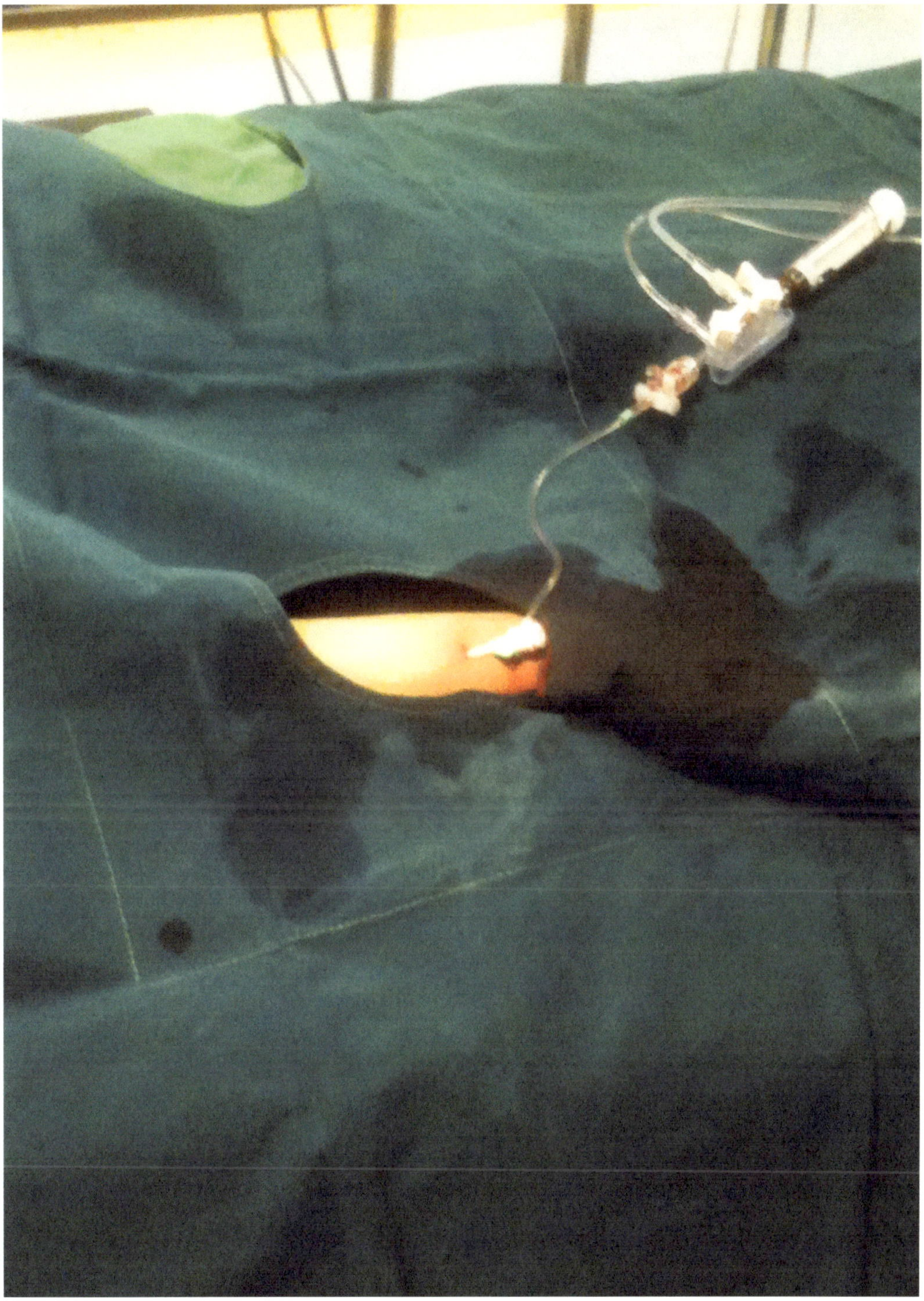

Fig. 8. The 6 Fr arterial sheath is connected to pressure transducer

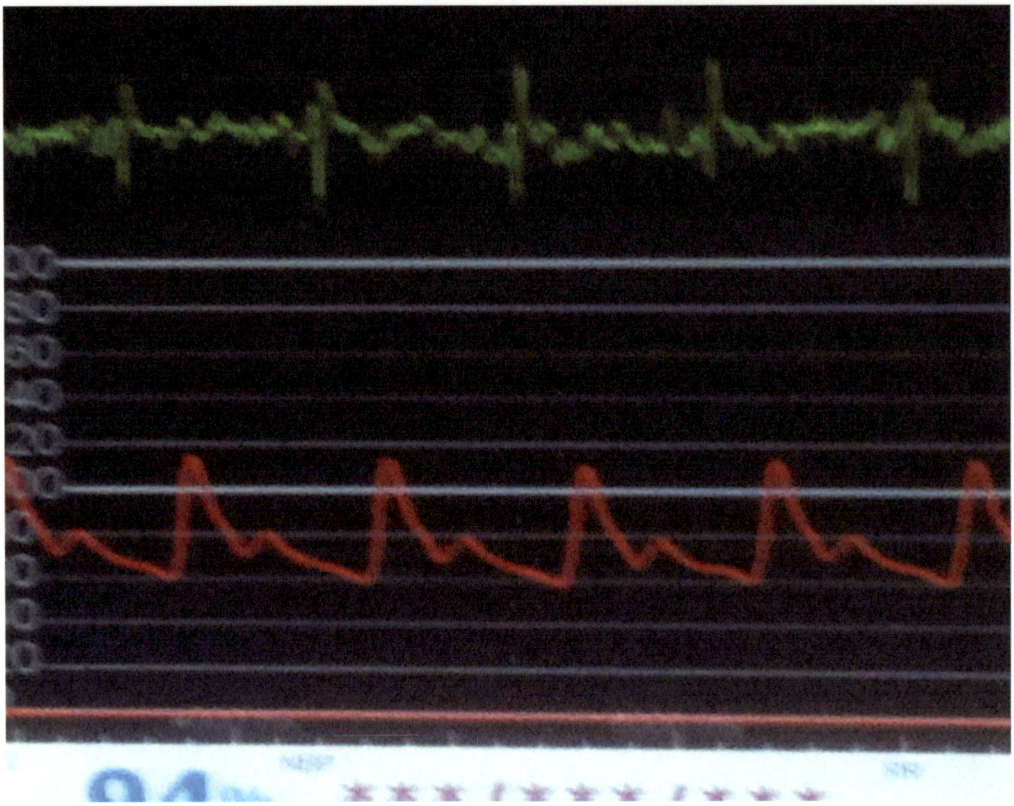

Fig. 9. Good radial artery waveform seen suggesting sheath is in intra luminal

observed with ischemic complications and reinfarction. Bleeding complications and transfusions have been identified as independent predictors of adverse outcomes in the recent OASIS-5 (Organization for the Assessment of Strategies for Ischemic Syndromes) and ACUITY (Acute Catheterization and Urgent Intervention Triage Strategy) trials (9-12). The HORIZONS AMI, a large randomized study comparing bivalirudin with a combination of heparin and Glycoprotein 2b/3a inhibitors also documented that significantly less major bleeds with the former led to reduced mortality at 30 days and at the end of one year (13).

The underlying mechanism for increased mortality accompanying major bleeds is unclear. The working hypothesis is that gastrointestinal or retroperitoneal bleeding during FA causes rapid loss of blood volume and oxygen carrying capacity that at times necessitates blood transfusion. Hypotension leads to reduced perfusion and the tendency to stop oral anti-platelets renders the bleeding patient more vulnerable to stent thrombosis. Moreover transfusion itself is associated with increased mortality probably due to the fact that stored red blood cells lose their flexibility and thereby their ability to negotiate the small sized capillaries in the microcirculation. Red cells also have depleted nitric oxide stores and are therefore unable to facilitate vaso dilatation in the capillaries. The net effect is aggravation of ischemic complications.

Bleeding in patients with ACS is a powerful determinant of fatal and non-fatal outcomes Approximately 5% of ACS patients develop major bleeds and suffer increased mortality by 5 times in the next 30 days.

Femoral punctures may result in local hematoma, pseudo aneurysm, arterovenous fistula, and worse retroperitoneal hemorrhage. The single most effective method of avoiding these complications is to employ TRA for diagnostic angiography and PCI. A systemic review of randomized trials has shown reduction of access site complications by 80% when the radial route instead of the femoral artery was employed (p=0.0001) (20).

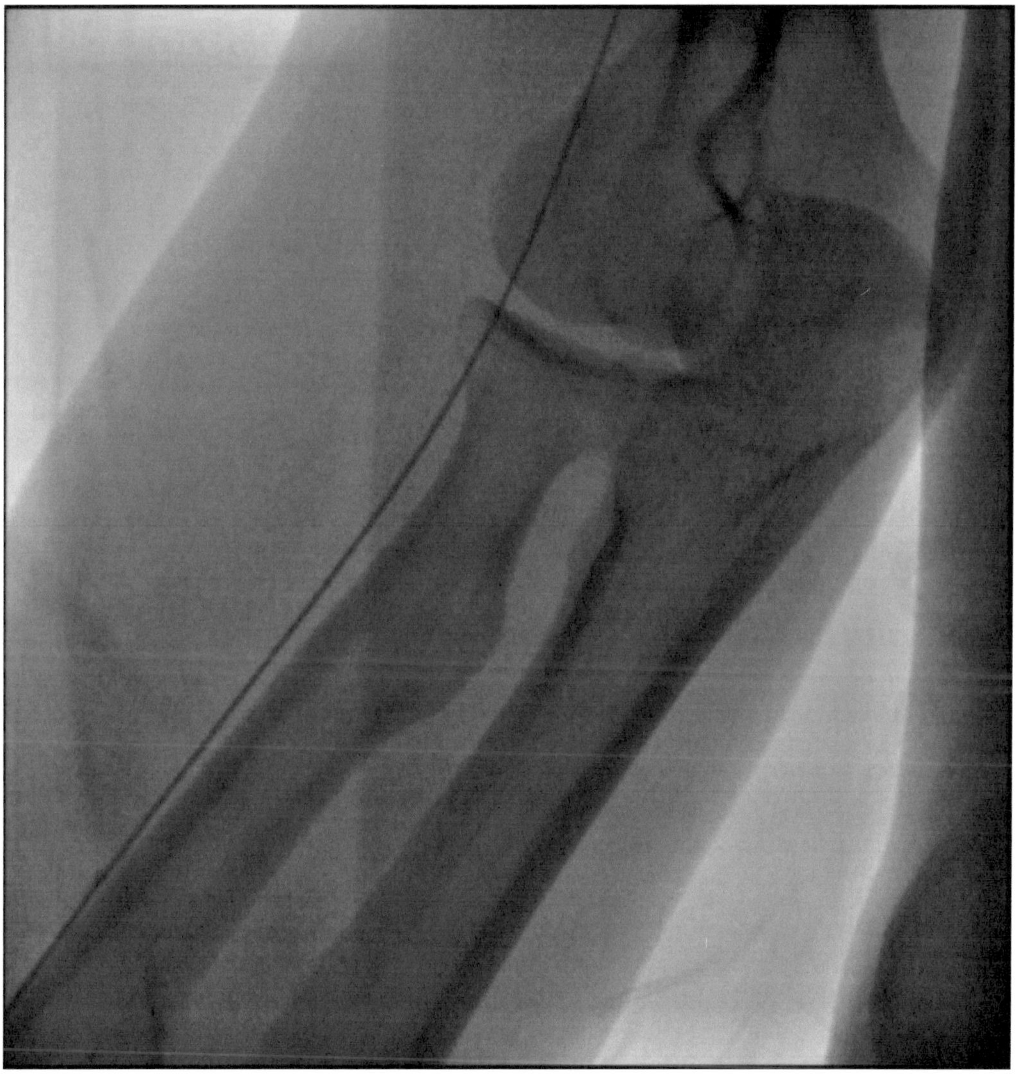

Fig. 10. Guide wire is being navigated through right brachial artery under fluoroscopy

The MORTAL (Mortality Benefit of Reduced Transfusion after PCI via the Arm or Leg) study retrospectively studied both approaches in 32,000 patients who underwent PCI in British Columbia from 1991 to 2005. Radial access approach resulted in 50% reduction in blood transfusion rate and a relative reduction in 30-day and 1-year mortality rates of 29% and 17% respectively (p<0.001)(15).

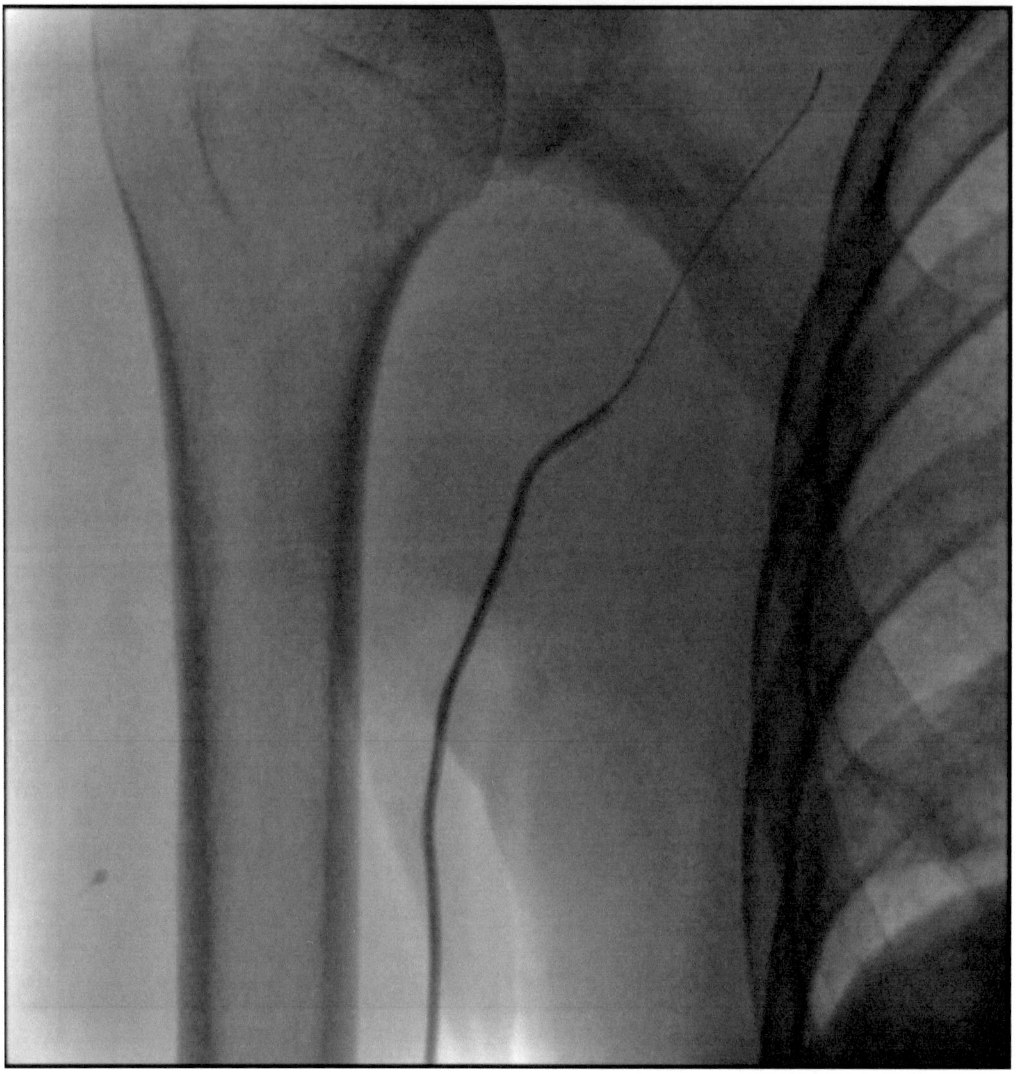

Fig. 11. Guide wire with Tiger II diagnostic catheter is now in right axillary artery

The MORTAL data was endorsed by the RIVIERA (Registry on Intravenous Anticoagulation in the Elective and Primary Real World of Angioplasty), a prospective international registry that reported reduction in bleeds and transfusions with the radial approach resulted in reduced PCI related mortality (16).

The Radial Access versus conventional Femoral Puncture: Outcome and Recourse Effectiveness in a Daily routine Practice (RAPTOR) trial explored whether it is feasible for an interventional center with operators experienced with FA to convert to RA routinely in a real world strategy. This was a prospective randomized trial comparing radial access with FA in an unselected population. Exclusion criteria included an abnormal Allen's test, end stage renal disease, planned coronary bypass surgery, pregnancy and hyperthyroidism. The mean age was 65 years and failure to gain access occurred in 3.4% of femoral patients and in 3.6% of the radial patients (non significant difference).

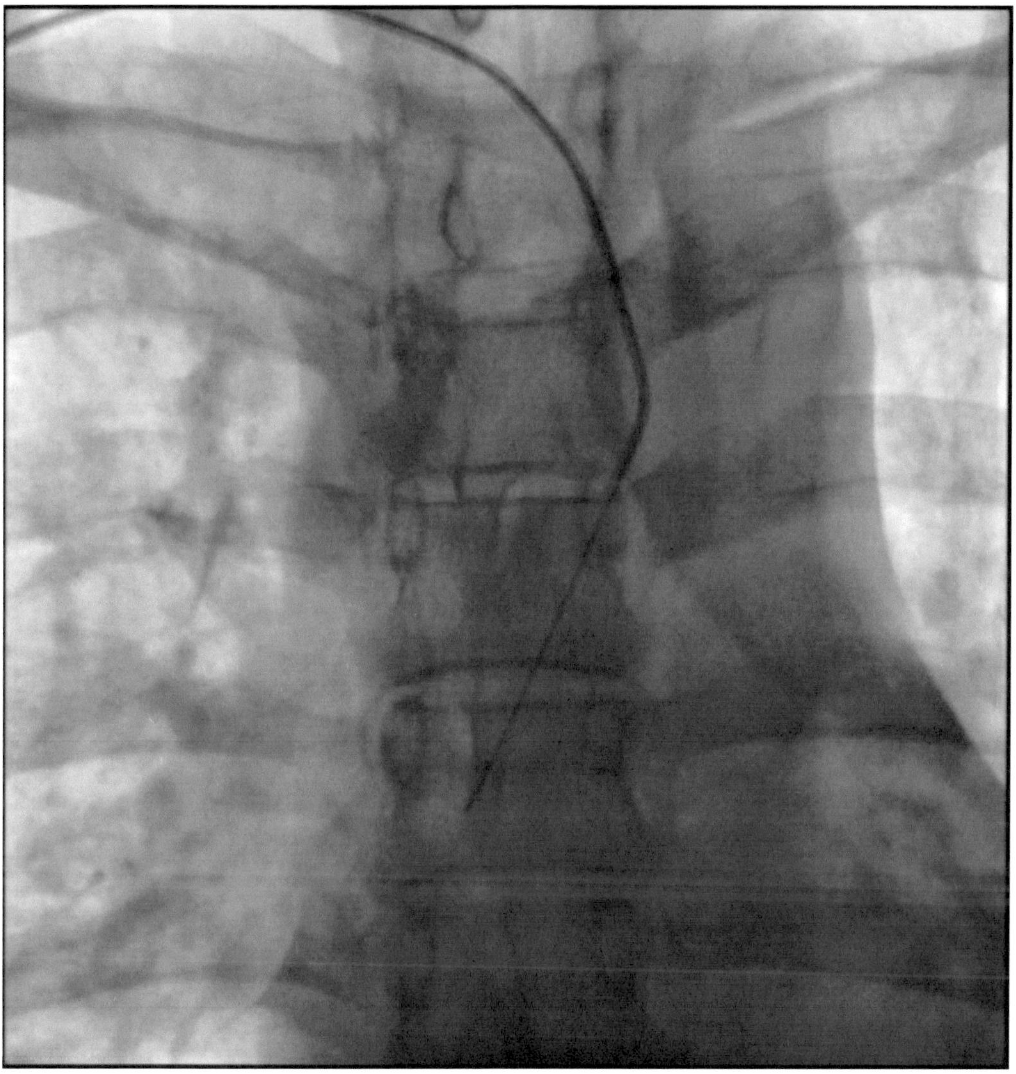

Fig. 12. Diagnostic catheter being negotiated into ascending aorta

It took 3 more minutes to get RA than the FA and 2 more minutes to perform diagnostic coronary angiogram. However time taken for PCI was almost similar by both routes (37 min by FA versus 34 min by RA; $p=0.2$). Radiation times and doses were significantly more in patients undergoing RTA during diagnostic coronary angiography (6.4 minutes versus 4.4 minutes, and 30 Gy cm sq versus 23 Gy cm sq; $p<0.01$)) but similar with PCI in both approaches. The RAPTOR study underscored the fact that experienced interventional cardiologists could convert to the RA approach quite comfortably and easily on a routine basis (17).

Every study describing RA technique for coronary angiography and coronary intervention has highlighted the substantial reduction in local vascular complications and bleeding. There is also the added advantage of patient comfort but neither the TRA nor the FA can be used in 100% of patients. There will always be difficulties with one of them necessitating converting to the other approach.

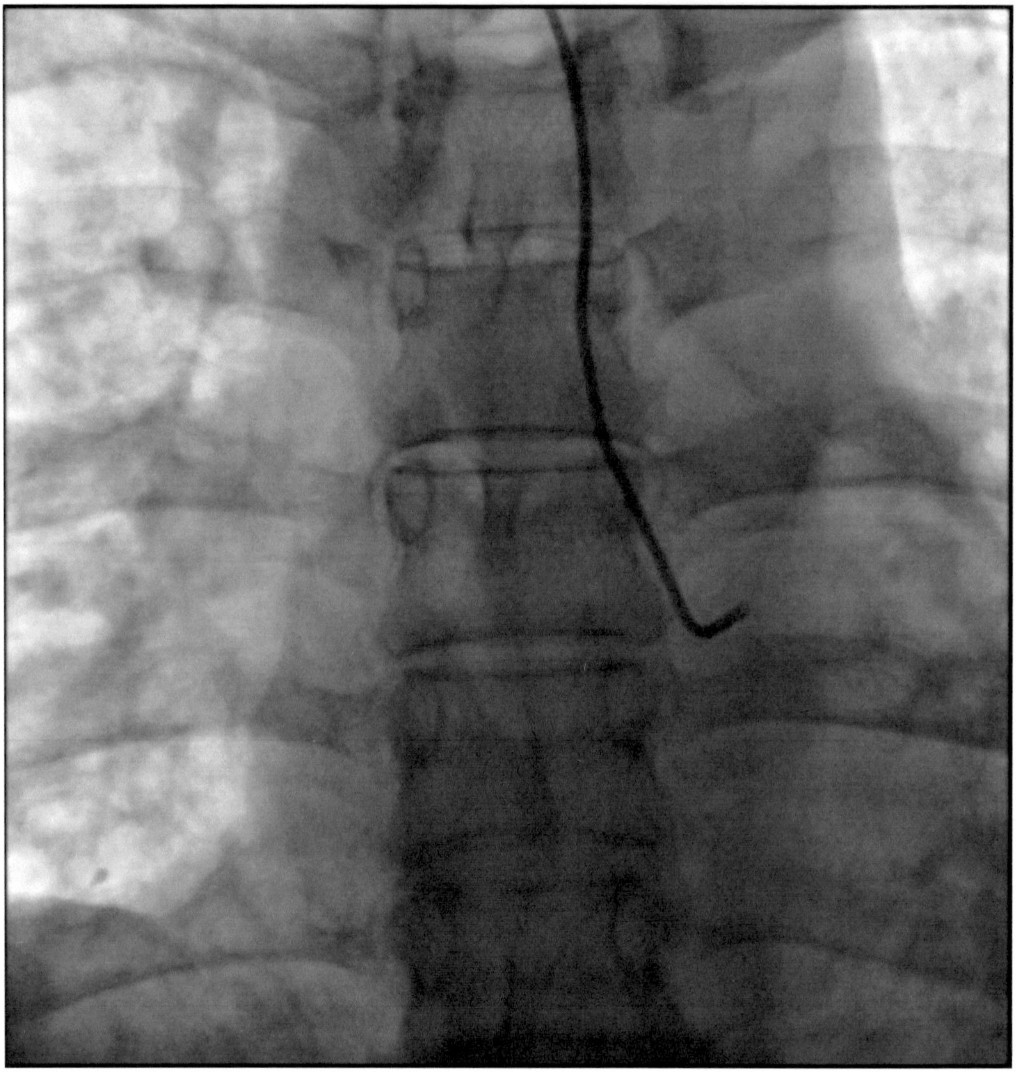

Fig. 13. Tiger II diagnostic catheter about to engage left coronary artery

Brueck et al in a randomized study comparing the 2 approaches showed that the femoral approach had 6 times the vascular access site complications (3.7% vs.6%, p=0.0008) compared to the radial group. Femoral access had slightly higher procedural success rates (99.8% transfemoral vs. 97% TRA, p<0.001) and lesser radiation exposure (42Gycm.sq vs. 38 Gycm.sq)(21).

Jolly et al in a meta-analysis of randomized trials reported that PCI with radial artery access reduced major bleeding 73% compared to FA (0.05% vs. 2.3%, p<0.01) and also demonstrated a trend in reduction in the composite of death, myocardial infarction and stroke (2.5% vs. 3.8%, p=0.058). There was no difference in mortality between the 2 techniques but TRA reduced hospital stay by 0.4 days (20).

The largest multi-centric randomized study to date is the radial versus femoral access for coronary angiography and intervention in patients with acute coronary syndromes (RIVAL).

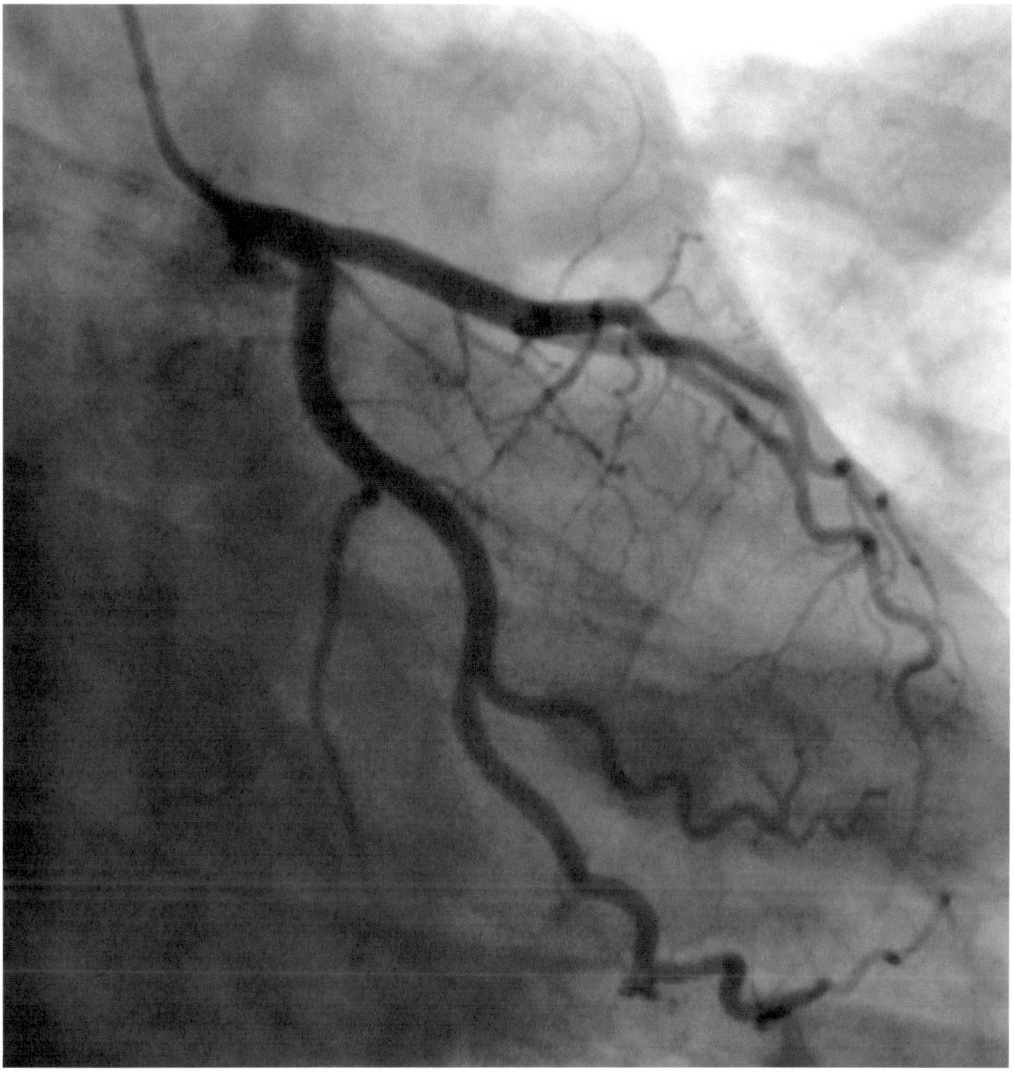

Fig. 14. Normal left coronary artery seen in right anterior oblique/caudal view

Patients were randomly assigned (1:1) to radial or femoral access. The primary outcome was a composite of death, myocardial infarction, stroke, or non -CABG related bleeding at 30 days. Patients were enrolled from 158 hospitals in 32 countries. The primary outcome occurred in 128 (3.7%) of 3507 patients in the radial access group compared to 139 (4%) of 3514 in the femoral access group (hazard ratio HR 0.92, 95% CI 0.72-1.17; p=0.5).Interestingly of the 6 pre-specified subgroups, there was significant interaction for the primary outcome with benefit for radial access in highest tertile volume radial centers (HR 0.49, 95% CI 0.28=0.87; p=0.015) and in ST-segment elevation myocardial infarction (HR 0.60, CI 0.38-0.94; p=0.026). The rate of death, myocardial infarction, or stroke at 30 days was 112(3.2%) in the RA group compared to 114(3.2%) in the FA group. The rate of non CABG related major bleeds at 30 days was 24(0.7%) in the RA group as compared to 33(0.9%) in the FA group (p=0.23). Large hematoma were significantly less in the RTA group (HR 0.73, 95%

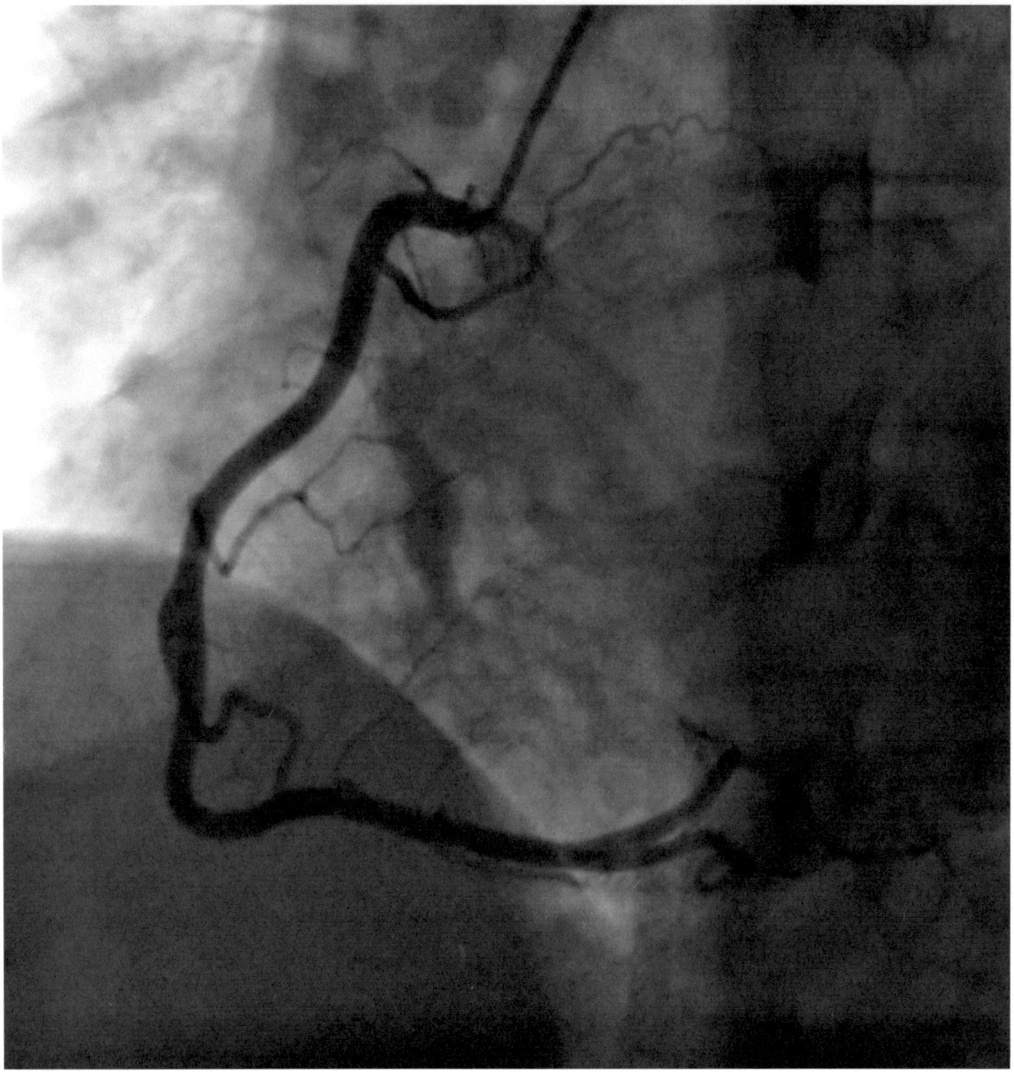

Fig. 15. Normal right coronary artery flow seen in left anterior oblique view

CI 0.28-0.57; $p<0.0001$) as also pseudoaneurysm requiring closure were significantly less again in the RTA group (HR 0.30, 95% CI 0.13-0.71; $p=0.006$).

The RIVAL study concluded that both radial and femoral approaches are safe and effective for PCI but the radial approach may be preferred because of significantly less local vascular complications (22).

Recently Swedish authors reviewed all ST-segment elevation myocardial infarction procedures conducted in Sweden (SCAAR registry) between 2005 and 2010. The radial approach for STEMI patients increased from 12% to 50%. Both 30-day and 1-year mortality were significantly lower in the radial group in a study cohort of 21,339 patients (29). Both serious bleeding and hospital stay were also lessened significantly by the radial approach. The radial access approach had the best results in patients of STEMI above 70 years and in women.

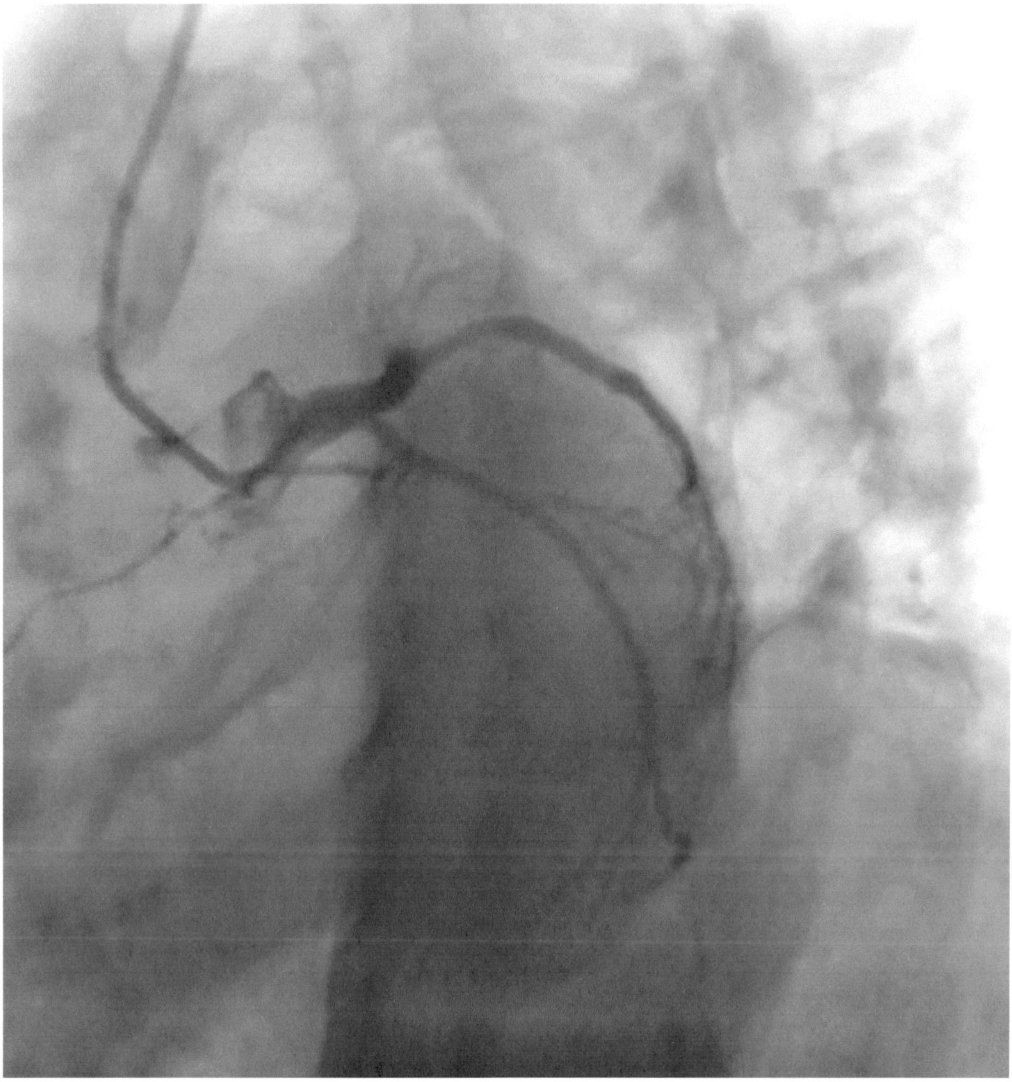

Fig. 16. Totally occluded proximal left anterior descending artery in a patient of acute anterior STEMI seen in left anterior oblique/ caudal view (Tiger diagnostic catheter)

Most complex PCI's can be easily performed by TRA because the 6 Fr guide catheters permit rotablators, intravascular ultrasound, pressure wire, "kissing balloon" left main and also coronary graft stenting. Primary PCI for STEMI can be easily managed by radial access with superior results as compared to the femoral route (24-27) and reiterated by the RIVAL study and SCAAR registry. Superior results with RTA in patients with acute ST elevation myocardial infarction (STEMI) are understandable because these patients receiving maximum quantum of antiplatelets plus antithrombotics in order to attain the best anti ischemic outcomes are paradoxically most vulnerable to local vascular and internal bleeds (Figures 16 -21)

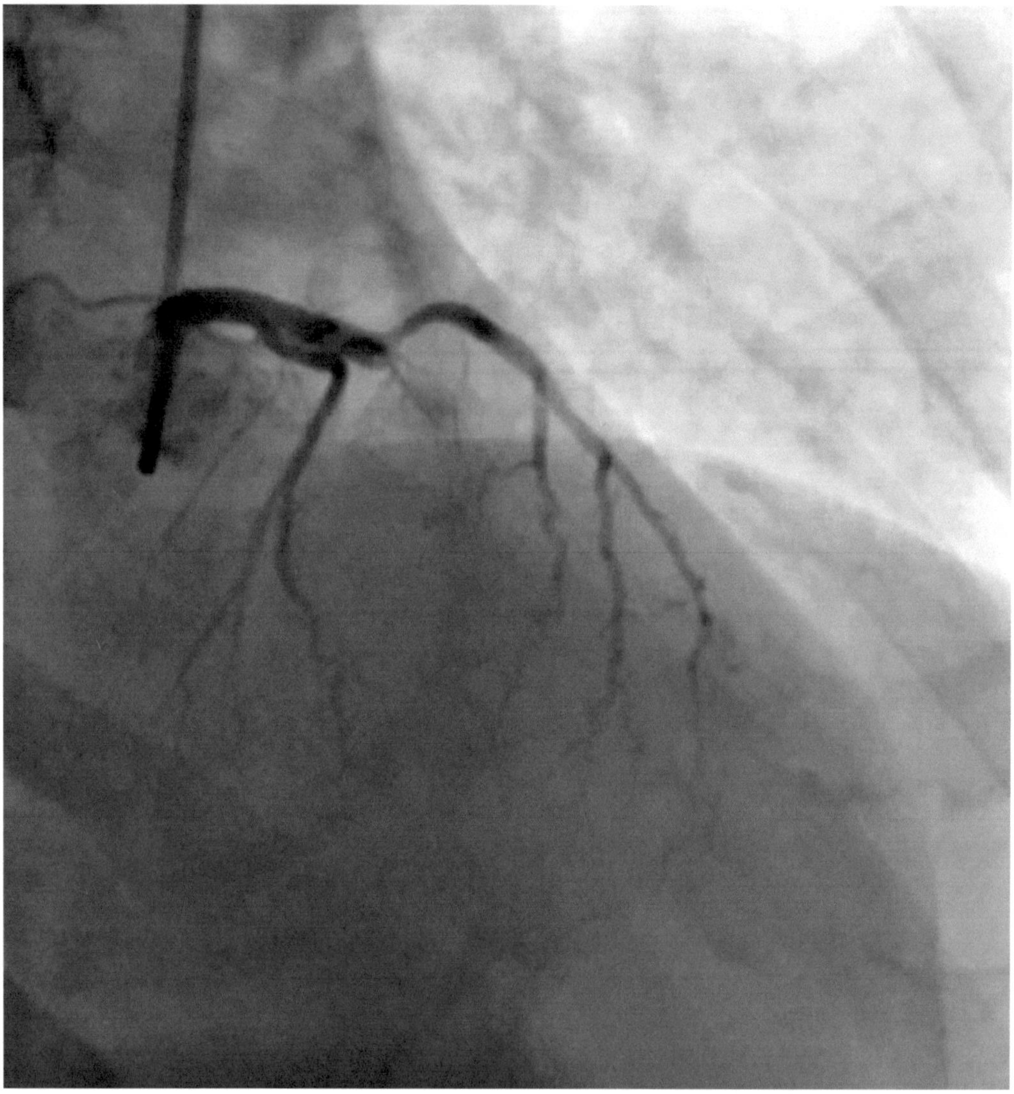

Fig. 17. Totally occluded proximal left anterior descending artery confirmed in right anterior oblique view.

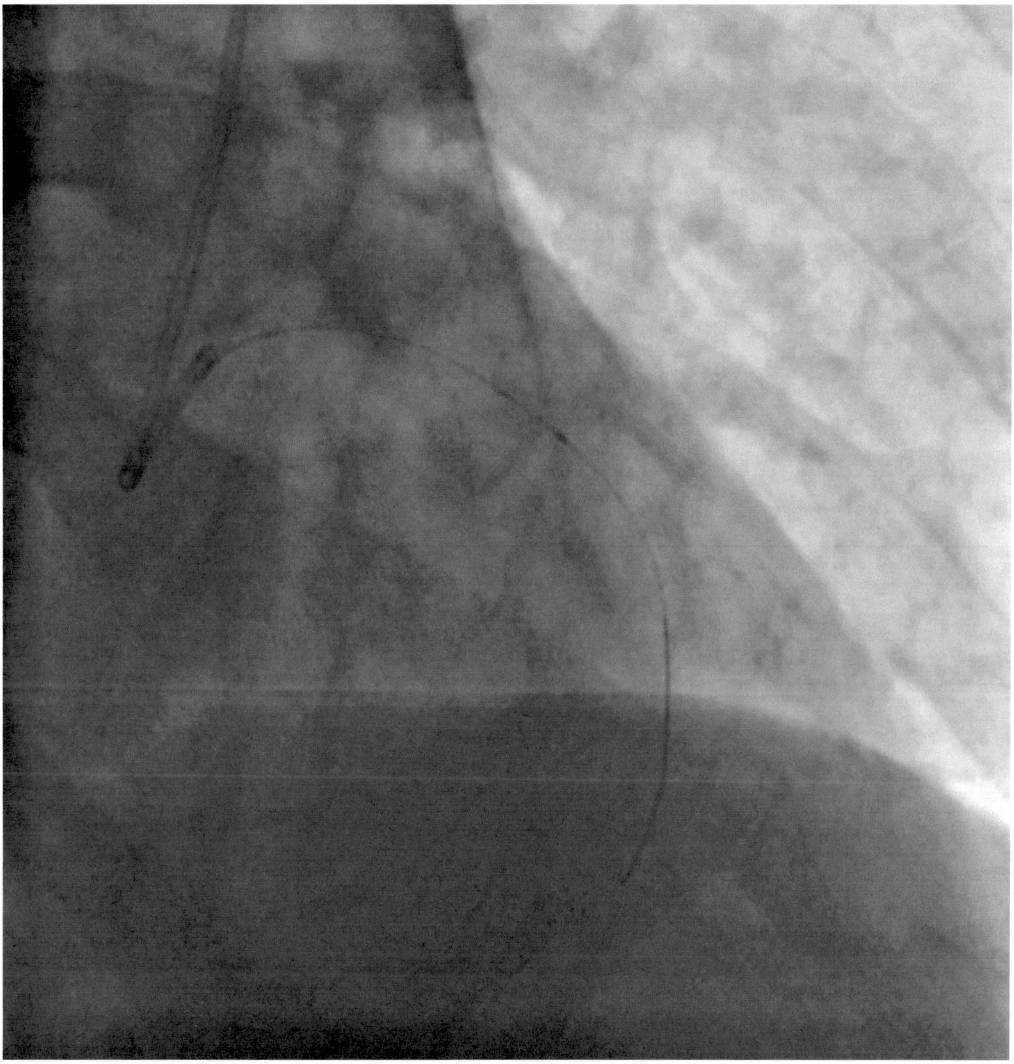

Fig. 18. A 0.012-inch guide wire is put across lesion and manual thrombo-suction being done by Export catheter via a 6 Fr EBU guide catheter

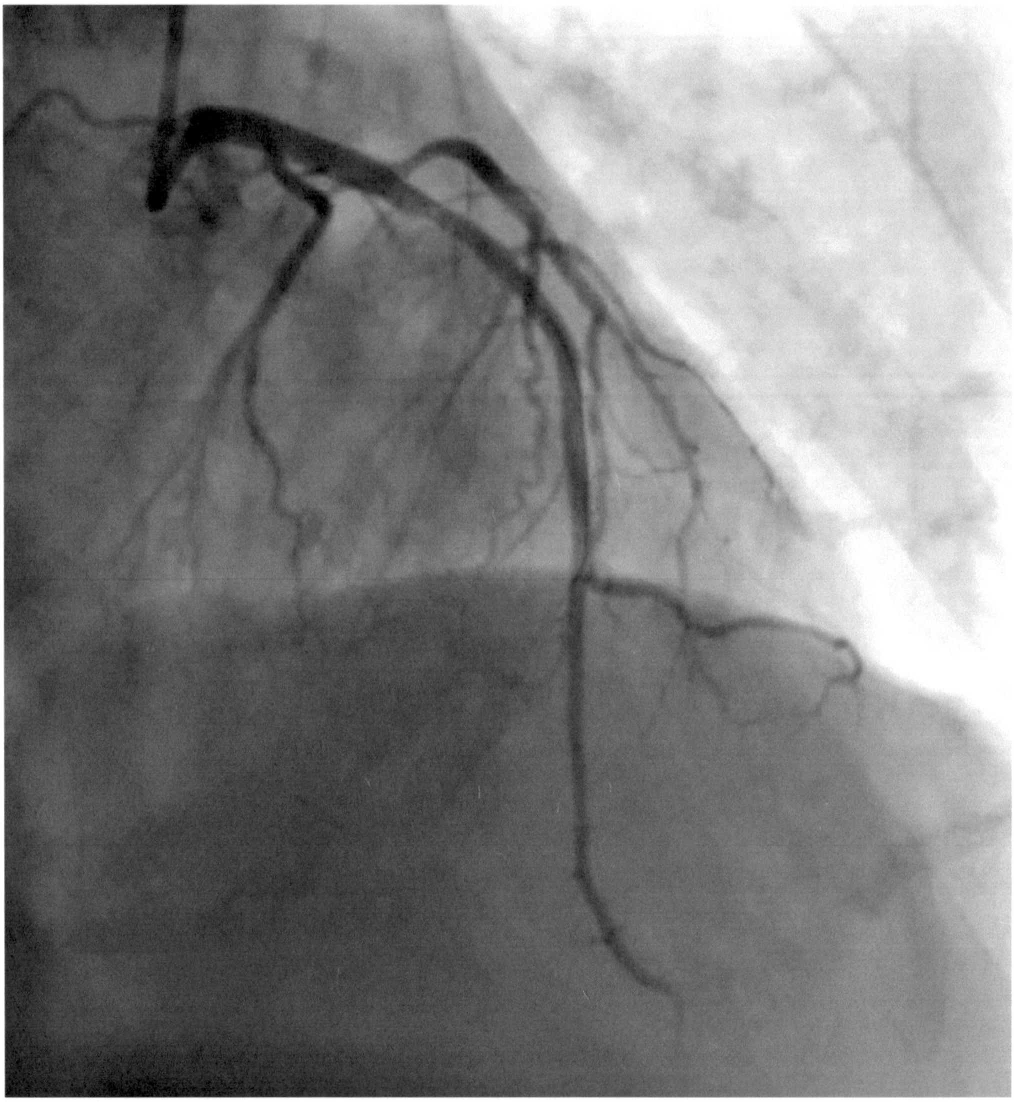

Fig. 19. Good ante grade flow post manual thrombo-suction and intracoronary Tirofiban bolus of 25 mcg/Kg.

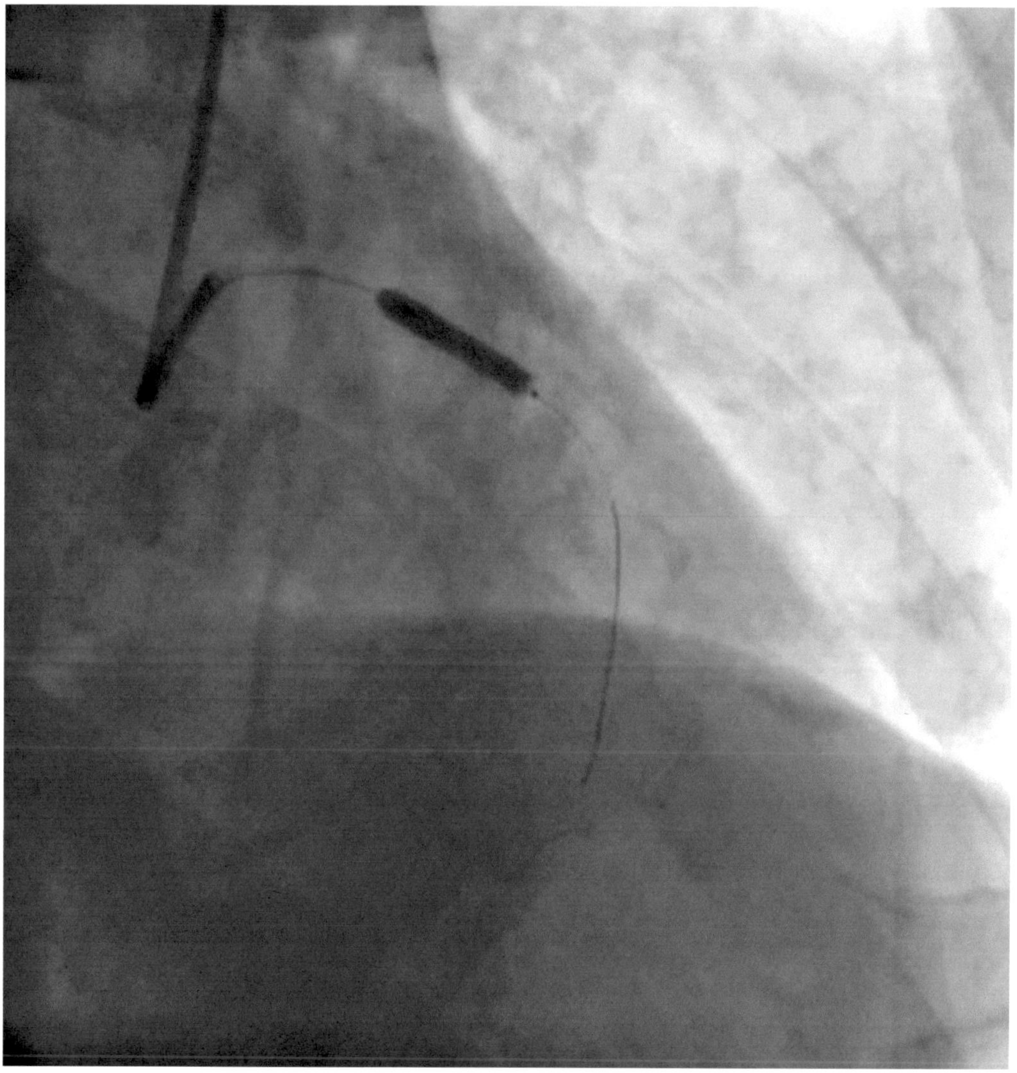

Fig. 20. Coronary stent being deployed at lesion site

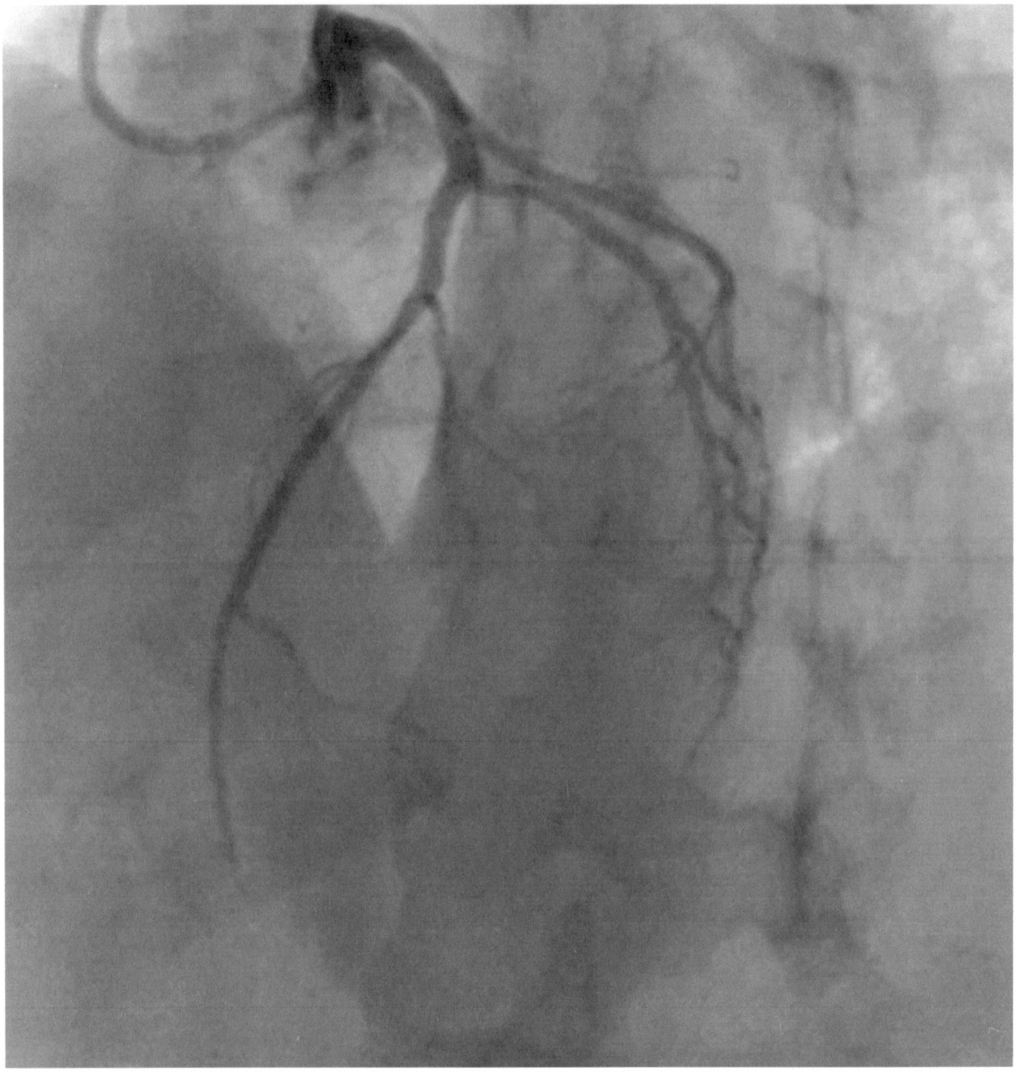

Fig. 21. Check angiogram showing brisk TIMI 3 flow with no residual stenosis

The incidence of complications when using radial access is negligible even in patients treated aggressively with anti-thrombotic and anti-platelet regimens. Patients have the added advantage of mobilization almost immediately post procedure and quicker discharge from hospital. The learning curve for the radial approach is exaggerated and most operators rapidly get comfortable and skillful with this technique (28).

The results of the first large international survey on global TRA practices were summarized as follows: 1) TRA is used by interventional cardiologists all over the world. 2) 23.4% of interventional cardiologists do not assess dual hand circulation before PCI using TRA. 3) In case of first attempt failure of TRA almost 50% resort to FA. 4) The catheters used for diagnostic coronary angiography and PCI are largely similar to the catheters used in the FA. 5) Heparin is used by more than 95% to thwart radial artery blocks. 6) Heparin remains the most employed anti thrombotic for diagnostic coronary angiography and PCI (30).

8. Conclusions

It is imperative that modern interventional cardiologists be trained in both radial and femoral artery puncture techniques. The radial artery can be used for most coronary procedures as also in patients treated with maximum antithrombotic regimens (such as patients of acute coronary syndrome) because of substantial mitigation in local vascular complications. Reduction in bleeding may account for the recent superior results in patients with STEMI. Rapid mobilization with earlier discharge adds considerably to patient comfort. The radial approach is preferred in the presence of aorto iliac disease, marked obesity and high bleeding risk.

For best results one needs to be skilled in both approaches and fortunately such a trend continues to evolve in most countries.

9. References

[1] Radner S. Thoracal aortography by catheterization from the radial artery; preliminary report of a new technique. Acta Radiol 1948; 29:178-80.

[2] Campeau L. Percutaneous radial artery approach for coronary angiography. Cathet Cardiovasc Diagn 1989;16:3-7.

[3] Campeau L. Entry sites for coronary angiography and therapeutic interventions: from the proximal to the distal radial artery. Can J Cardiol 2001;17:319-25.

[4] Kiemeneij F, Laarman GJ.Percutaneous transradial artery approach for coronary stent implantation. Cathet Cardiovasc Diagn 1993; 30:173-8.

[5] Kiemeneij F, Laarman GJ, Odekerken T,et al. A randomized comparison of percutaneous transluminal coronary angioplasty by the radial,brachial and femoral approaches-the access study. J Am Coll Cardiol 1997;29:1269- 1275.

[6] Allen EV. Thrombangiitis obliterans: Methods of diagnosis of chronic occlusive arterial lesions distal to the wrist with illustrative cases. J Med Science 1929;178-237.

[7] Benit E, et al. Frequency of a positive modified Allen's test in 1000 consecutive patients undergoing cardiac catheterization. Cath Cardiovasc Diagn. 1996;38:352-354.

[8] Ghuran AV,Dixon G, Holmberg S,etal. Transradial coronary intervention without pre-screening for a dual palmar blood supply. Int J Cardiol 2007; 121:320-2.

[9] Kinnaird TD,Stabile E, Mintz GS,et al. Incidence,predictors,and prognostic implications of bleedingand blood transfusion following percutaneous coronary interventions. Am J Cardiol 2003;92:930-935.

[10] Fei T, Voeltz MD, Attubato MJ,et al.Predictors and impact of major hemorrhage on mortality following percutaneous coronary intervention from REPLACE-2 Trial. Am J Cardiol 2007;100:1364-1369.

[11] Yusuf S, Mehta SAR, Chrolavicius S,etal.Comparison of fondaparinuxand enoxaparin in acute coronary syndromes. N Engl J Med. 2006;354:1464-1476.

[12] Stone GW, McLaurin BT, Cox DA,et al. Bivalirudin for patients with acute coronary syndromes. N Engl J Med 2006;355:2203-2216.

[13] Stone GW, Witzenbichler B, Guagliumi G,wt al. Bivalirudin during primary PCI in acute myocardial infarction. N Engl J Med 2008; 358:2218-2230.

[14] Agostoni P, Biondi GG, de Benedictis ML,et al. Radial versus femoral approach for percutaneous coronary diagnostic and interventional procedures; systemic overview and meta analysis of randomized trials. J Am Coll Cardiol 2004; 44: 349-356.

[15] Chase AJ, Fretz EB, Warburton WP, et al. Association of the arterial access site at angioplasty with transfusion and mortality: the MORTAL study (Mortality benefit

of Reduced Transfusion after percutaneous coronary intervention via the Arm or Leg). Heart 2008; 94:1019-1025.

[16] Montalescot G, Ongen Z, Guindy R, et al. Predictors of outcome in patients undergoing PCI. Results of the RIVIERA study. Int J Cardiol 2007; 129: 379-387.

[17] Schaufele TG. Radial Access versus conventional Femoral Puncture : Outcome and Recourse Effectiveness in a daily routine.(Raptor) trial. American Heart association (AHA) 2009 Scientific Sessions.

[18] Lefevre T, Thebault B, Spaulding C, et al. Radial artery patency after percutaneous left radial artery approach for coronary angiography.The role of heparin.Eur Heart J 1995;16:293.

[19] Varenne O, Jegou A, Cohen R, et al. Prevention of arterial spasm during percutaneous coronary interventions through radial artery: the SPASM study. Cathet Cardiovasc Diagn 2006; 68:231-5.

[20] Jolly SS, Amlani S, Hamon M, Yusuf S, et al. Radial versus femoral access for coronary angiography or intervention and the impact on major bleeding and ischemic events: a systemic review and meta analysis of randomized trials. Am Heart J 2009; 157: 132-40.

[21] Brueck M, Bandorski D, Kramer W, et al. A randomized comparison of transradial versus transfemoral approach for coronary angiography and angioplasty. J am Coll Cardiol 2009;2: 1047-54.

[22] Jolly SS, Yusuf S, Cairns J, et al. Radial versus femoral access for coronary angiography and intervention in patients with acute coronary syndromes (RIVAL): a randomized, parallel group, multicentre trial. Lancet 2011; 377: 1409-1420.

[23] Bertrand OF, De Larochelliere R, Rodes- Cabau J, etal. Eraly Discharge After Transradial Stenting of Coronary Arteries (EASY). A randomized study comparing same-day home discharge and abciximab bolus and infusion after transradial coronary stent implantation. Circulation 2006: 114: 2636-43.

[24] Saito S, Tanaka S, Hiroe Y,et al. Comaparative study on transradial approach vs transfemoral approach in primary stent implantatio for patients with acute myocardial infarction: results of the Test for Myocardial infarction by prospective Unicenter Randomization for Access sites (TEMPURA) trial. Catheter Cardiovasc Interv 2003; 59:26-33.

[25] Cantor WJ, Puley G, Natarjan MK, et al. Radial versus femoral access for emergent percutaneous coronary intervention with adjunct glyco-protein IIb/IIIa inhibition in acute myocardial infarction- The RADIAL- AMI pilot randomized trial. Am Heart j 2005; 150: 543-9.

[26] Hetherington SL, Adam Z, Morlet R, et al. Primary percutaneous coronary intervention for acute ST-segment elevation myocardial infarction: changing patterns of vascular access,radial versus femoral artery. Heart 2009;95:1612-18.

[27] Natarajan D and Vohra S. PCI via Radial Route for impending Anterior MI. 2009; http://www.tctmd.com

[28] Goldberg SL, Renslo R, Sinow R,et al. Learning curve in the use of the radial artery as vascular access in the performance of percutaneous transluminal coronary angioplasty. Cathet Cardiovasc diagn 1998; 44:127-52.

[29] Olivercona G. SCAAR registry: Transradial PCI cuts mortality in STEMI. 2011: EuroPCR.

[30] Bertrand OF, Rao SV, Pancholy S, et al. Transradial Approach for Coronary Angiography and Interventions : Results of the First International Transradial Pracvtice Surevey. J Am Coll Cardiol 2010;30: 1022-31.

4

An Infected Drug-Eluting Stented Coronary Aneurysm Forming Intracardiac Fistula

Ken Kishida
Department of Metabolism and Atherosclerosis, Graduate School of Medicine, Osaka University, Osaka
Japan

1. Introduction

Many cardiologists have usually operated percutaneous coronary intervention (PCI) for coronary artery disease practically. Sometimes, complications following stent implantation rarely include thrombosis, rupture, sepsis and infected coronary aneurysm [Baddour, 2004; Berkalp, 1999]. Particularly, infected coronary aneurysm causes fatal outcome. In addition to contamination at the time of catheterization, there are other mechanisms how stents can become infected, including transient bacteremia from skin flora via access-site hematomas, pseudoaneurysms, delayed bleeding, prolonged arterial sheath insertion, and several procedures performed from the same access site over a short time period [Baddour, 2004]. Previous report demonstrated that 18% of patients who underwent complex PCIs had detectable bacteremia [Ramsdale, 2004]. However, prophylactic antibiotics administarations are not conducted routinely prior to coronary stenting in the current PCI procedures, because the incident rate of stent infections was reported to be less than one in 10,000 cases [Myles, 2000].

The drug-eluting stent (DES) era was ushered in with the first published human study by Sousa *et al.* in 2001, showing a nearly complete abolition of neointimal hyperplasia by use of sirolimus-eluting stent (SES) [Sousa, 2001]. The role of DES is very questionable, because of long term anticoagulant therapy, but in the patients with comorbidity (diabetes mellitus) DES are recommend. Despite the dramatic capacity of SES to reduce the restenosis rate after PCI, several SES-related problems have been raised [Ong & Serruys, 2005]; 1) the requirement of a prolonged dual anti-platelet regimen to avoid the risk of DES thrombosis [McFadden, 2004], 2) the occurrence of acquired late malapposition 3) the late formation of coronary artery aneurysm (SES having an antiproliferative action may be responsible for the delayed and inappropriate healing, which should lead to weakening of the arterial wall and delayed aneurysm formation) [Abreu, 2005; Degertekin, 2003], 4) a severe localized hypersensitivity consisting predominantly of T lymphocytes and eosinophils, which was caused by the metallic stent, polymer, or sirolimus [Virmani, 2004; Nebeker, 2005; Stabile, 2004].

2. Case report

A 70-year-old man with hypertension, type 2 diabetes mellitus, mild renal dysfunction and old cerebral infarction, was admitted to our hospital with sustained angina. The patient suffered an inferior wall ST-depression unstable angina that required immediate PCI with two SESs (Cypher®, Cordis Johnson & Johnson, Japan) in the proximal right coronary artery (RCA) (Figure 1). Satisfactory angiographic results were obtained with smooth luminal outline, and then the arterial sheath was removed (Figure 1). The patient had other significant stenosis lesions in the proximal left anterior descending artery (LAD) and the middle circumflex artery (LCX).

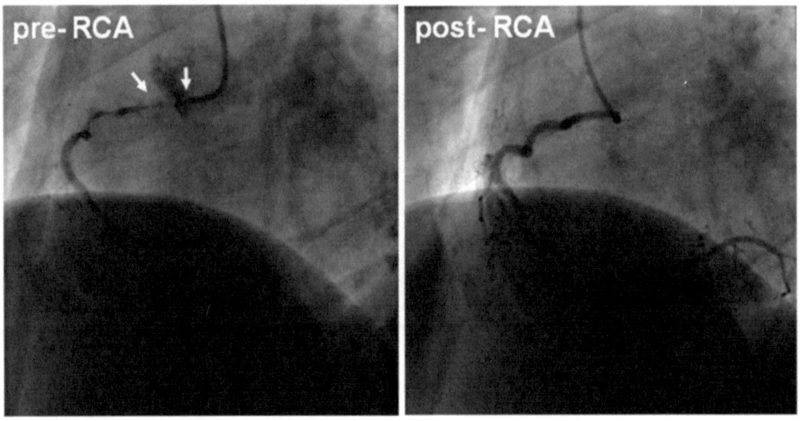

Fig. 1. Right coronary artery angiogram performed during the initial procedure. Preangioplasty (left anterior oblique (LAO) view): the RCA was affected with severe stenosis in the proximal site (arrow) (A). The RCA was opened and SESs was inserted (B). Satisfactory angiographic results were obtained with smooth luminal outline. No contrast extravasation outside the vessel wall was noted on the image [Reproducted Kishida, 2007].

Next day after the procedure, this patient had fever without suppuration on the access site, and grew *Staphylococcus aureus* on repeat blood cultures. Despite exhaustive screenings for a potential source of the infection, no infectious focus was detected. The patient was treated with intravenous adapted antibiotics, however, remained poor.

Three weeks after PCI, the patient had fever, convulsion and syncope attack with the torsades de pointes in ECG. The causes were considered due to trouble of the residual left coronary arteries (LCAs) lesions, and the patient was successfully implanted two SESs in the target LAD stenosis and a SES in the target LCX stenosis. The postprocedural course was uneventful, and the inflammatory sings were improved by the treatment with adapted antibiotics.

Two months later, the patient has recurrence fever with eosinophilia and an inferolateral wall ST-depression angina. Coronary angiography revealed no obvious changes in the LCAs, but an occluded proximal RCA stent, a large aneurysm off the stent, and a fistula into the right ventricular chamber with rapid clearance (Figure 2). A 16-slice multidetector computed tomographic angiogram scan confirmed both an occluded proximal RCA, and the aneurysm (50x30 mm in size) forming fistula (10 mm in size) into right ventricle (Figure 3).

The patient underwent a resection of the RCA stents and aneurysm, and a reconstruction of the right ventricular wall without coronary bypass grafting. Microscopic specimen from the resected aneurismal wall revealed an extensive inflammatory reaction with a predominance of neutrophils consisten with the micro-abscessn (Figure 4). The patient is doing well 5 years after operation [Kishida, 2007].

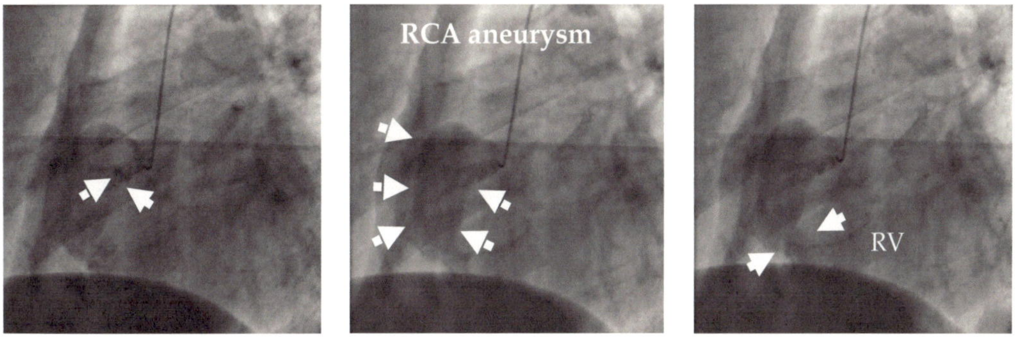

Fig. 2. Right coronary artery angiogram performed at the fever period

Angiography of the RCA demonstrated occlusion of proximal stent site, an entry point to aneurysm, and the saccular aneurysm in the area of proximal stents and its coronary artery fistula originating from the RCA stents, with contrast spillage into the right ventricular chamber through the fistula. Rapid clearance of contrast was observed, with none in the pericardial space [Reproducted Kishida, 2007].

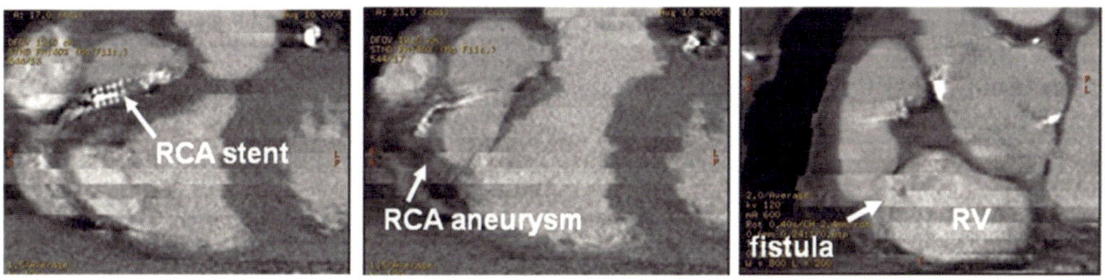

Fig. 3. The 16-slice multidetector computed tomographic angiogram disclosed huge RCA aneurysm (10x10 mm in diameter) and draining image into right ventricular chamber via fistula [Reproducted Kishida, 2007].

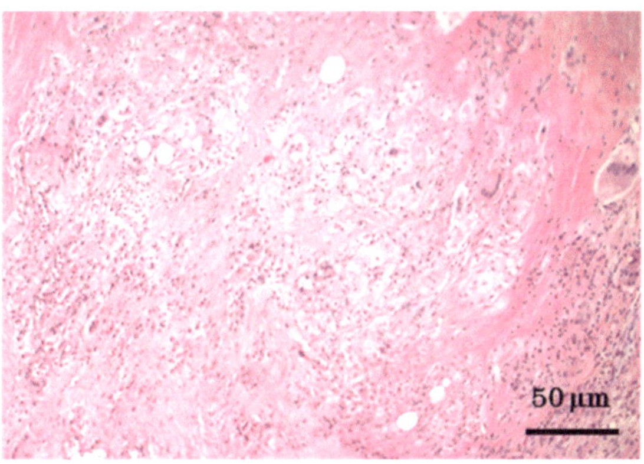

Fig. 4. Histopathology from pseudoaneurysm after surgical excision. Its histopathologic examination revealed marked inflammatory reaction with a predominance of neutrophils cocistent with an abscess. Hematoxylin and eosin staining. (original magnification, x200) [Reproducted Kishida, 2007].

2.1 Comments for case report

To date, there have been only 7 reported cases of infected drug-eluting stented coronary aneurysm, including our case [Kishida, 2007; Marcu, 2005; Alfonso, 2006; Singh, 2005; Jang, 2007; Le, 2007; Furutado, 2011] (Table 1). In six cases Staphylococcus aureus and one Pseudomonas aeruginosa bacteremia was responsible for causing mycotic stent complications. Of these cases, there were two cases of an infected drug-eluting stented coronary aneurysm forming fistula to cardiac chamber. The mechanism of infection at the site of drug-eluting stenting is not well understood. Potential caused for drug-eluting coronary stent infections include local suppression of immune response and endothelialization which should lead to weakening of the arterial wall and delayed aneurysm formation [Degertekin, 2003]. The potential role of SES in locally blunting the innate response to bacterial agents may be considered. Formation of mycotic aneurismal fistula in our case may be partly accounted for by this mechanism.

Case	Vessel	Stent	Fistula	Organism	Days	Max size	Ope	Outcome	Reference
55yo Male	LAD	P	—	*S. aureus*	90	15	+	Alive	2005 Marcu
47yo Male	RCA	S	—	*S. aureus*	2	—	—	Dead	2006 Alfonso
56yo Male	LAD	S	—	*S. aureus*	30	28	+	Alive	2005 Singh
70yo Male	RCA	S	RV	*S. aureus*	120	50	+	Alive	2005 our case
54yo Male	RCA	P	RA	*S. aureus*	120	—	+	Alive	2007 Jang
73yo Male	LCX	S	—	*S. aureus*	90	5	+	Dead	2007 Le
62yo Male	LAD	S	—	*P. aeruginosa*	20	20	+	Alive	2011 Furtado

P: paclitaxel eluting stent, S: sirolimus eluting stent, RA: right atrium, RV: right ventricle, S.:*Staphylococcus.*, P.: *Pseudomonas.*, Days:onset of aneurysm, Max size (mm): max diameter of aneurysm, Ope: surgical operation

Table 1. Infected drug-eluting stented coronary aneurysm

3. Conclusion

Infections specificity, related to the use of intracoronary DESs, is exceedingly rare. However, stent infection should be considered in the differential diagnosis of patients presenting unexplained fever and relapsing bacteremia at any time following drug-eluting stenting.

4. References

Baddour LM, et al. (2004) Nonvalvular cardiovascular device-related infections. *Clinical Infectious Diseses.* Vol.38, No.8, (April 2004), pp.1128-1130

Berkalp B, et al. (1999) Coronary artery aneurysm formation after balloon angioplasty and stent implantation. *International Journal of Cardiology.* Vol.69, No.1, (April 1999), pp.65-70

Ramsdale DR, et al. (2004) Bacteremia following complex percutaneous coronary intervention. *The Journal of Invasive Cardiology.* Vol.16, No.11, (Nov 2004), pp. 632-634

Myles O, et al. (2000) Infected endovascular stents managed with medical therapy alone. *Catheterization and Cardiovascular Interventions.* Vol.51, No.4, (Dec 2000), pp.51: 471-476

Sousa JE, et al. (2001) Lack of neointimal proliferation after implantation of sirolimus-coated stents in human coronary arteries: a quantitative coronary angiography and three-dimensional intravascular ultrasound study. *Circulation.* Vol.104, No.17, (Oct 2001), pp.192-195

Ong AT & Serruys PW. (2005) Drug-eluting stents: current issues. *Texas Heart Institute Journal.* Vol.32, No.3, pp372-377

McFadden EP, et al. (2004) Late thrombosis in drug-eluting coronary stents after discontinuation of antiplatelet therapy. *Lancet.* Vol.364, No.9444, (Oct 2004), pp1519-1521

Abreu L, et al. (2005) Coronary artery aneurysm one year and five months after sirolimus-eluting stent placement. *Arquivos Brasileiros de Cardiologia.* Vol.85, No.8, (Nov 2005) pp.340-342

Degertekin M, et al. (2003) Long-term follow-up of incomplete stent apposition in patients who received sirolimus-eluting stent for de novo coronary lesions: an intravascular ultrasound analysis. *Circulation.* Vol.108, No.22, (Dec 2003) pp.2747-2750

Virmani R, et al. (2004) Localized hypersensitivity and late coronary thrombosis secondary to a sirolimus-eluting stent: should we be cautious? *Circulation.* Vol.109, No.6, (Feb 2004) pp.701-705

Nebeker JR, et al. (2005) Hypersensitivity cases associated with drug-eluting coronary stents: a review of available cases from the Research on Adverse Drug Events and Reports (RADAR) project. *Journal of the American College Cardiology.* Vol.47, No.1, (Jan 2006), pp175-181

Stabile E, et al. (2004) Marked malapposition and aneurysm formation after sirolimus-eluting coronary stent implantation. *Circulation.* Vol.110, No.5, (Aug 2004), pp47-48

Kishida K, et al. (2007) Successful surgical treatment of an infected right coronary artery aneurysm-to-right ventricle fistula after sirolimus-eluting stent implantation. *Internal Medicine.* Vol.46, No.12, (Jun 2007), pp865-871

Marcu CB, et al. (2005) Post-infectious pseudoaneurysm after coronary angioplasty using drug eluting stents. *Heart Lung & Circulation.* Vol.14, No.2, (Jun 2005), pp85-86

Alfonso F, et al. (2006) Mycotic aneurysms after sirolimus-eluting coronary stenting. *Catheterization and Cardiovascular Interventions.* Vol.67, No.2, (Feb 2006), pp327-328

Singh H, et al. (2005) Mycotic aneurysm of left anterior descending artery after sirolimus-eluting stent implantation: a case report. *Catheterization and Cardiovascular Interventions.* Vol.65, No.2, (Jun 2005), pp282-285

Jang JJ, et al. (2007) Images in cardiovascular medicine. Pseudoaneurysm and intracardiac fistula caused by an infected paclitaxel-eluting coronary stent. *Circulation.* Vol.116, No.14, (Oct 2007), pp364-365

Le MQ & Narins CR. (2007) Mycotic pseudoaneurysm of the left circumflex coronary artery: a fatal complication following drug-eluting stent implantation. *Catheterization and Cardiovascular Interventions.* Vol.69, No.4, (Mar 2007), pp508-512

Furtado AD, et al. (2011) Infected pseudoaneurysm involving a drug-eluting stent. *Interactive Cardiovascular and Thoracic Surgery*. Vol.12, No.4, (Apr 2011), pp636-638.

This research was supported in part by a Grant-in-Aid for Scientific Research on Innovative Areas No. 22126008.

5

Acute Coronary Syndromes in Women - Gender Specific Changes in Coronarography

Anna Polewczyk, Marianna Janion and Maciej Polewczyk
II Kliniczny Oddział Kardiologii Wojewódzki Szpital Zespolony, Kielce
Poland

1. Introduction

Cardiovascular diseases (CVD) are one of the leading cause of mortality in both men and women in the world. According to a WHO report, about 55% of deaths in European women are related to CVD, including 23% caused by coronary artery disease (CAD) and 18% due to stroke. Conversely, in men, CVD is the cause of 43% of deaths, including CAD (21%) and stroke (11%). These statistics are alarming — in Europe, one woman dies of CVD every 6 minutes.

In respect of above data is very important to perform randomized clinical trials with women treated for acute coronary syndromes (ACS). This operation was initiated relatively not long ago. In the past 40 years, the attention of cardiologists regarding the treatment of coronary artery disease (CAD) has been focused mainly on the group of male patients, markedly less on the female population.

In the meantime, to the best of our knowledge, despite of apparent similarity of ACS clinical course in men and women, differences in the pathophysiological mechanisms, prevalence and profile of risk factors, angiographic changes, kind of treatment and prognosis are found. These observations are particularly important up against constantly rising cardiovascular morbidity and mortality among women.

2. Comparison of clinical course in women and men treated from ACS

2.1 Coronary risk factors in female and male

Acute coronary syndromes in women are the real challenge for clinical and invasive cardiologists. The ACS diagnosis and therapy in female are more difficult than in male. It is connected with ACS women older age, major coronary risk factors number, differences in pathophysiology and clinical course and complication during procedures. The coronary risk factors in women and men are the same, but their influence on female, especially during menopause is different than in male. This effect results from female specific hormone constellation during menopausal period. Generally, in ACS women population, the coronary risk factors are more often found than in ACS male group and this is the inverse phenomenon compared to population without myocardial infarction.

In majority of currently ACS registries these observations were affirmed. According to data from Polish ACS Registry (26035 patients with ACS STEMI hospitalized between 2005-2006; 8989 (34,5%) females) women were older than men by 7.7 years on average and this was statistically significant. In women, the well established risk factors were significantly more prevalent than in men: hypertension: 67,0% vs 56,1%, diabetes: 28% vs 16,6%, obesity: 23,7% vs 13,4% (p<0,001 for all groups). Only the prevalence of hypercholesterolemia was similar in both sexes and smoking was less often in female.

Analysis of Swedish registry: ACS-AMIS Plus Registry evaluated over 20- thousands ACS population (28% female) hospitalized between 1997-2006 also showed older women age by 7,5 years on average and more often presence of hypertension and diabetes in women.

Similar observation can be run into worldwide registries.

According to data from Chinese ACS Registry (CRACE) - 1301 ACS patients, 24,4% women treated from 2001 to 2004, female subjects were also significant older than male patients (67.23 years vs 61.80 years, P < 0.0001). The incidence of diabetes mellitus and hypertension in the female group was higher than in male group (30.8% vs 18.6%, p < 0.0001 and 66.4% vs 56.8%, p = 0.001 respectively), conversely, the incidence of smoking was less in female group than men group (6,6% vs 66,2%, p<0,001).

Longstanding observation of female and male population hospitalized from ACS in USA in years 1997-2006 demonstrated significantly frequent prevalence of hypertension, diabetes mellitus, heart failure and cerebrovascular diseases in women from all aging categories.

Beside of greater number of risk factors in women than in men, stronger impact some of them to woman organism is again and again suspected. First of all, this finding affects smoking. The risk of acute coronary syndrome in smoking women is about six fold higher compared to no- smoking female, whereas in smoking men only three fold risk increase is observed. The cause of this effect is probably adverse influence nicotine for hormonal profile in women. It is proved that smoking women have lower estrogen level.

The similar observation regard impact of diabetes for ACS risk in female. The prevalence of diabetes frequently correlates with acute coronary syndromes in women than in men.

The next differences are connected with lipid profile. Stronger prognostic impact of higher LDL level in men is indicated, whereas in women the big importance of low HDL level is emphasized. Low HDL-C levels in women have been shown to be a risk factor for CHD and premature atherosclerosis independent of serum LDL-C and triglyceride levels. In female with established coronary disease, low HDL-C levels may be a better predictor of subsequent coronary events than high levels of LDL-C. The Nurses' Health Study estimates that a 17 mg/dL elevation in HDL-C reduces the risk of CHD development in postmenopausal women by approximately 40%. Generally, the risk of CHD decreases by 3% for every 1 mg/dL increase in HDL-C in women, but only by 2% in men. Similarly, the presence of diabetes tends to confer a more negative effect on HDL-C and triglycerides (TG) in diabetic women compared to men.

Angiographic and ultrasound evidence demonstrate that low plasma levels of HDL-C are associated with major severity of CHD in females and males, as indicated by an increase in the number and extent of coronary vessel involvement. Furthermore, among men and women with angiographic evidence of CHD but with normal total cholesterol levels, patients with HDL-C levels <35 mg/dL had significantly more cardiovascular events than those with higher levels. Then, the correlation between lipid profile in female and male are complicated. The further observations are necessary to confirm these interdependences.

2.2 Clinical characteristic of acute coronary syndrome process in women and men

Studies compared ACS clinical symptoms in women and men demonstrate different results. According to part of them myocardial infarction clinical course is similar in female and male. In contrast, other observations convince of significant differences in ACS gender manifestation.

Myocardial infarction symptoms in men are usually typical: strong retrosternal pain with typical radiation, without reaction or with transient abating after nitroglycerin usage.
Women with acute coronary syndrome more often complain for atypical disorders: back pain, neck pain, nausea or vomiting, dyspnea, palpitation or strong weakness. In women more often indolent myocardial infarction course was also affirmed.
The interesting meta- analytic evaluation of ACS gender differences confirmed these observations. Review of articles and dissertation from 1966 to 2007 demonstrated that above gender differences of moderate or larger magnitude were evident and women were more likely than men to report non-specific symptoms. For most symptoms, the magnitude of effects did not vary across different symptom-assessment strategies.
Additionally, majority contemporary studies showed that ACS women were admitted to hospital later then ACS men and, this fact also suggests more often presence atypical complains in female.
Data from Polish ACS Registry (over 20 thousands ACS women) demonstrated that women especially during the first 3 hours from symptom onset, presented to hospital significantly less often and that the delay of > 12 hours occurred more often in this patients.
Likewise, Swedish ACS Registry showed that female patients came to hospital later then men- median difference 60 minut. The delay on admission with atypical ACS symptoms in women may cause worse effect of therapy.
The five month analysis over 6 thousands group of consecutive patients presenting with ACS showed that patients with atypical presentation were significantly less likely to receive evidence-based therapy and coronary angiography and suffered worse in-hospital outcomes. After adjustment for confounders, the absence of typical chest pain was associated with higher mortality rate (odds ratio 2.0, 95% confidence intervals 1.29-2.75).
On the other hand women even though presenting the typical ACS symptoms, often are treated worse than men. First of all, to this time, myocardial infarction is perceived as "male disease ". Female and doctors often ignore important disorders, in contrast, paradoxically, typical symptoms are the strongest ACS predictors in women. Chest pain has consistently been underestimated in women because of the disappointing results of evaluations of this symptom in the past.
In women, more often than in men, despite the clinical and biochemical ACS characteristic, changes in coronary angiography aren't found. In the CASS (Coronary Artery Surgery Study), 30% of women with typical angina and 64% with atypical angina had normal coronary angiograms, but this was observed in only 7% and 34% of men, respectively.
Syndrome X, which was defined as symptoms and signs of myocardial ischemia in the presence normal coronary angiograms, predominates in women, but this syndrome may represent microvascular disease or endothelial dysfunction, which are more often observed in women.
Recently, data from WISE (Women's Ischemia Syndrome Evaluation) and WTH (Women Take Heart) studies demonstrated, that rates of cardiovascular events were highest for symptomatic women with nonobstructive coronary artery disease compared to symptomatic women with normal coronary arteries; on the other hand, symptomatic women with normal coronary arteries had almost three-fold higher rates of events when compared to asymptomatic women. These facts suggest that in women, as in men, chest pain compatible with angina deserves careful evaluation.
The following observations of ACS clinical course in women demonstrate worse clinical presentation on admission. It is probably a consequence of older female age and more risk factors.

Analysis of contemporary European and American ACS Registries confirm higher frequency of heart failure in Killip-Kimball class III-IV in female compared with male.
Presumably atypical ACS symptoms, delay from onset pain to admission and worse clinical presentation on admission contribute to still emphasized less often women qualifications to invasive procedures. According to Polish ACS Registry primary PCI was performed in 47,8% women and 57,4% men (p<0,001).
In Swedish AMIS Plus Registry reperfusion strategy was used in 27,2% women and 36,6 % men (p<0,001).
Data from in the American College of Cardiology-National Cardiovascular Data Registry also showed lower utilization rates of emergent PCI for women than for men across all ethnic subsets.
The next problem, mentioned above, is specific coronary angiography changes in women presenting ACS. The reasons for more often presence of normal coronary arteries or non critical narrows in coronary artery angiography performed in ACS women are unclear. The mostly accepted conception is phenomenon of atherosclerotic plaque erosion with thrombus formed on apparently undamaged artery wall. These findings were obtained on the basis postmortem examinations patients died from ACS - in 37% women the surface plaque damage without significant coronary artery injury was demonstrated.
Other studies with widely intravascular technique (IVUS) usage showed in women without significant changes in coronary angiograms a presence of atherosclerotic process in ACS responsible arteries.
Additionally, female and male unstable angina consecutive studies demonstrated qualitative and quantitative gender differences between morphology of atherosclerotic plaques. Women atherosclerotic plaques indicated lower optical density and less expressed calcification than men plaques.
However, presently there are the disagreements in reports estimated atherosclerotic plaques morphology. The contemporary analysis of plaque components in 362 ACS patients (254 men, 108 women) showed no differences between female and male atherosclerotic plaques. In this study more often occurrence of diabetes and high hsCRP level in ACS women than men was emphasized and with these factors more female plaques instability was related.
These contradictions in studies, order to searching another reasons of specific coronary changes in women.
The next conception posits the differences in plaque reaction for response to hormonal factors and thrombogenic stimulation.
According to epidemiological data the protective role of endogenic estrogens in young women is widely known. It is directly connected with impact of these hormones to coagulation system.
In young, premenopausal women the lower fibrinogen and VII coagulation factor's level was affirmed. Women in each age with family premature coronary diseases review, demonstrate excessive platelet aggregation. Following the excessive thrombocytes aggregation in these patients the bigger number of fibrinogen molecules are indicated - perhaps invisible during coronary angiography atherosclerotic changes undergoing action of stronger prothrombic factors in some women.
Moreover, in connection with higher prothrombic inclination, probably we can more often observe a distal microvessels embolisation effect imperceptible during routine coronary angiography. Therefore, the differences in coronary angiography changes between female and male could be more complicated than earlier suspected.

3. Specific ACS coronary angiography changes in women during pregnancy and postpartum period

3.1 Epidemiology of acute coronary syndromes during pregnancy and postpartum period

Myocardial infarction in pregnant women is an extremely rare event. The frequency of ACS in this period is difficult to estimate. According to the scarce epidemiological studies, in the United States the incidence of AMI in pregnancy ranges from 2.81 to 6.22 cases per 100,000 deliveries. No data are available for Europe or other countries. In addition, these studies do not differentiate between AMI with and without ST-segment elevation.

Currently we can observe increased frequency of acute coronary syndromes during pregnancy or postpartum period. This effect is probably connected with old age of pregnant women, and, generally increasing morbidity of coronary diseases among young women.

Presently, women at first more often give the time for professional career, holding off maternity for later years of life. In the meantime, the risk of complication during pregnancy significantly increased with aging - it is emphasized, that myocardial infarction during pregnancy usually occurs in pregnant women after 33 years old.

The analysis of literature demonstrated, that in older pregnant, multiparas, more often the typical, atherosclerotic substrate of acute coronary syndrome was indicated. Majority of them have occurred in III pregnancy trimester.

However, in younger mothers, primiparas, the ACS pathogenesis is often atypical with often occurrence's during postpartum period.

3.2 Hemodynamic, hormonal and biochemical transitions during pregnancy affecting to cardiovascular system

Pregnancy isn't termed as coronary risk factor, although in this period a lot of changes in circulatory system, hormonal and coagulation parameters transformations are demonstrated. During pregnancy the increase of ejection volume and acceleration of cardiac activity is indicated. Both changes cause growth of oxygen cardiac muscle demand.

Additionally, the physiological anemia and decrease of systolic and diastolic pressure contribute for limitation in oxygen delivery to cardiac muscle's cells.

Moreover, increase of volume blood circulating and ejection fraction causes intensification of the shearing forces action for big arteries walls -these effects can provoke coronary arteries dissection.

Hormonal changes during pregnancy relies on increased progesterone production leading of impairment vascular wall through losing of normal elastic fibers structure, reticuline fibers fragmentation and decrease of acid mucopolisacharides. These effects also aggravate the risk of arteries dissection.

Changes in coagulation system during pregnancy are connected with increment of fibrinogen and factors VII, VIII, IX, X, XII and von Willebrand factor's concentration. In result of increase concentration of inhibitors of plasminogen activator PAI-1 and PAI-2, the serum fibrinolytic activity is decreased. It caused hipercoagulation state, which worsening during delivery when the great of PAI- 1 amount is released from placenta.

The essence above changes is often occurrence atypical ACS patophysiology during pregnancy and postpartum period.

3.3 Coronary angiography changes during acute coronary syndromes in pregnancy based on pathophysiological substrate

According to current reports, the most often cause of acute coronary syndrome in pregnant women, similarly to overall population, is sudden atherosclerotic rupture. Atherosclerotic changes was indicated in 40% pregnant women, in majority ACS symptoms occurred in antepartum period (54%).

According to mentioned above high ACS risk in older pregnant women, in these population the higher number of coronary risk factors is indicated.

The myocardial infarction risk during pregnancy rises 2,4 fold in women with hypertension, 4,9 fold in smoking and 6,9 fold in diabetics.

Idiopathic coronary artery dissection rarely appeares in general population, whereas during pregnancy, the frequency of this effect may approximate even 27%. Usually it is observed in peripartum (50%) or postpartum (34%) period - in connection with described earlier changes in arteries walls construction and hemodynamic disorders. Some of authors suggest that coronary artery dissection in pregnant women is even more often, though the artery wall undergoes essential healing and if the coronary angiography is performed after acute ACS phase, the image of angiogram may be correct. Relatively often, the coronary dissection in these women is found in more than one artery. It suggests existence of generalized arteries pathology.

Another possible pathophysiological cause of acute coronary syndrome in pregnant women is angiospasm. The recognition of coronary artery spasm as the reason of myocardial infarction is difficult, because the angiospasm may be transient with quick idiopathic return of normal coronary flow.

In Roth's analysis coronary spasm only in 2% women was documented and only during antepartum period. Nonetheless in 13 % these patients angiograms were normal, perhaps in part of them the angiospasm occurred before the procedure had been performed.

Normal coronary angiogram occurrs in equal proportion during all pregnancy periods. The potential reason of acute coronary syndrome in women without significant angiographic changes beside of healing dissection or transient angiospasm may be thrombus or embolus, which were resolved.

In 8% women the cause of myocardial infarction was exactly thrombus. It can be connected with mentioned above tend to hipercoagulation state.

Angiography changes are usually localized in only one of coronary artery, extremely rarely we can find multivessel disease in pregnancy. The single case of multivessel atherosclerotic changes in 41- years old postpartum woman come from own observation. In the literature we can meet also single multivessel dissection description.

3.4 Coronary interventions during pregnancy

Currently, the most effective therapy of acute coronary syndrome's is primary coronary intervention. This procedure during pregnancy is connected with dangerous fetus exposure to radiation. It can cause genetic disorders, height inhibition, different malformations.

Bithell and Stuart demonstrated that children exposed to radiation during fetal life are characterized major cancer development risk. The dose of radiation until 1 rad is considered as no dangerous for fetus. This doses is simultaneously enough to performed diagnostic and therapeutic procedures.

However, in case of complications, longer radiation time may be necessary- exposition time may rises above 5 rads. Because of lack of unequivocal directions, in this situation, the pregnancy termination could be imperative.

To the maximum security, usage of leaden protection for stomach, pelvis and lumbo-sacral region is recommended.
According to data from literature, 55-89% women undergoing coronary angiography have received stents. During pregnancy we don't possess certain data relevant to safety usage drug eluting stents, the bare metal stents in this situation are rather recommended.
The great doubts are connected with coronary angioplasty during coronary artery dissection as a cause of acute coronary syndrome. According to European- American Guidelinesses from 2003 year, PCI is recommended in this situation. Nonetheless, numerous reports demonstrate that in case of stable patient state, the conservative treatment is also effective and in postpartum period the idiopathic healing is noticed.
On the other hand, Roth indicate that during coronary angiography the risk of iatrogenic coronary artery dissection is increased, that's why particular caution in qualification for invasive procedures in this period should be recommended.
The reports concern of possible complications of invasive treatment during pregnancy are very rare. The single cases of contrapulsation aortic balloon usage during complications of extensive anterior wall myocardial infarction were described.
Similarly, our knowledge about remote results of acute coronary syndromes invasive treatment in pregnant women is poor, but at present, this is a method from choice.
Coronary artery bypass grafting (CABG) is the procedure performed extremely rarely during pregnancy.
According to James's et al. analysis, CABG was done in 51 pregnancy women (6% analyzed group), but pregnancy period and results of the treatment data weren't released.
Another analysis by Roth and Elkayam 5 women underwent CABG during antepartum period. One of them died after 3 months and after delivery (healthy child was born), in the second pregnant the fetal death in utero came up.
The most often direction of CABG is ineffectiveness or complications after PCI. During surgery the fetal monitoring is necessary, because hypothermia and extracorporeal circulation can cause fetal arrhythmias.
The single reports about CABG in women during pregnancy suggest, that these procedures are connected with high risk for mother and child.

4. The valuation of coronary arteries in menopausal women treated for acute coronary syndromes

4.1 Impact of pathophysiological transformations during menopause on coronary risk

Menopause is considered as a single, strong coronary risk factor. In this period in woman organism multidirectional changes are achieved. These transformations concern of lipid profile (increase of LDL, TGL, apolipoprotein B, apolipoprotein (a) level; decrease HDL and apolipoprotein AI level), coagulation factors production (significant increase of fibrinogen level, increase of factor VII, antithrombin III and inhibitor tissue activator of plasminogen (PAI-1) activity), insulinoresistance's and abdomen's obesity development. Disadvantageous is also impact of menopause for endothelium function.
Though the current understanding of the role of menopause in cardiovascular diseases (CVD) is controversial, studies suggest that menopause does not exacerbate CVD independent of aging, and hormone replacement therapy is not effective for secondary prevention of CVD.

According to long-term 16 years observation over 11 thousands Italian population, menopause wasn't found an independent cardiovascular risk factor.
Despite above divergences, there is a fact, that cardiovascular women morbidity significantly rises during menopausal period.
Inhibition of estradiol distribution during menopause constitutes of biological challenge for woman organism, especially for women aggravated other circulatory risk factors. The next years after menopause, on account of lack of estrogen coordinated in numerous metabolic transformations, are characterized intensification of existing diseases and another exposure. We can suspect that required of adaptation a new metabolic balance causes worse process and prognosis in menopausal women with coronary artery diseases.
Presently, more often the differences in artery stiffness in female and male are emphasized. The genders differ in large artery biomechanical properties throughout the lifespan with females displaying higher stiffness than males during the prepubertal years and a dramatic increase after menopause. Males on the other hand experience an increase in arterial stiffness postpuberty and a linear increase thereafter, suggesting that females have intrinsically stiffer large arteries than males, but that such effects are mitigated by sex steroids during the reproductive years. These factors may contribute in part to the observed gender differences in the pathophysiology and clinical manifestations of cardiovascular disease.
On the other hands, hormonal replacement therapy (HRT) usage to decreased of circulatory diseases risk in menopausal women is presently not recommended.

4.2 Influence of hormonal replacement therapy on coronary artery state

Reports relevant HRT are controversial. Until 1988 year, the knowledge about benefit effects of hormonal replacement therapy was based on only retrospective studies. Metaanalyses demonstrated 30-40% decreased of coronary disease's risk mostly in women received conjugationed estrogens (less often together with progestagenes) and particularly good effects was observed in women with earlier recognized coronary disease.
In 1998 year, the results of the first randomize, multicenter study- HERS were published. In this study the HRT effect in secondary prevention was assessed. In years 2002 and 2004 the next study results were presented- WHI I and WHI II- evaluated HRT implementation in primary prevention. In these studies the unambiguous evidences affirmed HRT benefits in circulatory diseases were expected. Adverse results were a big shock. The more amount of cardiovascular events in the first year of therapy, more numerous thromboembolic events and more often breast cancer were documented.
From this time, the American Heart Association and European Cardiac Society recommended not initiating and no continuing hormonal replacement therapy in circulatory system diseases prevention. Repeated analysis of mentioned above studies demonstrated, that the important point is the period of HRT inclusion. It is suspected that earlier usage of HRT, in the beginning of menopause is probably more favourable than in later years. This effect is connected with HRT impact for not yet damaged endothelium.
The therapy inception in the later years can favour of impairment's of coagulation and inflammation mechanisms and in consequence's can be responsible for thromboembolic complications and unstability of atherosclerotic plaque.
The greatest thromboembolic disorders risk was indicated in the first year of HRT therapy, particularly during oral treatment, because of first liver passage effect, which caused thrombotic processes stimulation. Transdermal estrogenes, deprived of first passage effect, don't affect also for increased of CRP, fibrinogen and prothrombin level.

The results of Danish observation study (700 thousands healthy women) affirmed the beneficial effect of transdermal estrogens for cardiovasculatory system with myocardial infarction reduction and without the increased thromboembolic risk.
Despite of optimistic reports, currently still doesn't exist evidence that hormonal replacement therapy improve of survival and doesn't indicate of side effects. Therefore, HRT indications still contain only clinical menopausal symptoms, not cardiovascular prevention.

4.3 Coronary artery changes in menopausal women treated from acute coronary syndromes

To this time, there are very little studies estimated the specific coronary angiography changes in menopausal women. One of sparse comparative analysis concerned assessment of these changes in pre- and postmenopausal women demonstrated more frequent involvement of triple vessels in postmenopausal CAD patients (33.8% vs 20.4%, p=0), and single vessel in premenopausal (43,2 % vs 26,9%, p=0) which indicated more serious CAD in postmenopausal patients. There was no significant difference in left main and double vessels involvement in the two groups.
In postmenopausal group more lesion of middle left anterior descending (LAD), left circumflex artery (LCX) and right coronary artery (RCA) were found (all p value <0.05) compared to much more severe lesions (≥90%) at left main (2.9% vs 1.1%, p=0.048) and proximal LAD (28.2% vs 16.6%, p=0) in the premenopausal CAD group.
As for lesion length, there were more local lesions at the posterior descending artery (PDA) (6.4% vs 2.5%, *P*=0.014), diffuse lesion at diagonal 1 (7.1% vs 3.6% *P*=0.036), middle and distal RCA (13.5% vs 8.6%, *P*=0.033; 5.8% vs 2.1%, *P*=0.014) in the postmenopausal CAD group. But tubular lesion seemed to be located more at middle and distal LAD (19.6% vs 9.0%, *P*=0; 12.1% vs 7.9%, *P*=0.036) in the premenopausal CAD group.
Other items with regard to lesion length were comparable without a significant difference between the two groups.
Probably, above observation confirm the different dynamism of atherosclerotic processes, connected with hormonal state. Additionally in mentioned study, in both of groups: pre- and postmenopausal women, the significant more often prevalence of prior myocardial infarction, hypertension, diabetes mellitus and dyslipidemia in CAD women compared to non CAD patients was documented. Furthermore, the frequency of coronary risk factors was higher in CAD postmenopausal group compared to premenopausal CAD women. Then, the high number of coronary risk factors in women probably correlates with more often multivessel coronary atherosclerotic changes.

5. Comparison of efficacy percutaneous coronary interventions and coronary artery bypass grafts in women and men during acute coronary syndromes

5.1 Review of clinical studies assessed gender differences in coronary interventions during acute coronary syndromes NSTEMI and STEMI

Percutaneous Coronary Intervention (PCI) is the preferred technique for the treatment of acute coronary syndrome with or without ST-segment elevation according to the Guidelines. The available data concerned gender differences in qualification and PCI effects are still conflicted.
Historically, the first PCI effects analysis coming from the end of XX century, in majority demonstrated a fewer qualification and worse prognosis in women treated by invasive

strategy. This effect was visible in all acute coronary syndromes types: ACS STEMI, NSTEMI and unstable angina.

In FRISC II study, women PCI benefits weren't indicated in comparison to conservative ACS NSTEMI treatment, whereas the definitely better PCI results in men were observed.

In spite of more optimistic results of TACTICS TIMI 18 study, in which the benefits from invasive therapy with widely stents and inhibitor GP IIb/IIIa usage were evident also in women, in the next study RITA 3, the positive effects of early invasive strategy during NSTEMI indicated the strongly advantage in male compared to female.

The reports concerned ACS STEMI were similar - there were documented an improvement of myocardial infarction therapy results in women, but, beside of better and better PCI techniques usage, greater PCI effects in men were demonstrated.

In Stent PAMI study the ACS STEMI female mortality after six month observation was significantly higher than in male.

The later study - CADILLAC also indicated higher STEMI population women after 30 days and 1 year, independent of kind of interventional technique's.

These worse results of procedures in women were tried to assign of major risk factors account (the more often prevalence of hypertension, diabetes and hiperlipidemia in female were confirmed in above studies), however in multivariable analysis the female sex was independent predictors of one - year more frequency of adverse events and mortality.

The causes of this phenomenon aren't still explained. Responsible could be the ACS clinical factors: delayed in disease's onset detection, older age, hormonal factors and comorbidities (hypertension, diabetes mellitus)- more often found in women. Nonetheless, gender differences in efectivenesses of coronary interventions were visible despite of allowing in studies and registries mentioned above factors.

The impact of specific coronary angiography changes in women to coronary interventions results are also often named as a cause of worse effect of therapy. Especially, smaller coronary artery size can be the reason of more often dissection or vascular perforation after PCI.

Based on reports from 1990 year, the frequency of vascular complications in women underwent of coronary interventions were about 3 fold higher than in men. This effect is assigned to difficulties in tailoring catheters size's to generally lower coronary arteries caliber in female.

Other authors suggested that the higher mortality seen in women after an AMI might be explained by less aggressive treatment, and if women had access to the same quality of care as men, their survival would be the same.

5.2 Current effects of coronary interventions in women

Current studies evaluated of differences between female and male PCI effectiveness are still controversial.

The analysis of the great PCI Registry (over 22 thousands procedures; 31,8% women) showed, that compared with men, women were older, had a higher prevalence of comorbidities, and had a significantly higher frequency of adverse outcomes after PCI. After adjustment for baseline demographics, comorbidities, clinical presentation, and lesion characteristics, female gender was associated with an increased risk of in-hospital death, vascular complication, blood transfusion, stroke, and major adverse cardiac events (MACE). The relationship between female gender and increased risk of death and MACE was no longer present after further adjustment for kidney function and low body surface area.

Authors concluded that differences in mortality rates between men and women no longer exist after PCI.

This study included different clinical presentations of coronary artery disease with a mixed of ST- segment elevation myocardial infarction, non ST-segment elevation myocardial infarction (NSTEMI), unstable and stable angina, a heterogeneity which could minimize a difference to some extent.

Current analysis of Polish ACS Registry, assessed population of 26,035 patients with ACS STEMI (34,5% women) was evidently demonstrated higher in-hospital (15% vs 9%, p<0,001) and one-year (22% vs 14,1%, p<0,001) women mortality. Coronary angiography was carried out significantly less often in female (47,8% vs 57,4% , p<0,001). In women receiving interventional treatment, primary angioplasty was performed significantly less often within 12 hours from symptom onset (35,8% vs 44,0%, p<0,001). The pharmacological treatment was less aggressive in women: GPIIb/IIIa inhibitor was administered in 12,2 % women vs 16,8 % men (p<0,001). Foregoing results were assigned the worse ACS clinical female presentation.

According to the Switzerland Registry included also over 20 thousands population hospitalized from ACS in 1997-2006 years (28% women) female gender was an independent factor for undergoing PCI less frequently. Although performed less often than in men, women benefited similarly from PCI and it was associated with lower in-hospital mortality, whether or not ACS was associated with ST-segment elevation.

Very interesting information comes from currently conducted observations concerned evolution of PCI effects in female and male in connection with improvement of PCI techniques.

According to retrospective analysis compared by gender two PCI populations: one of them consisted of patients underwent PCI between 1979-1995 (28% female), the second- between 1996-2004 (31 female), PCI was successful in 89% of women and 90% of men. In the recent group, 30-day mortality was significantly reduced compared with that in the early group in women (2.9% vs. 4.4%, p = 0.002) and men (2.2% vs. 2.8%, p = 0.04). However, long-term survival was similar between the early and recent groups among both men and women. After adjustment for risk factors, there was no difference between men and women from 1994 onward for either 30-day or long-term outcomes. Traditionally, compared with men, women undergoing PCI were older and more likely to have diabetes mellitus, hypertension, or hypercholesterolemia.

Authors suggested that the 30-day mortality after PCI in men and women has decreased in the past 25 years. After accounting for baseline risks, no differences in short-term or long-term mortality were observed between men and women.

The next problem is the prevalence of coronary interventions complications. According to majority observations in women more often than in men the periprocedural arteries damages and bleeding complications were found.

Argulian et al. analyzed process of 4768 percutaneous coronary interventions performed between 2001-2004.

The baseline characteristics, periprocedural complications, angiographic success, procedural success, and major in-hospital complications (death, myocardial infarction, and emergency coronary artery bypass graft surgery) after PCI were compared between men and women. Women were more likely older, with a significantly greater prevalence of hypertension and diabetes mellitus compared with men. After adjusting for baseline characteristics and coronary artery size, the incidence of coronary vascular injury complications was higher in

women than in men, particularly in patients <or=55 years (odds ratio [OR] 2.74, 95% confidence interval [CI] 1.49 to 5.04).
The difference was less when comparing women and men >55 years (OR 1.32, 95% CI 0.87 to 1.99, p = 0.047 for gender-age interaction).
The bleeding complications were also more often demonstrated in women than in men (<or=55 years OR 5.39, 95% CI 2.26 to 12.8, >55 years OR 2.55, 95% CI 1.68 to 3.87, p = 0.121 for gender-age interaction).
No significant gender differences were present in a combined end point of death, myocardial infarction, and emergency coronary artery bypass graft surgery.
Authors suggest, that among patients who have undergone PCI, women, particularly younger women, are more likely than men to experience coronary vascular injury and bleeding complications unaccounted for by coronary artery size and other patient characteristics. No differences were found in major in-hospital complications by gender.
The next analysis of Northern New England PCI Registry (13563 women underwent PCI in years 2002-07; 6,4% STEMI, 10,4% NSTEMI, 40,1 % unstable angina) demonstrated significantly improved rates of bleeding or vascular complications (VC) in women undergoing PCI during the past 6 years. The incidence of bleeding/VC decreased >50% in both men and women during the study period. Although these results are encouraging, this study demonstrates that women continue to be more than twice as likely as men to have significant bleeding/VC after PCI.
Authors conclude that the persistence of the gender gap may suggest a role of inherent biological or anatomical differences between women and men, which have yet to be identified.
The next retrospective analysis of current PCI Registry (8 thousands ACS STEMI population; 29% women) confirm that female sex was associated with a higher unadjusted in-hospital mortality (6.02% vs 3.45%, odds ratio [OR] 1.79, 95% CI 1.45-2. P < .0001) and higher risk of contrast-induced nephropathy (OR 1.75, P < .0001), vascular complications (OR 2.13, P < .0001), and postprocedure transfusion (OR 2.84, P < .0001). The gap in sex-specific mortality narrowed over time. In a propensity-matched analysis, female sex was associated with a higher rate of transfusion (OR 1.88, 95% CI 1.57-2.24, P < .0001) and vascular complications (OR 1.65, 95% CI 1.26-2.14, P < .0002); but there was no difference in mortality (OR 1.30, 95% CI 0.98-1.72, P = .07).
Authors suggest that these differences are explained by older age and worse baseline comorbidities among women.
Lower observational studies increasingly suggest evanescence of gender differences among patients undergoing primary PCI during ACS. These researches suspects that improvement of coronary intervention effectiveness's is connected with usage of more intensive pharmacotherapy.
The prospective analysis of 297 consecutive patients presenting with STEMI (27,6% women) treated by PCI with additional bare metal stent implantation and a GP IIb/IIIa inhibitor demonstrated that the incidence of major adverse cardiac events (MACE, defined as death, re-myocardial infarction, target lesion revascularization and coronary artery bypass graft) during long-term follow-up was similar in women and men (20% vs 26%, p = 0.29). In this study, female gender did not emerge as an independent predictor for MACE, but women presenting with STEMI had a higher cardiovascular risk profile; this emphasizes the need for a more extensive therapeutic strategy. Authors conclude that combination therapy with primary PCI and GP IIb/IIIa inhibitors might mitigate gender-related differences in clinical outcomes.

Above mentioned study results are affirmed by another observational reports.
The retrospective analysis of 468 consecutive patients underwent PCI for ACS (29.3% female) demonstrated no significant gender differences in the short-term adverse event rate at 30 days despite of several important differences between female and male patients. Authors emphasizes women older age, smaller size of stent and first of all noticed that female patients were less likely to be treated with optimal medical therapy, with lesser use of glycoprotein IIb/IIIa inhibitors and beta-blockers.
Therefore, we can suspect that further improvement of PCI technique and usage of respectively aggressive pharmacotherapy in women treated from acute coronary syndromes perhaps completely eliminate ACS gender gap.

5.3 Evaluation of coronary artery bypass grafting effects in female compared to male

The surgical treatment effects of acute coronary syndromes in women are still differently assessed.
In the previous years, when the coronary artery bypass grafting (CABG) was only one possibility of invasive strategy of advanced coronary artery diseases therapy, the Cardiosurgical Centers demonstrated increased mortality women underwent CABG.
Despite the lapse of the time, these observations are affirmed through the successive clinical reports.
There are the differences between studies results, because women constitute the lower group of patients undergoing CABG (20-30%). According to the great database of Society of Thoracic Surgeons (STS Database) - CABG was performed in 28% female patients hospitalized in years 1994-1996.
Currently studies assessed prognosis in women and men after CABG still demonstrate conflicted results.
The analysis over 70 thousands population of patients undergoing CABG in years 2003-2005 reaffirmed a significant effect modification by gender in 39 hospitals; the adjusted odds ratios showed significant increased risk for females. Authors suggest that the highest in-hospital mortality of females is frequently explained by gender physiological differences related to technical issues in surgery.
The smaller size of coronary arteries in women as compared with men has been often indicated as potentially increasing periprocedure and postprocedure complications in women. Actually, the influence of vessel size on gender differential mortality after CABG surgery remains controversial. Two studies used the body size as an indicator of vessel size. One found that gender differential mortality persists after adjustment for measures of body size, while another study showed that, both in men and women small body size does not increase the risk of operative mortality.
The next current analysis of 3441 patients (21,3% women) undergoing CABG between 2004-2008 years showed significantly higher 30-days (5,2% vs 2,5%, p=0,01) and one year (8,7% vs 4,8%, p=0,0008) women mortality. Moreover, these differences decline in patients operated using off-pump coronary artery bypass (OPCAB) technique. Authors suggest that female gender is a strong independent predictor and risk factor of increased postoperative mortality rates when extracorporeal circulation is used. OPCAB significantly reduces early and midterm postoperative mortality in women and may therefore be proposed as the preferred revascularization technique among female patients.
In the literature we can meet also observation indicated lack of significant differences between female and male prognosis after CABG, independent of surgical technique.

The analysis of group 954 patients undergoing CABG (19,7% women) in 2004-2009 years demonstrated no gender differences in the clinical outcomes after surgery (only the cerebrovascular event rate was higher in females compared with that in males (4.3% vs 1.6%; P=0.0432).

In spite of conflicted reports concerned PCI and CABG effects in women, admittedly that review of currently literature demonstrates absolute benefits of reperfusion therapy of acute coronary syndromes in female and male. Majority of above analyzed studies confirms baseline worse clinical ACS women presence, particularly older age, major coronary risk factors number and more often occurrence of advanced heart failure, shock and cardiac arrest. Undoubtedly these factors, in significant way affects for worse early and distant prognosis.

Certainly, relatively short time of ACS gender differences observation and generally lower women participation in clinical studies prevent unequivocal conclusions.

The further studies are necessary with particular acknowledgement coronary anatomy and acute coronary syndromes pathophysiology in female and male.

6. Analysis of selected cases of acute coronary syndromes in women

In every day clinical practice we can see a lot of very interesting cases of specific acute coronary syndromes proceeding in female. According to earlier documentation, these contraries of ACS process are the most often presented during one of two particular women life periods: pregnancy and menopause.

6.1 Acute myocardial infarction in a 29-year-old woman during postpartum period - specific coronary changes

The case of acute coronary syndrome STEMI in 29-years old woman in postpartum period illustrate of atypical ACS pathophysiology.

29- years old woman, three months after natural delivery was admitted to Cardiology Ward due to two- hours strong retrosternal pain. Heretofore patient was healthy, periodically complained for migraine and didn't indicate any coronary risk factors. During pregnancy she received hormonal therapy- luteine. Physical examination didn't demonstrate any abnormalities. In ECG- ST elevation in II, III, aVF, V5-V6 leads was revealed. Fig.1.

Biochemical testes demonstrated significantly increased of TnT's level (1,42 ng/ml). Echocardiography showed only descreet akinesis of apical segment lateral left ventricle wall with normal ejection fraction (EF- 65%). Coronary angiography revealed marginal branch aneurysm with prevalence of thrombus. Remaining coronary arteries were normal. Fig.2.

On account of small size of marginal branch, patient was disqualified from coronary revascularization. The typical pharmacological ACS therapy was used: low molecular weight heparin, double antiplatelet treatment, ACE-inhibitor, beta blocker and statin. After these treatment, the patient clinical state was improved.

Diagnostic process descoped congenital coagulation disorders as a cause of arterial thrombosis. Mutation prothrombin's gene G 20210 was excluded. Antiphospholipid antibodies level was negative. Only fibrinogen level and fibrinogen degradation products level were significantly increased.

During hospitalization any complications weren't observed. In ECG the negative T waves in II, III, aVF leads occurred, without pathological Q waves.

After ten days patient was discharged with further pharmacological treatment recommendation (ASA, Clopidogrel, beta blocker and statin). Only ACE-I was interrupted because of hypotension.

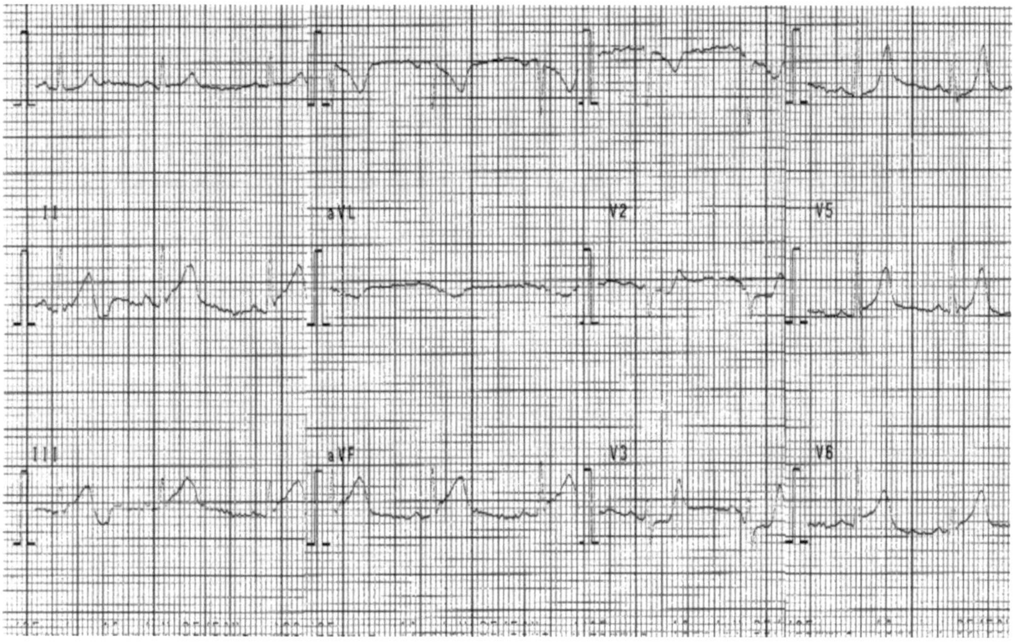

Fig. 1. ECG on admission. The description in the text.

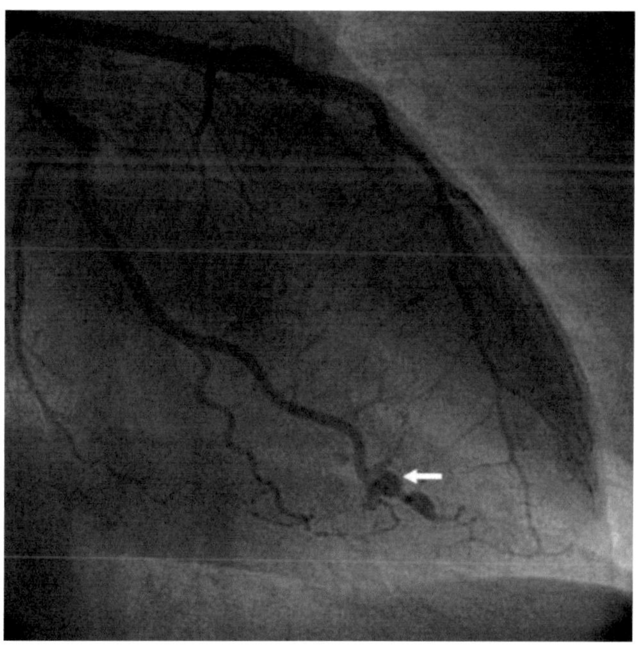

Fig. 2. Aneurysm with thrombus in marginal branch

One year later, after ceasing of Clopidogrel therapy, woman was again admitted to Cardiology Ward with the same complaints. In ECG the ST elevation in the same leads were observed, troponin T level was again increased (0,8 ng/ml). Coronary angiography image was also similar. The decision about further pharmacological treatment (double antiplatelet therapy) was maked.

During long-term, three years observation, patient is in good condition, but over the time takes medication: ASA, Clopidogrel, beta blocker, statin.

This case of myocardial infarction in postpartum women with aneurysm of coronary artery is an extremely rare and it is the real diagnostic and therapeutic challenge. Particularly, it is difficult to explain the coincidence's between both effects and make a decision about prevented of recurrences.

Probably, the base of acute coronary syndrome in this case wasn't typical, atherosclerotic. Perhaps the coronary artery aneurysm was a congenital malformation and in this particular postpartum period was favoured to initiation of thrombotic process. It is commonly allowed, that aneurysm prevalence increases the thrombosis risk and that during pregnancy and postpartum period this risk is still higher. It is a result of mentioned above coagulation system changes. Additionally, it is possible, that development of coronary artery dilatation could occur during pregnancy as an effect of progesterone influence's on arterial wall. Then, the initial cause could be the arterial dissection.

In conclusion, this case show very complicated pathogenesis of acute coronary syndromes during postpartum period. The problem is the great, because of lack of any experiences in the treatment.

6.2 Analysis of two cases of women treated from acute coronary syndromes during menopausal period

6.2.1 Case 1

54-years old woman, treated from hypertension, with hypercholesterolemia in review, was admitted to Cardiology Department due to typical exercise angina pectoris. Patient has never smoked, BMI was correct-24 kg/m2. The last menstruation was two years ago, patient didn't receive hormonal replacement therapy.

Distance of angina accounted for 300 meters on plane terrain, the disorders had intensified during three months before hospitalization.

On admission, patient was in good condition. Physical examination, ECG and biochemical parameters were normal. Echocardiography showed hypokinesis of inferior and lateral left ventricular wall without worsening global ejection fraction- EF-60%.

Exercise test (10,3 METs) revealed significant depression of ST segment in II, III, aVF, V4-V6 leads (Fig.3) with typical, retrosternal pain during exercise.

Patient was qualified to further conservative treatment. The pharmacological therapy: ASA, beta blocker, ACE-I and statin was included (Clopidogrel was 7 years ago not yet commonly used in only conservative treatment). Patient was discharged in good condition. During 1-year observation, patient was stable.

Therefore, she was admitted to hospital due to acute coronary syndrome NSTEMI (typical, rested retrosternal pain, ST depression, TnT level-0,19 ng/ml). Coronary angiography again revealed noncritical, the same 40% LAD stenosis, without another atherosclerotic changes in remaining coronary arteries. This time, probe of conservative treatment was ineffective-patient complained for recurrence retrosternal pain. After a few days, the PCI of proximal LAD stenosis with metal stent implantation was performed. The pharmacological treatment was continued with Clopidogrel added after coronary intervention.

In seven years observation patient is in good condition, without angina.

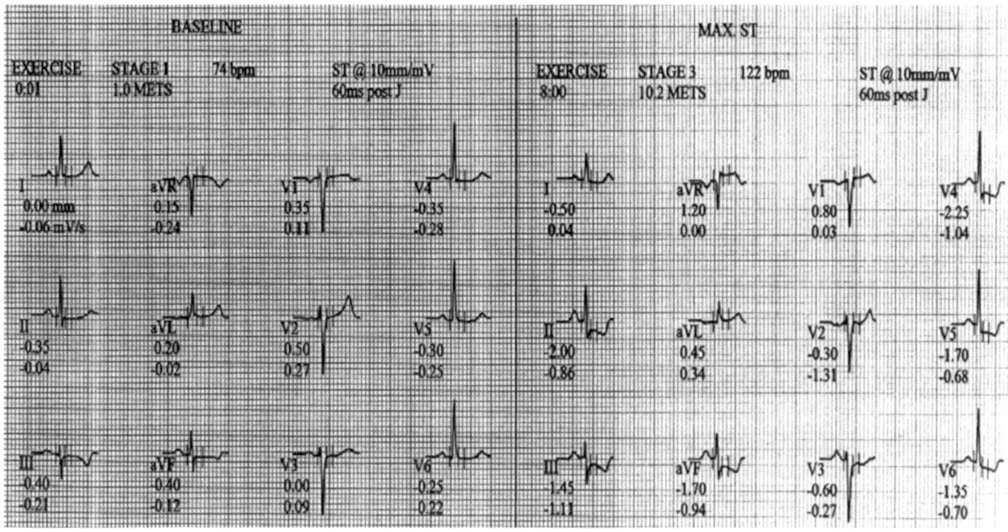

Fig. 3. Exercise test- visible ST segment depression in II, III, aVF, V4-V6 leads.

Patient was qualified to coronary angiography due to unstable angina. Coronarography revealed noncritical 40% stenosis of proximal left anterior descending (LAD) artery segment. The remaining coronary arteries were normal. Fig.4.

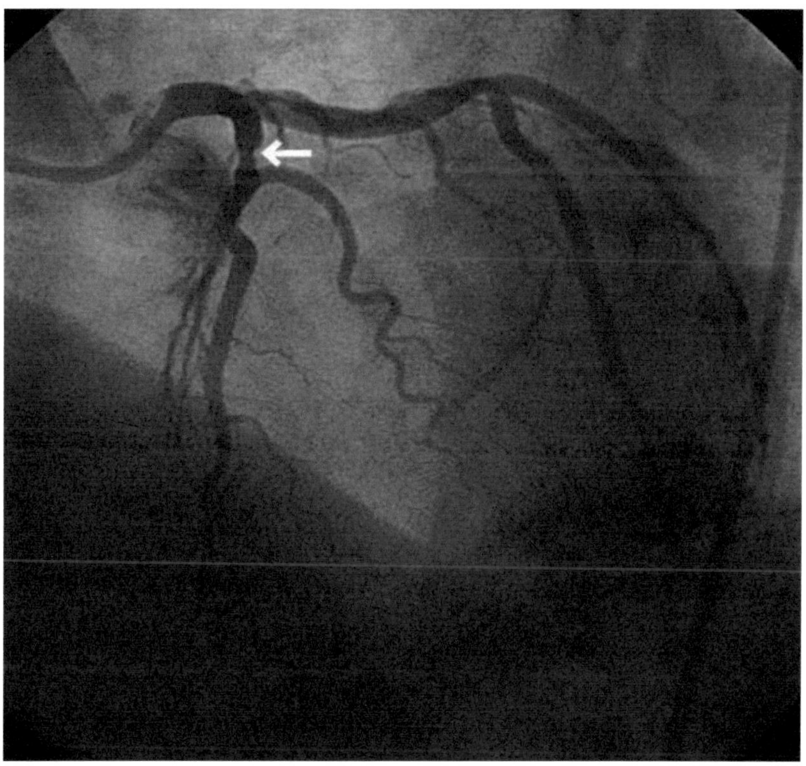

Fig. 4. Coronary angiogrogram. 40% LAD stenosis.

6.2.2 Case 2

52-years old women with overweight (BMI-29 kg/m2), hypertension, smoking, hypercholesterolemia and TIA in review, was admitted to hospital due to unstable angina. The last menstruation was one year earlier, patient has never received hormonal replacement therapy.

Three months ago patient was hospitalized due to ACS NSTEMI. Coronary angiography revealed non critical, 50% stenosis of right ventricular artery (RCA) without atherosclerotic changes in remaining arteries. Fig.5.

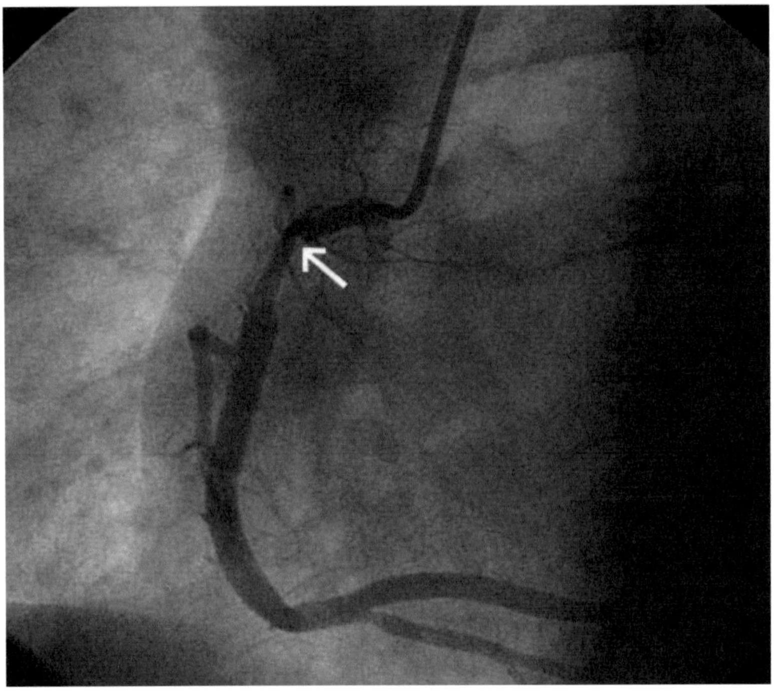

Fig. 5. Coronary angiogram- 50% stenosis of RCA is visible

After that, the typical pharmacoteraphy to stabilization atherosclerotic plaque was included (ASA, beta blocker, ACE-I, statin) and patient was discharged without complaints. Clopidogrel wasn't popularly used to conservative ACS treatment 7 years ago

After three months patient was again hospitalized due to recurrence retrosternal pain with radiation to the lower jaw, more often during the rest, in the night. On admission patient state was stable. Physical examination and TnT level were normal. In ECG the negative T vawe in II, III, aVF leads was visible. Echocardiography showed hypokinesis of basal and middle segments of left ventricular inferior wall's and hypokinesis of interventricular septum with normal ejection fraction (EF-55%).

Exercise test (9,2 METs) didn't revealed ST segment changes, it was finished after seven minutes due to patient fatigue. After pharmacological stabilization, patient was again discharged in good condition.

One month later patient was again admitted to Cardiologic Intensive Care Unit due to inferior all acute coronary syndrome STEMI. In ECG- the typical ST elevation in II, III, aVF leads were revealed. Fig 6.

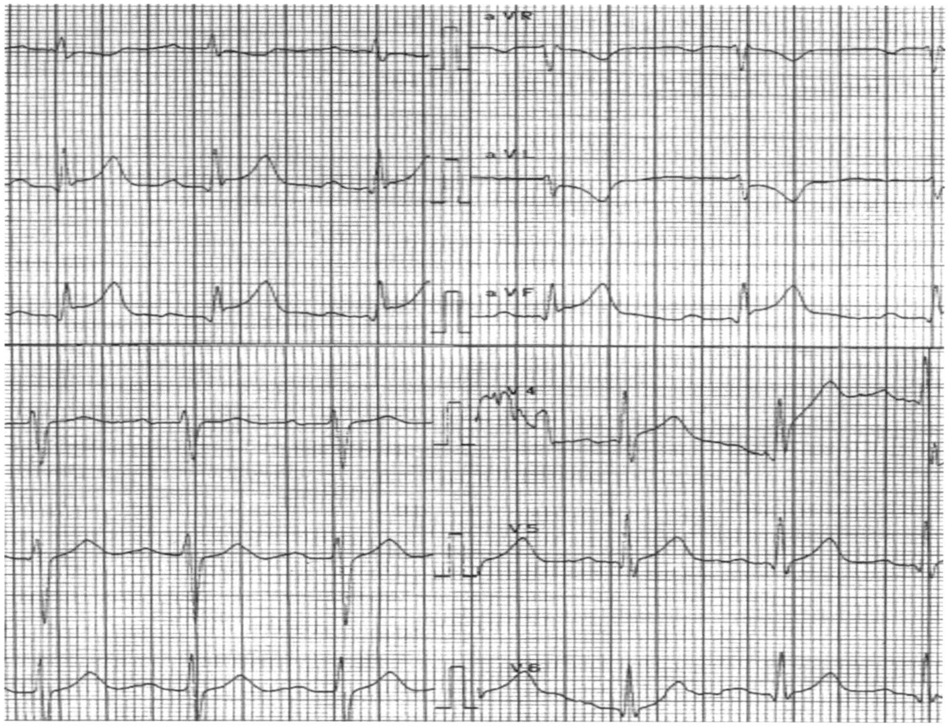

Fig. 6. ECG on admission- ST elevation in II, III, aVF leads.

Coronary angiography reaffirmed only prevalence of 50% stenosis of middle RCA segment. This time, PCI- RCA with bare metal stent implantation was performed. Coronary intervention was complicated by RCA dissection with thrombus involved. After intracoronary GP IIb/IIIa served, TIMI III flow was attained.

Further hospitalization was not complicated. Patient was again discharged in good condition.

In 7- years observation patient state is stable.

These cases of acute coronary syndromes in menopausal women are very specific. In both situations, despite typical symptoms, electrocardiographic and biochemical changes, coronary angiography didn't revealed critical stenosis of infarction responsible artery. Only the recurrence of complaints caused the interventional treatment.

It is important that ACS was presented during menopause in women with coronary artery risk factors. The essential is also fact the typical angina in both women, but noninvasive exercise test in second woman was doubted.

Noninvasive diagnostic process in women with coronary disease is difficult. Anatomical conditions aggravate imagination diagnostic and small exercise tolerance is a barrier in exercises testing.

Account of these facts, qualification to invasive diagnosis and treatment is more difficult than in men. Additionally, the coronary angiography changes are often nonspecific.

There are a lot of studies demonstrating that coronary angiograms in ACS women are often normal, or reveal noncritical stenosis. Presumably, the cause of acute coronary syndrome is mentioned above the plaque erosion with thrombus forming on undamaged artery wall. The another possibility is coronary artery spasm or dissection with idiophatic healing.

These effects occur exceptionally often in women during pregnancy and menopause in connection with hormonal changes in these periods.
Treatment of these cases is very difficult and should be empirical.

7. Conclusions

Women cardiovascular diseases are currently even more problematic than earlier. Mostly, the present data indicate, that female cardiovascular morbidity still rises. This effect is connected with a lot of factors.
Modern women have professional and housewife responsibilities, consume excess of fat and carbohydrates, smoke, do not exercise regularly and do not have enough time to rest. This situation leads to overweight, dyslipidemia, arterial hypertension, impaired glucose tolerance and diabetes.
Women do not often participate in preventive studies and, probably still undergo less intensive and invasive evaluation and treatment for chest pain when compared to men.
However, currently studies are more optimistic. Much of them show that in this era the gender gap will evanescence.

8. References

Ahmed B, Piper WD, Malenka D et al. Significantly improved vascular complications among women undergoing percutaneous coronary intervention: a report from the Northern New England Percutaneous Coronary Intervention Registry. Circ Cardiovasc Interv. 2009 Oct;2(5):423-9.

Ani C, Pan D, Martins D, et al. Age- and sex-specific in-hospital mortality after myocardial infarction in routine clinical practice. Cardiol Res Pract. 2010 Dec 28;2010:752765.

Argulian E, Patel AD, Abramson JL, et al. Gender differences in short-term cardiovascular outcomes after percutaneous coronary interventions. Am J Cardiol. 2006 Jul 1;98(1):48-53.

Berthillot C. Stephan D, Chauvin M et al. In-hospital complications after invasive strategy for the management of Non STEMI: women fare as well as men. BMC Cardiovasc Disord. 2010; 10: 31. Published online 2010 June 24.

Chin-Leng Poh, Chi-Hang Lee. Acute Myocardial Infarction in Pregnant Women. Ann Acad Med Singapore 2010;39:247-53.

Dou KF, Xu B, Yang YJ ,et al. Clinical and angiographic characteristics of premenopausal women with coronary artery disease. Chin Med J (Engl). 2008 Dec 5;121(23):2392-6.

Duvernoy CS, Smith DE, Manohar P et al. Gender differences in adverse outcomes after contemporary percutaneous coronary intervention: an analysis from the Blue Cross Blue Shield of Michigan Cardiovascular Consortium (BMC2) percutaneous coronary intervention registry. Am Heart J. 2010 Apr;159(4):677-683.e1.

Eapen DJ, Kalra GL, Rifai L, et al. Raising HDL cholesterol in women. Int J Womens Health. 2010 Aug 9;1:181-91.

Eifert S, Kilian E, Beiras-Fernandez A et al. Early and mid term mortality after coronary artery bypass grafting in women depends on the surgical protocol: retrospective analysis of 3441 on- and off-pump coronary artery bypass grafting procedures. J Cardiothorac Surg. 2010 Oct 25;5:90.

El-Menyar A, Zubaid M, Sulaiman K, et al. Gulf Registry of Acute Coronary Events (Gulf RACE) Investigators. Atypical presentation of acute coronary syndrome: A significant independent predictor of in-hospital mortality. J Cardiol. 2011 Mar;57(2):165-171.

Fukui T, Takanashi S. Gender differences in clinical and angiographic outcomes after coronary artery bypass surgery. Circ J. 2010 Oct;74(10):2103-8. Epub 2010 Aug 3.

Hong YJ, Jeong MH, Choi YH et al. Gender differences in coronary plaque components in patients with acute coronary syndrome: virtual histology-intravascular ultrasound analysis) J Cardiol. 2010 Sep;56(2):211-9.

Jackson EA, Moscucci M, Smith DE et al. The association of sex with outcomes among patients undergoing primary percutaneous coronary intervention for ST elevation myocardial infarction in the contemporary era: Insights from the Blue Cross Blue Shield of Michigan Cardiovascular Consortium (BMC2). Am Heart J. 2011 Jan;161(1):106-112.e1.

Janion M. Kardiologia. Wyd. Stachurski. Kielce 2005.

Janion M, Sadowska- Janion A. Zawał serca u kobiet w ciąży. Przewodnik Lekarza 2010; 13 (4):105-111.

Janion, M, Polewczyk A, Sielski J et al. Odmienności przebiegu choroby niedokrwiennej serca u kobiet - analiza przypadków klinicznych. Kardiol Pol 2006; 64: 628-636.

Johannes J, Bairey Merz CN. Is cardiovascular disease in women inevitable?: preparing for menopause and beyond Cardiol Rev. 2011 Mar-Apr;19(2):76-80.

Kralev S, Hennig O, Lang S, et al. Sex-based differences in clinical and angiographic outcomes in patients with ST-elevation myocardial infarction treated with concomitant use of glycoprotein IIb/IIIa inhibitors. Cardiol J. 2010;17(6):580-6.

Maraschinia A, Seccarecciaa F, D'Errigoa P et al. Role of gender and age on early mortality after coronary artery bypass graft in different hospitals: data from a national administrative database. Interact Cardiovasc Thorac Surg. 2010 Nov;11(5):537-42. Epub 2010 Aug 13.

Mirelis JG, Fernandez-Diaz JA, Goicolea J, Myocardial Infarction during Pregnancy: Whose Responsibility? J Invasive Cardiol. 2007 Nov;19(11):E343-5.

Radomska E, Polewczyk A, Sadowski M et al. Ostry zawał serca w przebiegu wykrzepionego tętniaka tętnicy wieńcowej u 29-letniej kobiety w okresie poporodowym. Kardiol Pol 2008; 66: 1302-1305.

Radovanovic D, Erne P, Urban P, et al. Gender differences in management and outcomes in patients with acute coronary syndromes: results on 20290 patients from the AMIS Plus Registry. Heart. 2007 November; 93(11): 1369–1375.

Rossi P, Francès Y, Kingwell BA, et al. Gender differences in artery wall biomechanical properties throughout life. J Hypertens. 2011 Feb 22. Epub ahead of print.

Sadowski M, Gąsior M, Gierlotka M et al. Clinical characteristics of Polish women with ST–segment elevation myocardial infarction. Kardiologia Polska 2010; 68, 6: 627-634.

Shaw LJ, Shaw RE, Merz CN et al. Impact of ethnicity and gender differences on angiographic coronary artery disease prevalence and in-hospital mortality in the American College of Cardiology-National Cardiovascular Data Registry. Circulation. 2008 Apr 8;117(14):1787-801.

Shin JY, Martin R, Suls J. Meta-analytic evaluation of gender differences and symptom measurement strategies in acute coronary syndromes. Heart Lung. 2010 Jul-Aug;39(4):283-95.

Solimene MC. Coronary heart disease in women: a challenge for the 21st century. Clinics (Sao Paulo) 2010;65(1):99-106.

Song XT, Chen YD, Pan WQ, et al CRACE investigators. Gender based differences in patients with acute coronary syndrome: findings from Chinese Registry of Acute Coronary Events (CRACE). Chin Med J (Engl). 2007 Jun 20;120(12):1063-7.

Stramba-Badiale M, Fox KM, Priori SG et al. Cardiovascular diseases in women: a statement from the policy conference of the European Society of Cardiology. Eur Heart J, 2006; 27: 995–1005.

6

Tako-Tsubo Cardiomyopathy: A Recent Clinical Syndrome Mimicking an Acute Coronary Syndrome

Montassier Emmanuel[1], Segard Julien[1], Arnaud Martinage[1],
Nicolas Piriou[2], Philippe Le Conte[1], Gilles Potel[1] and Jean Pierre Gueffet[2]
[1]*Emergency Department, Hotel Dieu Teaching Hospital*
[2]*Cardiology, Laennec Teaching Hospital, Nantes*
France

1. Introduction

Tako-Tsubo cardiomyopathy (TTC), first described in 1990 by Sato in Japan (Sato et al., 1990), has recently gained increasing consideration when reported in non-Japanese patients, including the United States and Europe (Hachamovitch et al., 1995; Sharkey et al., 2005; Desmet et al., 2003; Bybee et al., 2004; Dec, 2005; Kurowski et al., 2007)

Typical presentation mimics acute coronary syndrome, with acute chest pain and/or dyspnoea, associated to electrocardiographic changes and moderate cardiac biomarkers release, but in which coronary angiography reveals no coronary arteries lesions. Echocardiography and left ventriculography show the characteristic abnormalities: a reversible left ventricle systolic dysfunction (Pilgrim et al., 2008; Prasad et al., 2008; Wittstein et al., 2005). These transient regional wall motion abnormalities, involving typically the left ventricle, usually extend beyond a single vessel territory (Sato et al., 1990; Dote et al., 1991).

An expert consensus panel proposes a definition of TTC: "TTC is a recently described clinical entity characterised by acute but rapidly reversible left ventricle systolic dysfunction in the absence of atherosclerotic coronary artery disease, triggered by profound psychological stress. This distinctive form of ventricular stunning typically affects elderly women and preferentially involves the distal portion of the left ventricle chamber (apical ballooning), with the basal left ventricle hypercontractile. Although presentation often mimics ST-segment Elevation Myocardial Infarction, outcome is favourable with appropriate medical therapy" (Maron et al., 2006).

The classical, first described, variant of TTC manifests as ballooning of the apical segment and compensatory hypercontraction of the middle-to-basal segments of the left ventricle during systole, similar to the Japanese octopus-trap pot, called Tako-Tsubo (Sato et al., 1990; Dote et al., 1991). Several variants of TTC have been reported recently, involving any part of the heart, but most commonly the left ventricle (Hahn et al., 2007; Kurowski et al., 2007; Pilliere et al., 2006; Reuss et al., 2007; Hurst et al., 2006).

The incidence of TTC, also known as stress-induced cardiomyopathy, transient apical ballooning or broken heart syndrome, is estimated to be present in 1.7% to 2.2% of the patients with suspected acute coronary syndrome (Wittstein et al., 2005; Akashi et al., 2010;

Pavin et al., 1997; Brandspiegel et al., 1998; Flavahan 2006). TTC typically occurs in postmenopausal women, with a mean age ranged between 58 to 75. The condition is frequently precipitated by emotional or physical stress but a triggering event may not be identified (Bybee et al., 2004; Gianni et al., 2006).
Prognosis is good, in contrast to acute coronary syndrome, provided that the patients survive the possible life-threatening acute presentation, with correction of the left ventricle dysfunction within several days or weeks (Bybee et al., 2004; Gianni et al., 2006; Nef et al., 1993; Prasad et al., 2008; Krishnan et al., 2009; Pernicova et al., 2010).

Search strategy

The review was based on a thorough search of evidence-based sources of information, including the Cochrane Database of systematic Reviews and the electronic database Medline with the MeSH terms "Tako-Tsubo cardiomyopathy", "Tako-Tsubo syndrome", "stress cardiomyopathy", "apical ballooning syndrome", "catecholamines". Papers cited include English and French-language articles.

Table 1. Search strategy and review criteria.

2. Clinical Features

2.1 Clinical presentation

The clinical presentation of TTC is similar to an acute coronary syndrome, usually indistinguishable from an acute coronary syndrome and resembling an ST Elevation Myocardial Infarction. Acute phase includes substernal chest pain and/or dyspnoea (Bybee et al., 2004; Gianni et al., 2006). 70 to 90% of the patients exhibit chest pain at rest, referring it as the most common symptom. Mild to moderate congestive heart failure is common. Non specific symptoms including syncope, weakness and nausea have also been reported (Hurst et al., 2010). Moreover, few patients were described as asymptomatic, often admitted for non cardiac illnesses, and TTC was suspected on electrocardiogram or cardiac biomarkers.
Life-threatening initial symptoms are uncommon and out-hospital cardiac arrest due to cardiac rupture has also been very rarely recorded (Akashi et al., 2004; Ohara et al., 2005). However, hemodynamic compromise may occur, related to acute complications such as ventricular tachycardia, ventricular fibrillation, severe congestive heart failure or left ventricular outflow tract obstruction (Valbusa et al., 2008; Prasad et al., 2008).

2.2 Population

The cardiomyopathy usually affects women over 50 years of age, with a mean age ranged between 58 to 75 years, with approximately 3% of the cases in patients under 50 years of age (Prasad et al., 2008). TTC was rarely described in the male population, representing less than 10% of all the cases (Bybee et al., 2004; Tsuchihashi et al., 2001; Sharkey et al., 2005; Akashi et al., 2008; Kurowski et al., 2007). In this population, cardiac risk factors seem to be less described, whereas highest prevalence of anxiety or depression was reported (Kurowski et al., 2007; Vidi et al., 2009; Mudd et al. 2007; Pace et al., 2011).

2.3 Incidence

TTC is an infrequent cardiomyopathy, representing 0,7 to 2,2% of the patients with suspected acute coronary syndrome admitted to the hospital (Wittstein et al., 2005; Akashi et al., 2010; Pavin et al., 1997; Brandspiegel et al., 1998; Flavahan, 2006; Bybee et al., 2004; Gianni et al., 2006). A similar prevalence was reported from a registry of patients with troponine-positive acute coronary syndrome (Kurowski et al., 2007). The annual incidence of TTC was estimated to be 0,00006 to 0,05% (Klinčeva et al., 2007; Pilliere et al., 2006). Recently, Italian multicenter studies have showed a variation in TTC occurrence with a summer and morning peak. Moreover, they have also described a weekly variation with a significant Monday peak in the working population (Manfredini et al., 2010; Gallerani et al., 1992). However, other series found differing results in terms of peak of occurrence (Mansencal et al., 2010).

3. Precipitating events

3.1 Preceding stressful event

A main feature of the TTC is that it usually follows an identifiable emotional or a physical stressful event. This condition is found in approximately two thirds of the TTC patients (Sharkey et al., 2010; Elesber et al., 2007; Gianni et al., 2006).

In the case of seasonal, weekly, circadian variations of TTC occurrence, stress caused by resuming working activities after a break was suggested as a triggering factor (Manfredini et al., 2010). A recent study has showed that in TTC patients, a high-anxiety trait is common but not significantly higher as compared with ST Elevation Myocardial Infarction patients. Moreover high-anxiety trait is not a predictor of TTC in patients with suspected acute coronary syndrome (Pace et al., 2011).

3.2 Emotional stressful event

Numerous emotional factors have been noted: being informed of the death of a loved one, receiving tragic news, public speaking, heated argument, marital discord, spousal departure, accidents and financial loss, unexpected bill, surprise birthday party, babysitting grandchildren, assault, loved one hospitalisation, car accident, catastrophic medical diagnosis, jellyfish sting, natural disaster: earthquarke, Xynthia tempest (Bielecka-Dabrowa et al., 2010; Wittstein et al., 2005 ; Watanabe et al., 2005; Hurst et al., 2010; Bybee et al., 2004; Parodi et al., 2007; Prasad et al., 2008; Sharkey et al., 2005; Trebouet et al., 2011; Movaheda et al., 2007, Montassier et al., 2009).

3.3 Physical stressful event

3.3.1 General anesthesia

Numerous cases of TTC related to general anesthesia have been described, involving various surgical procedures such as digestive surgery (cholecystectomy, hepatectomy, colectomy, hernia repair), cardiothoracic surgery, orthopedic surgery, eye surgery. In such cases, several mechanisms may represent the triggering event: preoperative anxiety, stress of surgery, induction of anesthesia, laryngoscopy, perioperative hemodynamic instability, perioperative administration of vasopressors agents, extubation, and postoperative pain (Liu et al., 2010; Lentschener et al., 2006; Gavish et al., 2006; Takayama et al., 2004; Liu S et al., 2008; Ramakrishna et al., 2005; Takigawa et al., 2003; Mizutani et al., 2002; Itoh H et al., 2007; Littlejohn et al., 2008; Jabaudon et al., 2007).

3.3.2 Other physical stressful events

Gastrointestinal triggers have been commonly reported (high-intensity vomiting, diverticulitis, pelvic abscess, acute cholecystitis, pancreatitis, pseudomembranous colitis) but other physical stressful event have been showed to act as triggering events, such as cardiac stress test, severe pain, asthma or chronic obstructive airway exacerbation, sepsis, acute intracranial events (intracranial bleeding, head trauma, ischemic stroke, epileptic seizure), thyrotoxicosis (Dorfmann al., 2007; Rossor et al., 2007; Ionescu et al., 2010; Sharkey et al., 2005; Bybee et al., 2004; Gianni et al., 2005; Rajani et al., 2010).

Several cases have been reported after administration of pharmacologic agents: beta-agonist bronchodilator, epinephrine, norepinephrine, dobutamine. All these are exogenous cathecolaminergic agents (Abraham et al., 2009; Cherian et al., 2008; Winogradow et al. 2011). Several cases have been noted to be connected to cocaine use, opiate withdrawal or excessive alcohol consumption (Daka et al., 2007; Rivera et al., 2006).

TTC has also been described following a normal vaginal delivery or after caesarean delivery (Teh et al., 2010; Zdanowicz et al., 2011; Citro et al., 2010; Crimi, 2008; Muller et al., 2007; Parodi et al., 2007; Hawthorne et al., 1997). These cases in premenopausal women highlight the potential role of estrogens in TTC etiopathogenesis and the interaction of the latter with catecholamines.

Recently, several cases have been reported in postmenopausal women underlying malignancies (Fazio et al., 2010; Abe et al., 2003; Kawai et al., 2000). In these conditions, precipitating factors could be the context of a stressor or paraneoplastic phenomenon, but the link remains unclear.

4. Electrocardiogram and cardiac biomarkers

4.1 Electrocardiogram findings

As clinical presentation, TTC is indistinguishable from an acute coronary syndrome based on ECG analysis and ECG findings may vary at presentation. Most frequently, the ECG characteristics of the TTC are consistent with ST-segment elevation, mimicking an ST-elevation myocardial infarction, typically in the anterior precordial leads (Bybee et al., 2007; Ogura et al., 2003; Kurisu et al., 2004; Tsuchihashi et al., 2001). Inferior or lateral leads could also be involved. ST-segment is reported in approximately 30 to 50% of the TCC patients (Sharkey et al. 2010; Abe et al., 2003; Akashi et al., 2005; Kurisu et al., 2002; Elesber et al., 2007; Sato et al., 2006; Tsuchihashi et al., 2001; Dib et al., 2009). Moreover, transient ST-segment isolated elevation in lead aVR has also been described in the TTC patients (Rostoff et al., 2009).

The next most common ECG characteristic in TTC are deep T wave inversions, especially in precordial leads, and frequently associated with corrected QT interval prolongation. These ECG abnormalities have been reported in several series (Krishnan et al., 2009; Kim et al., 2010; Silva et al., 2009). Furthermore, these corrected QT interval prolongations have been noted to be correlated with highest occurrence of ventricular fibrillation and extent of wall motion abnormalities in acute coronary syndrome patients (Yunus et al., 1996; Stajer et al., 1993).

Transient pathological Q waves may rarely develop in TTC patients (Rostoff et al., 2009; Krishnan et al., 2009; Kim et al., 2010; Silva et al., 2009). Moreover, a new bundle-branch block or a normal ECG may be found at presentation (Prasad et al., 2008; Bybee et al,. 2007; Ogura et al., 2003; Kurisu et al., 2004; Tsuchihashi et al., 2001; Sharkey et al. 2010).

Atrial and ventricular arrhythmias may occur, but ventricular tachycardia and fibrillation are rarely reported, occurring in 1% to 6% of the patients (Matsuoka et al., 2003; Denney et al., 2005; Bonello et al., 2008). Moreover, despite the frequent corrected QT interval prolongation, the occurrence of torsades de pointes is rarely described (Elkhateeb et al., 2008; Dib et al., 2008).

4.2 Cardiac biomarker

The majority of the patients had a moderate cardiac troponin T release, with a peak within 24 hours (Sharkey et al., 2005; Bybee et al., 2004; Desmet et al., 2003). The discrepancy between the minor elevation in cardiac biomarkers and the extent of the wall motion abnormities is a hallmark of the TTC (Prasad et al., J 2008; Kurisu et al., 2004). Thus, this modest rise in cardiac biomarker may possibly help to distinguishes it from acute coronary syndrome.
Brain Natriuretic Peptide level is usually elevated. Furthermore, its rise, higher than that the one seen in acute coronary syndrome, is purely correlated with the left ventricle systolic dysfunction (Akashi et al., 2004).

5. Coronary angiography and cardiac imaging

As the clinical features of TTC are indistinguishable from the acute coronary syndrome, TTC, defined as a reversible left ventricle systolic dysfunction, may be diagnosed by coronary angiogram, echocardiography or cardiac magnetic resonance (Pilgrim et al., 2008; Prasad et al., 2008; Sharkey et al., 2005; Wittstein et al., 2005).
Classically, at presentation, transthoracic echocardiography and left ventriculography show the characteristic regional wall motion abnormalities involving hypokinesis or akinesis of apex and mid segments of the left ventricle with hyperkinesis in basal segment.
Thus, the classical abnormality is revealed as an apical ballooning of the apex with systole, in the shape resembling to a traditional Japanese jar used for catching octopus, which was named "Takotsubo". The name of the syndrome is derived from this fisherman's device (Sato et al., 1990; Dote et al., 1991; Pilgrim et al., 2008; Pilgrim et al., 2008; Prasad et al., 2008; Sharkey et al., 2005; Wittstein et al., 2005).

5.1 Echocardiography

Clearly, the widespread use of echocardiography, especially in critical care patients, is responsible for the recent increased frequency of TTC recognition (Sharkey et al., 2005; Park et al., 2005; Haghi et al., 2006). However, in the acute phase, echocardiography may not help to distinguish TTC from acute coronary syndrome in view of regional wall motion abnormalities. Thus, diagnosis is frequently made by cardiac catheterization (Bybee et al., 2004; Hurst et al., 2010).

5.2 Coronary angiography

It is worth noticing that the wall motion abnormalities involving more than one particular coronary artery territory are a hallmark of TTC (Prasad et al., 2008; Krishnan et al., 2009). This TTC characteristic is most frequently identified during left ventriculography. Moreover, in patients with TTC, coronary angiography shows normal coronary arteries or coronary arteries with no significant disease (<50% luminal stenosis) (Pilgrim et al., 2008; Prasad et al., 2008; Sharkey et al., 2005; Bybee et al., 2004; Gianni et al., 2006). Thus, when the coronary anatomy is free of significant atherosclerotic lesions with wall motion abnormalities of the left ventricle, usually of the apex, and unrelated to a single coronary

artery territory, the diagnosis of TTC may be postulated. As the patients are supposed to suffer from an acute coronary syndrome, the diagnosis of TTC is currently made during left ventriculography, showing the typical regional wall motion abnormalities.
In the acute phase, severe left ventricle systolic dysfunction is frequently noted, with ejection fraction decreasing from 10% to 30%. In a review of several series, the mean ejection fraction ranged from 20 to 49% (Bybee et al., 2004; Gianni et al., 2006).

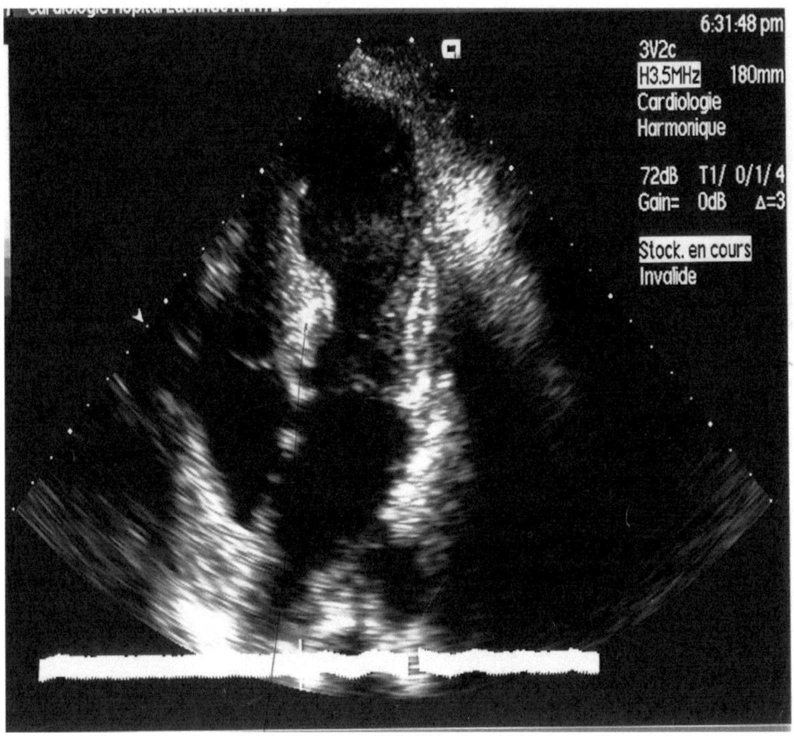

Fig. 1. Echocardiography showing hypokinesis of the apex with hyperkinesis of the base of the left ventricle.

Several variants of TTC have been described, related to a variety of angiographic presentations, involving different areas of the left ventricle. Indeed, based on anatomic location, four different types of TTC are described in literature. All these patients have initially the same clinical presentation. The classic type, previously reported, is described as apical ballooning, with depressed contractile function of the mid and apical segment of the left ventricle and with compensatory hyperkinesis of the basal segments. This type is the most encountered in literature (Bybee et al., 2004; Gianni et al., 2006; Prasad et al., 2008; Abe et al., 2003). The second type is the reverse type in which patients present hyperdynamic apex, with hypokinesis or akinesis of the basal left ventricle segments. Given its distinct basal involvement with apical and mid-ventricular sparing, this type of TTC was considered to be atypical or inverted (Van de Walle et al., 2006; Abdulla et al., 2006; Mansencal et al., 2010). In a recent study, its prevalence was estimated to be 24% of all left ventricle variants of TTC (Mansencal et al., 2010). The third type involves the mid left ventricle wall, with sparing of the basal and apical segments. It is also called "midventricular ballooning"

(Ohtsubo et al., 2005; Hurst et al., 2006; Tamura et al., 2007; Yasu et al., 2006). The fourth type is characterised by a localized wall motion abnormality affecting a segment of the left ventricle wall, usually the anterior wall (Suzuki et al., 2004; Lamm et al., 2007; Mazzarotto et al., 2005; Strunk et al., 2006). These variants of TTC have similar prognoses.

Furthermore, involvement of the right ventricle is commonly associated to left ventricle systolic dysfunction in TTC, revealed in 30% of the patients (Elesber et al., 2006; Haghi et al., 2006; Novak et al., 2007). In these patients, the presence of right ventricle dysfunction seems

Fig. 2. Ventriculography in systole showing apical ballooning.

to be associated with worse left ventricle systolic dysfunction, longer hospitalization and a higher possibility of development of severe complications, particularly occurrence of congestive heart failure (Prasad et al., 2008; Silva et al., 2009; Elesber et al., 2006; Haghi et al., 2006; Novak et al., 2007; Nef et al. 2010). A report described a case of TTC characterized by biventricular ballooning, pulmonary hypertension and hemodynamic compromise associated with prolonged hospitalisation, highlighting the fact that initial management should evaluate left ventricle function but also detect right ventricle involvement (Citro et al., 2010). In another series, association between right ventricle involvement and lower ejection fraction has not been shown (Teh et al., 2010). However, this condition should be immediately known as it possibly impacts outcome.

5.3 Cardiac magnetic resonance

Cardiac magnetic resonance is interesting in order to appreciate the extent of the regional wall motion abnormalities and the variety of depressed contractile function patterns. TTC is characterized by lack of delayed hyper-enhancement following gadolinium injection. Thus, this procedure may help differentiate TTC from acute coronary syndrome or myocarditis (Mitchell et al., 2007; Deetjen et al., 2006). Furthermore, cardiac magnetic resonance is the most accurate procedure in order to assess the right ventricle involvement in the cardiomyopathy (Haghi et al., 2007; Sharkey et al., 2010; Haghi et al., 2006). In addition, cardiac magnetic resonance may help identify ventricular thrombi not visualised by echocardiography (Sharkey et al., 2010). Thus, cardiac magnetic resonance is the best diagnosis procedure after the acute phase, when the patient's condition is stabilised.

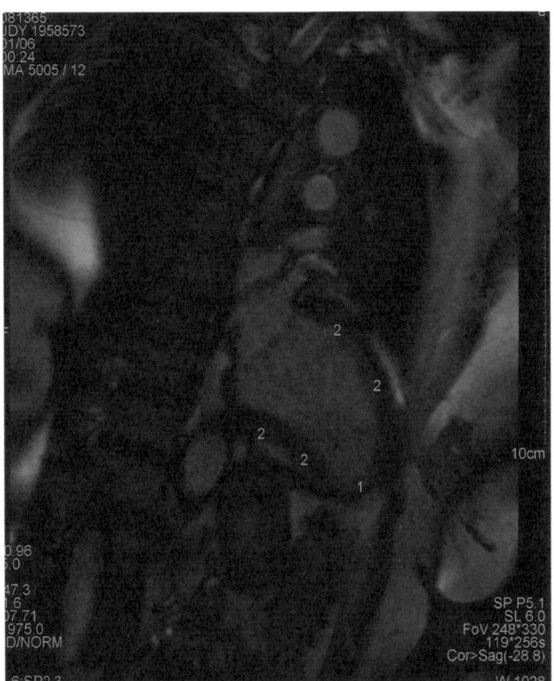

Fig. 3. Cardiac magnetic resonance image showing preserved contraction of the base of the ventricle and apical ballooning.

6. Diagnosis

Two guidelines have been proposed for the diagnosis of TTC, based on a consensus of experts, because there is no diagnosis test of the condition. The first one was proposed by the Mayo Clinic in the United States and the other by the Tako-Tsubo Cardiomyopathy Study Group in Japan (Bybee et al., 2004; Prasad et al., 2007; Kawai et al., 2007).

The Mayo Clinic proposed criteria for the diagnosis of TTC included: (1) new electrocardiographic abnormalities (either ST-segment elevation or T wave inversion) or modest elevation in cardiac troponin, (2) transient hypokinesis, akinesis or dyskinesis of the LV mid segments with or without apical involvement, with wall motion abnormalities extending beyond a single epicardial vascular distribution, with a stressful triggering factor often, but not always, present, (3) absence of obstructive coronary disease or angiographic evidence of plaque rupture, (4) absence of pheochromocytoma or myocarditis.

The Mayo Clinic criteria were initially proposed by Bybee et al. and were secondly revised by Prasad et al (Bybee et al., 2004; Prasad et al., 2007). In the second modified version of the criteria for TTC, patients with intracranial bleeding were no longer excluded, including those with subarachnoid haemorrhage (Prasad et al., 2007).

For its part, the Japanese guideline calls the apical ballooning seen in cerebrovascular accidents and pheochromocytoma a Tako-Tsubo-like myocardial dysfunction (Kawai et al., 2007).

These guidelines include the different variants of TTC. Moreover, the most important feature of TTC is a documented correction of the ejection fraction. Thus, diagnosis of TTC may only be concluded after the recovery of the transient left ventricle systolic dysfunction, not only based on criteria at time of presentation.

1. New electrocardiographic abnormalities (either ST-segment elevation or T wave inversion) or modest elevation in cardiac troponin. 2. Transient hypokinesis, akinesis or dyskinesis of the LV mid segments with or without apical involvement, with wall motion abnormalities extending beyond a single epicardial vascular distribution, with a stressful trigger often, but not always, present, 3. Absence of obstructive coronary disease or angiographic evidence of plaque rupture 4. Absence of pheochromocytoma or myocarditis.

Table 2. Mayo Clinic proposed criteria for the diagnosis of Tako-Tsubo cardiomyopathy.

7. Diagnosis strategy

The differential diagnosis with an acute coronary syndrome is not yet possible in the acute phase based on clinical or laboratory features. Thus, the diagnosis should be considered in postmenopausal women, presenting with chest pain and/or dyspnoea, with no or few risk factors for coronary artery disease and history of recent stress associated to electrocardiographic abnormalities and a moderate cardiac troponin T release. Furthermore, the diagnosis should also be suspected in inpatients, especially in the intensive care unit population, with acute left ventricle systolic dysfunction associated to hemodynamic compromise, pulmonary oedema, electrocardiographic abnormalities consistent with an acute coronary syndrome or a cardiac troponin T release (Elesber et al., 2006; Haghi et al., 2006; Novak et al., 2007).

The diagnosis of TTC is most frequently made during coronary angiography, performed as recommended by guidelines for the management of acute coronary syndrome. In fact, patients with TTC, due to their initial presentation similar to an acute coronary syndrome, are usually referred for urgent reperfusion therapy. The absence of fixed epicardial coronary artery disease and no angiographic evidence of plaque rupture or intracoronary thrombus formation associated with characteristic regional wall motion abnormality, as previously described, leads to the diagnosis. Thus, in patients with TTC, coronary angiography shows normal coronary arteries or coronary arteries with no significant disease (<50% luminal stenosis). However, few patients exhibit a concomitant obstructive coronary artery disease in witch case cardiac magnetic resonance may be useful to distinguish TTC from acute coronary syndrome (Hoyt et al., 2009; Deetjen et al., 2006).

As briefly indicated above, in case of typical presentation of TTC, in a postmenopausal woman with chest pain related to a stressful event with no or few risk factors for coronary artery disease, coronary angiography should be considered as the first choice. Indeed, these patients may be exposed to inappropriate therapy such as thrombolysis, which may lead to serious complications, especially in this classical aged population (Kolkebeck et al., 2008). Thus, a good strategy seems to be to transfer a patient suspected of TTC to a cardiac catheterization laboratory for emergency coronary angiography and avoid the administration of fibrinolytic therapy. However, suspicion of the diagnosis of TTC is not sufficient to contraindicate fibrinolytic therapy if needed, as the great majority of patients with a ST-segment Myocardial Infarction will have an obstructive coronary disease. Basically, guidelines recommended managing these patients as usual, with urgent cardiac catheterization or with fibrinolytic therapy (Prasad et al., 2008; Reeder et al., 2010).

The diagnosis of TTC without cardiac catheterization is difficult and coronary angiography should be rapidly performed. Indeed, echocardiography realised in the acute phase may not help to distinguish the regional wall motion abnormalities of TTC from acute coronary syndrome, even if in case of TTC, the wall motion abnormalities involve more than one particular coronary artery territory. Moreover, the variants of the classical TTC pattern are harder to diagnose by echocardiography alone. However, sometimes, patients are contraindicated to undergo invasive strategy. In these patients, repeated echocardiography allows for the documentation of the correction of the left ventricle systolic dysfunction (Anand et al., 2010).

8. Complications

In the acute phase, complications may occur and life-threatening presentation is not rare. Indeed, acute complications have been shown in approximately 20% of the patients (Bybee et al., 2004; Bonello et al., 2008). Most of them are related to left ventricular heart failure, reported as follows (prevalence): pulmonary oedema (15%), cardiogenic shock (6,5%), left ventricle outflow tract obstruction (11%), mitral regurgitation (25%), ventricular mural thrombus formation (7%) (Pernicova et al., 2010; Donohue et al., 2005; Akashi et al., 2004; Nef et al., 2006; Nef al., 2009; Bonello al., 2008; Barrera-Ramirez et al., 2003; Zaroff et al., 2000). In case of left ventricular thrombus formation, thromboembolic complications, such as stroke, occur in 0,8% of the patients (de Gregorio et al., 2008).

Arrhythmias are also described, including atrial or ventricular arrhythmias. Incidence of atrial fibrillation has been quoted at 15%, ventricular tachycardia at 1,6% (Bielecka-Dabrowa et al., 2010; Ionescu et al., 2010). QT prolongation resulting in torsades de pointes is a

potential mechanism for ventricular arrhythmias (Bonello et al., 2008). This condition is involved in a large proportion of the syndrome mortality rate, as sudden cardiac death due to ventricular fibrillation was estimated to be 4% (Ionescu et al., 2010).
Other rare complications have been noted such as pneumothorax or left ventricular rupture (Bielecka-Dabrowa et al., 2010; Matsuoka et al., 2000; Sakai et al., 2005; Ohara et al., 2005). A TTC complicated by a ventricular septal dissection with a concomitant septal performation have been recently reported (Mariscalco et al., 2010). This patient never recovered a normal left ventricular systolic function. Furthermore, increase risk of bleeding has been noted secondary to anticoagulation prescribed in case of left ventricular thrombus formation or in case of inappropriate thrombolysis.

9. Prognosis and recurrence

9.1 Prognosis

Prognosis is favourable, provided that the patients survive the possible life-threatening acute phase, with full recovery of the left ventricular systolic function within several weeks, typically within 1 to 4 weeks (Bybee et al., 2004; Gianni et al., 2006; Nef et al., 2007; Prasad et al., 2008; Pernicova et al., 2010). Therefore, the correction of the left ventricle systolic dysfunction and the correction of the regional wall motion abnormalities during the electrocardiographic follow-up is a hallmark of the cardiomyopathy. However, a recent study has showed a more important delay in the correction of the left ventricular systolic dysfunction, with a normalisation in 2.5 to 12 months in 5% of their included patients (Sharkey et al., 2010).
As mentioned before, severe acute presentation may occur and in-hospital mortality rate is estimated to be 1.1% to 2%, mostly related to arrhythmias or mechanical complications (Mariscalco et al., 2010). Thus, this data highlight the fact that TTC is not entirely benign and that TTC may require early and aggressive management. In several reviews, long-term survival seems to be similar to the one expected in the general population (Elesber, et al., 2006; Gianni et al., 2006). Late sudden death is particularly uncommon (Fineschi et al., 2010). However, a recent study has showed that survival, in two-third of the patients with TTC, was worst than in the general age- and sex-matched population. In their patients, mortality has always been related to noncardiac diseases, and for the authors, TTC may be a marker for impaired health (Sharkey et al., 2010). Another study found that the long-term mortality rate was higher than the long-term mortality rate in the general population and mostly due to patients' comorbidities. Moreover, in this study, the severity of the initial presentation was not correlated to long-term outcome (Parodi et al., 2010). Thus, long-term outcome remains unclear in patients with TTC and larger studies are needed to confirm these recent findings.

9.2 Recurrence

As noted in several reviews, 3.5% to 10% of the patients have a recurrence during the first few years after the initial presentation (Bybee et al., 2004; Gianni et al., 2006; Nef et al., 2007; Prasad et al., 2008). A recent 4-year follow-up study described 11.4% recurrence of TTC (Elesber et al., 2007). Published data has also showed that the different variants of TTC may differ on recurrence (Blessing et al. 2007). This recurrence occurs in particularly similar circumstances, highlighting the importance to educate the patients in order to banish stress or physical triggering factors (Sharkey et al., 2010). Furthermore, chest pain and dyspnoea recurrence occurs frequently. Indeed, a study indicated a rate of rehospitalisation for cardiac complaints estimated at 30% (Ionescu et al., 2010).

10. Treatment

10.1 Acute phase

In the acute phase, the treatment of TTC is empirical and mainly supportive, adapted on clinical presentation (Prasad et al., 2008). The objective is to correct the left ventricle systolic dysfunction with standard medication for left ventricle systolic dysfunction. Moreover, as the differential diagnosis with an acute coronary syndrome is not initially possible, data suggest starting usual treatment for acute coronary syndrome, suspended upon confirmation of the diagnosis (Prasad et al., 2008; Silva et al., 2009).

Thus, initial management consists in administration of β-blockers, angiotensinconverting enzyme inhibitors, aspirin and heparin. Congestive heart failure is treated by diuretics (Bybee et al., 2004; Gianni et al., 2006). β-blockers are recommended in patients with left ventricle outflow tract obstruction and are contraindicated in case of congestive heart failure with low ejection fraction, hypotension or bradycardia. For their part, angiotensin-converting enzyme inhibitors are recommended in patients without a left ventricle outflow tract obstruction. The duration of the treatment remains unclear but it is commonly accepted to continue the treatment until the full recovery of the left ventricle systolic function.

10.1.1 Hemodynamic compromise

In the case of hemodynamic compromise due to pump failure, the use of an intra-aortic balloon pump is better than the use of inotropic agents, as these are known to enhance left ventricle outflow tract obstruction (Previtali et al., 2005). Therefore, echocardiography has to be done upon presentation in order to detect left ventricle outflow tract obstruction (Tsuchihashi et al., 2001; Bybee et al., 2004). In patients with hypotension due to pump failure without significant left ventricle outflow tract obstruction proven by echocardiography, a treatment with inotropic agents may be started with caution. Inotropic agents proposed are dobutamine or dopamine. Importantly, in patients with severe hypotension without significant left ventricle outflow tract obstruction but with severe left ventricular dysfunction, the use of an intra-aortic balloon pump is preferred to inotropic agents. Moreover, in patients with hypotension due to pump failure associated with a significant left ventricle outflow tract obstruction proven by echocardiography, a treatment with inotropic agents should not be started and the use of an intra-aortic balloon pump is recommended (Villareal et al., 2001; Sharkey et al., 2005). As mentioned above, β-blockers are recommended in patients with left ventricle outflow tract obstruction and fluid resuscitation is also recommended in the absence of congestive heart failure (Villareal et al., 2001; Bybee et al., 2004). In case of intolerance or inadequately response to β-blockers, use of an alpha agonist such as phenylephrine is proposed, used with caution and close monitoring due to its vasocontrictive effects (Reeder et al., 2010).

10.1.2 Left ventricular thrombus

Left ventricular thrombus must be detected in the acute phase. Short-term anticoagulation is indicated in this case and also in order to prevent its occurrence in patients with severe left ventricle systolic dysfunction. The anticoagulation is continued until left ventricular systolic function improves (Kimura et al., 2007; Haghi et al., 2008). Short-term anticoagulation is also prescribed in case of atrial fibrillation (Kimura et al., 2007).

10.2 Chronic treatment

Chronic treatment is rarely detailed and it also remains empirical. Chronic β-blockers are recommended in order to reduce the recurrence rate, in the absence of contraindications or intolerance (Prasad et al., 2008). However, several studies showed the partial efficacy of this therapy in order to prevent either the first episode or a recurrence of the TTC (Sharkey et al. 2010; Parodi et al., 2010). Aspirin is not maintained even if the patient had a coexisting coronary atherosclerosis and angiotensin-converting enzyme inhibitors are not continued if the patient recovers left ventricle systolic function (Prasad et al., 2008; Bybee et al., 2004).

11. Pathophysiology

Several hypotheses have been proposed to explain TTC, but the precise mechanisms remain unclear. These pathophysiological hypotheses include: direct toxic effects of catecholamine excess on cardiomyocytes, coronary artery vasospasm, diffused coronary microvascular dysfunction and left ventricle outflow tract obstruction (Wittstein et al., 2005; Akashi et al., 2010; Nef et al., 2007; Nef et al., 2007; Nef et al., 2009a; Nef et al., 2009b).

11.1 Catecholamine excess

Catecholamine excess following an emotional or physical stress is supposed to play an important role in the pathophysiology of the TTC and this mechanism is widely reported. Increased catecholamine levels promote microvascular spasm, damage and hypocontraction of the myocardial muscle responsible for the typical regional wall motion abnormalities. A mouse model demonstrated that catecholamine excess is responsible for a negatively inotropic effect (Heubach et al., 2004).

The analysis of endomyocardial biopsies showed contraction band necrosis and mononuclear cell infiltrate, typically consistent with catecholamine excess. The apex of the left ventricle has an increase density of adrenoreceptors accounting for the apex being the most exposed to the cardiomyopathy. Moreover, there is a difference in the distribution of these adrenoreceptors among persons, which could explain the different variants of TTC (Hurst et al., 2006; Lyon et al., 2008; Litvinov et al., 2009).

This neuro-hormonal hypothesis including catecholamine excess and exaggerated stimulation of the sympathetic nervous system is supported by several studies showing that patients with TTC have supraphysiologic and higher levels of plasma catecholamines than patients with acute coronary syndrome (Wittstein et al., 2005)

Moreover, several cases have been described after administration of exogenous cathecolaminergic agents such as dobutamine (Previtali et al., 2005; Abraham et al., 2009; Cherian et al., 2008; Winogradow et al., 2010). However, other studies have documented no significant elevation in plasma catecholamine levels in TTC patients (Bybee et al., 2004; Gianni et al., 2006; Nef et al., 2007; Tsuchihashi et al., 2001; Kawai et al., 2007; Elesber et al., 2007; Sharkey et al., 2008; Blessing et al., 2007; Sharkey et al., 2007; Fazio et al., 2008). Thus, this pathophysiological mechanism is still debated.

11.2 Coronary artery vasospasm

Early reports have showed that TTC may be explained by coronary artery vasospasm, based on studies realising an induction of multi-vessel coronary spasm secondary to intra-

coronary acetylcholine injection (Dote et al., 1991; Tsuchihashi et al., 2001). In fact, most of the patients in Japanese series exhibit a coronary epicardial spasm but it has been rarely described in the Caucasian population (Tsuchihashi et al., 2001; Kurisu et al., 2002; Bybee et al., 2004; Wittstein et al., 2005; Gianni et al., 2006).
However, the duration of the TTC compared to a classical vasospasm and the regional wall motion abnormalities usually extending beyond a single vessel territory limit this theory of causal mechanism. Indeed, recent reviews consider that this mechanism is unlikely to be the underlying cause of TTC (Prasad et al., 2008; Tsuchihashi et al., 2001; Desmet et al., 2003; Kurisu et al., 2002; Yoshida et al., 2007; Abe & Kondo, 2003).

11.3 Coronary microvascular dysfunction

Largely abnormal coronary microvascular function is another pathophysiological mechanisms proposed. Reduced blood flow rates using TIMI frame count and spontaneous improvement of coronary flow reserve suggest a possible involvement of the microvascular function in the pathophysiology of the TTC (Previtali et al., 2005; Kimura et al., 2007; Haghi et al., 2008; Nef al., 2007; Nef et al., 2009). However, it has not yet been clearly defined whether microvascular dysfunction is a primary or secondary phenomenon (Bybee et al., 2004; Yanagi et al., 2002; Barcin et al., 2003; Kume et al., 2005; Gibson et al., 1996). In fact, the coronary microvascular dysfunction could be the result of various causes, such as direct toxic effects of catecholamine excess and excessive sympathetic response or estrogen depletion (Kaski, 2006).
Anyway, highlighting this pathophysiological mechanism, a recent study has demonstrated the key role of myocardial vasoconstriction in the etiopathogenesis of the TTC. For the authors, the typical regional wall motion abnormalities appear to be secondary to microvascular dysfunction, secondary to coronary microvascular vasoconstriction (Galiuto et al., 2010).
However, data still remain controversial as another study showed that the akinetic territories involved were much larger than those affected by the coronary microvascular dysfunction. For the authors, even if coronary microvascular dysfunction is currently present during the acute phase of TTC, this may not be considered as the only pathophysiological mechanism of the cardiomyopathy (Fazio et al., 2010).

11.4 Left ventricle outflow tract obstruction

Left ventricle outflow tract obstruction has also been proposed to contribute to TTC pathogenesis. Published data showed that left ventricle outflow tract obstruction might be present in 11% of the TTC patients (Nef et al., 2010; el Mahmoud et al., 2008). Moreover, inotropic agents have been reported to induce or worsen left ventricle outflow tract obstruction.
Consequently, such findings support a possible role of the left ventricle outflow tract obstruction in the pathogenesis of the TTC, but this pathogenic mechanism is still under debate.

11.5 Myocarditis

Another hypothesis has been proposed as a pathophysiological mechanism: myocarditis. Indeed, some cases have been reported to be associated with cardiotropic viruses (Bahlmann et al., 2007). However, the biopsy analysis of the myocardial muscle and the viral serology do not emphasize this pathophysiological mechanism (Silva et al., 2009; Abe et al., 2003).

11.6 Hormonal environment

Last but not least, the cardiomyopathy usually occurs in postmenopausal women, highlighting the role of the hormonal environment and the protecting role of estrogens (Ueyama et al., 2003; Hinojosa-Laborde et al., 1999; & Celermajer, 2002; Connelly et al., 2006). A case of TTC was described in a young woman suffering from an estrogen deficiency due to Turner syndrome. The woman had a low level of estrogens, as noted in postmenopausal women, explaining why she was more susceptible to TTC (Sato et al., 2009). Moreover, an animal model with estrogen supplementation showed low occurrence of TTC (Ueyama et al., 2003).

12. Conclusion

Tako-Tsubo cardiomyopathy (TTC) is a syndrome which has recently gained increasing consideration. Typical presentation mimics acute coronary syndrome, with acute chest pain and/or dyspnoea, associated to electrocardiographic changes and moderate cardiac biomarkers release. The syndrome is characterized by a reversible left ventricle systolic dysfunction typically involving the apex, but in which coronary lesions are not involved. The transient regional wall motion abnormalities usually extend beyond a single vessel territory.

It is important to note that patients with TTC may exhibit life-threatening acute phase and may require early and aggressive initial management.

The pathophysiology of the syndrome remains still unclear and more research is needed in this area. The diagnosis of TTC is most frequently made during coronary angiography, performed as recommended by the guidelines for the management of acute coronary syndrome.

Patients with TTC may be exposed to inappropriate therapy such as thrombolysis, which may lead to serious complications, given the fact that coronary artery obstruction is not being involved. Thus, a good strategy seems to be the transfer of the patients suspected of TTC to a cardiac catheterization laboratory for emergency coronary angiography.

13. Acknowledgement

None of the authors have any conflicts of interest, financial or other disclosures to acknowledge.

14. References

Abe, Y.; Kondo, M.; Matsuoka, R.; Araki, M.; Dohyama, K. & Tanio, H. Assessment of clinical features in transient left ventricular apical ballooning. *Journal of the American College of Cardiology*, Vol.41, No.5, (2003), pp.737–742.

Abe, Y. & Kondo, M. Apical ballooning of the left ventricle: a distinct entity? *Heart*, Vol.89, No.9, (2003), pp. 974–976.

Abdulla, I.; Kay, S.; Mussap, C.; Nelson, GI.; Rasmussen, HH.; Hansen, PS. & Ward, MR. Apical sparing in Tako-Tsubo cardiomyopathy. *Internal Medicine Journal*, Vol.36, No.7, (2006), pp.414-418.

Abraham, J.; Mudd, JO.; Kapur, N.; Klein, K.; Champion, HC. & Wittstein, IS. Stress cardiomyopathy after intravenous administration of catecholamines and beta-receptor agonists. *Journal of the American College of Cardiology*, Vol. 53, No.15, (2009), pp. 1320–1325.

Akashi, YJ.; Tejima, T.; Sakurada, H.; Matsuda, H.; Suzuki, K.; Kawasaki, K.; Tsuchiya, K.; Hashimoto, N., Musha, H.,

Sakakibara, M.; Nakazawa, K. & Miyake F. Left ventricular rupture associated with Takotsubo cardiomyopathy. *Mayo Clinic Proceedings Mayo Clinic*,Vol.79, No.6, (2004), pp.821–824.

Akashi, YJ.; Musha, H.; Nakazawa, K. & Miyake, F. Plasma brain natriuretic peptide in Takotsubo cardiomyopathy. *QJM: montly journal of the association of physicians*, Vol.97, No.9, (2004), pp.599-607.

Akashi, YJ.; Musha, H., Kida, K.; Itoh, K.; Inoue, K.; Kawasaki, K.; Hashimoto, N. & Miyake, F. Reversible ventricular dysfunction takotsubo cardiomyopathy. *European Journal of Heart Failure*, Vol.7, No.7, (2005), pp.1171–1176.

Akashi, YJ.; Goldstein, DS.; Barbaro, G & Ueyama, T. Takotsubo cardiomyopathy: a new form of acute, reversible heart failure. *Circulation*, Vol.118, No.25, (2008), pp.2754-2762.

Akashi, Y.; Nef, H. M.; Möllmann, H. & Ueyama, T. Stress cardiomyopathy. *Annual Reviews of Medecine.* Vol.61, (2010), pp. 271–286

Anand, G.; Gong-Yuan, . & Dellsperger, KC. Echocardiography in stress cardiomyopathy and acute LVOT obstruction. *The International Journal of Cardiovascular Imaging*, Vol.26, No.5, (2010), pp.527–535.

Bahlmann, E.; Schneider, C.; Krause, K.; Pankuweit, S.; Harle, T. & Kuck, KH. Tako-Tsubo cardiomyopathy (apical ballooning) with parvovirus B19 genome in endomyocardial biopsy. *International Journal of Cardiology*, Vol.116, No.1, (2007), pp.18–21.

Barcin, C.; Denktas, AE.; Garratt, KN. ; Higano, ST.; Holmes, DR. & Lerman, A. Relation of Thrombolysis in Myocardial

Infarction (TIMI) frame count to coronary flow parameters. *The American Journal of Cardiology*, Vol.91, No.4, (2003), pp.466–469.

Barrera-Ramirez, CF.; Jimenez-Mazuecos, JM. & Alfonso, F. Apical thrombus associated with left ventricular apical ballooning. *Heart*, Vol.89, No.8, (2003), pp.927.

Bielecka-Dabrowa, A.; Mikhailidis, DP.; Hannam, S.; Rysz, J.; Michalska, M.; Akashi, JA. & Banach, M. Takotsubo cardiomyopathy — The current state of knowledge. *International Journal of Cardiology*, Vol.142, No.2, (2010), pp.120–125.

Blessing, E.; Steen, H.; Rosenberg, M.; Katus, H. & Frey, N. Recurrence of Takotsubo cardiomyopathy with variant forms of left ventricular dysfunction. *Journal of the American Society Echocardiography*, Vol.439, No.4, (2007), pp.11–12.

Bonello, L.; Com, O.; Ait-Moktar, O.; Theron, A.; Moro, PJ.; Salem, A.; Sbragia, P. & Paganelli, F. Ventricular arrhythmias during Takotsubo syndrome. *International Journal of Cardiology*, Vol.128, No.2, (2008), pp.50–53.

Brandspiegel, HZ.; Marinchak, RA.; Rials, SJ. & Kowey PR. A broken heart. *Circulation*, Vol.98, No.13, (1998), pp.1349.

Bybee, KA.; Prasad, A.; Barsness, GW.; Lerman, A.; Jaffe, AS.; Murphy, JG.; Wright, RS. & Rihal, CS. Clinical characteristics and thrombolysis in myocardial infarction frame counts in women with transient left ventricular apical ballooning syndrome. *The American Journal of Cardiology*, Vol.94, No.3, (2004), pp.343-346.

Bybee, KA. ; Kara, T. ; Prasad, A.; Lerman, A.; Barsness, GW.; Wright, RS.& Rihal, CS. Systematic review: transient left ventricular apical ballooning: a syndrome that mimics St segment elevation myocardial infarction. *Annals of Internal Medicine*, Vol.141, No.11, (2004), pp. 858-865.

Bybee, KA.; Motiei, A.; Syed, IS.; Kara, T.; Prassad, A.; Lennon, RJ.; Murphy, JG.; Hammill, SC.; Rihal, CS.& Wright, RS. Electrocardiography cannot reliably differentiate transient left ventricular apical ballooning syndrome from anterior ST-segment elevation myocardial infarction. *Journal of Electrocardiology*, Vol.40, No.1, (2007), pp.1-6.

Cherian, J.; Kothari, S.; Angelis, D.; Atef, A.; Downey, B.& Kirkpatrick, J. Atypical takotsubo cardiomyopathy: dobutamine-precipitated apical ballooning with left ventricular outflow tract obstruction. *Texas Heart Institute Journal*, Vol.35, No.1, (2008), pp.73-75.

Citro, R.; Pascotto, M.; Provenza, G.; Gregorio, G.& Bossone, E. Transient left ventricular ballooning (tako-tsubo cardiomyopathy) soon after intravenous ergonovine injection following caesarean delivery. *International Journal of Cardiology*, Vol.138, No.2, (2010), pp.31-34.

Citro, R.; Caso, I.; Provenza, G.; Santoro, M.; Gregorio, G. & Bossone, E. Right Ventricular Involvement and Pulmonary Hypertension in an Elderly Woman With Tako-Tsubo Cardiomyopathy. *Chest*, Vol.137, No.4, (2010), pp.973-975.

Connelly, K.; MacIsaac, A. & Jelinek, MV. The "tako-tsubo" phenomenon and myocardial infarction. *Southern Medical Journal*, Vol.99, No.1, (2006), pp.2-3.

Crimi, E.; Baqqish, A.; Leffert, L.; Plan-Smith, MC.; Januzzi, JL. & Jlang, Y. Acute reversible stress-induced cardiomyopathy associated with cesarean delivery under spinal anesthesia. *Circulation*, Vol.117, No.23, (2008), pp.3052-3053.

De Gregorio, C.; Grimaldi, P. & Lentini, C. Left ventricular thrombus formation and cardioembolic complications in patients with takotsubo-like syndrome: a systematic review. *International Journal of Cardiology*, Vol.131, No.1, (2008), pp.18-24.

Daka, MA.; Khan, RS. & Deppert, EJ. Transient left ventricular apical ballooning after a cocaine binge. *Journal of Invasive Cardiology*, Vol.19, No.12, (2007), pp.378-380.

Dec, GW. Recognition of the apical ballooning syndrome in the United States. *Circulation*, Vol.111, No.4, (2005), pp.388-390.

Deetjen, AG.; Conradi, G.; Mollmann, S.; Rad, A.; Hamm, CW. & Dill T. Value of gadoliniumenhanced magnetic resonance imaging in patients with Tako-Tsubo-like left ventricular dysfunction. *Journal of Cardiovascular Magnetic Resonance*, Vol.8, No.2, (2006), pp.367-372.

Denney, SD.; Lakkireddy, DR. & Khan, IA. Long QT syndrome and torsade de pointe in transient left ventricular apical ballooning syndrome. *International Journal of Cardiology*, Vol.100, No.3, (2005), pp.499-501.

Desmet, WJ.; Adriaenssens, BF. & Dens, JA. Apical ballooning of the left ventricle: first series in white patients. *Heart*, Vol.89, No.9, (2003), pp.1027-1031.

Dib, C.; Prasad, A.; Friedman, PA.; Ahmad, E.; Rihal, CS.; Hammill, SC. & Asirvatham, SJ. Malignant arrhythmia in apical ballooning syndrome: risk factors and outcomes. *Indian Pacing and Electrophysiology Journal*, Vol. 8, No. 3, (2008), pp.182–192.

Dib, C.; Asirvatham, S.; Elesber, A.; Rihal, C.; Friedman, P. & Prassad, A. Clinical correlates and prognostic significance of electrocardiographic abnormalities in apical ballooning syndrome (Takotsubo/stress-induced cardiomyopathy). *American Heart Journal*, Vol.157, No.5, (2009), pp.933–938.

Donohue, D. & Movahed, MR. Clinical characteristics, demographics and prognosis of transient left ventricular apical ballooning syndrome. *Heart Failure Reviews*. Vol.10, No.4, (2005), pp. 311-316.

Dorfman, T.; Aqel, R.; Allred, J.; Woodham, R. & Iskandrian AE. Takotsubo cardiomyopathy induced by treadmill exercise testing: an insight into the pathophysiology of transient left ventricular apical (or midventricular) ballooning in the absence of obstructive coronary artery disease. *Journal of the American College of Cardiology*, Vol.49, No.11, (2007), pp.1223–1225.

Dote, K.; Sato, H.; Tateishi, H.; Uchida, T. & Ishihara, M. Myocardial stunning due to simultaneous multivessel coronary spasms: a review of 5 cases. *Journal of Cardiology*, Vol.21, No.2, (1991), pp.203–214.

El Mahmoud, R.; Mansencal, N.; Pillère, R. ; Leyer, F. ; Abbou, N. ; Michaud, P. ; Nallet, O. ; Digne, F. ; Lacombe, P. ; Cattan, S. & Dubourg, O. Prevalence and characteristics of left ventricular outflow tract obstruction in Tako-Tsubo syndrome. *American Heart Journal*, Vol.156, No.3, (2008), pp.543–548.

Elesber, AA.; Prasad, A.; Bybee, KA.; Valeti, U.; Motiel, A.; Lerman, A.; Chandrasekaran, K.; & Rihal, CS. Transient cardiac apical ballooning syndrome: prevalence and clinical implications of right ventricular involvement. *Journal of the American College of Cardiology*, Vol. 47, No.5, (2006), pp.1082-1083.

Elesber, AA.; Prasad, A.; Lennon, RJ.; Wright, RS.; Lerman, A & Rihal, CS. Four-year recurrence rate and prognosis of the apical ballooning syndrome. *Journal of the American College of Cardiology*, Vol.50, No.5, (2007), pp.448–452.

Elkhateeb, OE. & Beydoun, HK. Recurrent long QT syndrome and syncope in transient apical ballooning syndrome (takotsubo cardiomyopathy). *The Canadian Journal of Cardiology*, Vol.24, No.12, (2008), pp.917–919.

Fazio, G.; Pizzuto, C.; Barbaro, G.; Sutera, L.; Incalcaterra, E.; Evola, G.; Azzarelli, S.; Palecek, T.; Di Gesaro, G.; Cascio, C.; Novo, G.; Akashi, YJ. & Novo, S. Chronic pharmacological treatment in Takotsubo cardiomyopathy. *International Journal of Cardiology*, Vol.127, No.1, (2008), pp.121–123

Fazio, G.; Sarullo, FM.; Novo, G.; Evola, S.; Lunetta, M.; Barbaro, G.; Sconci, F.; Azzarelli, S.; Akashi, Y.; Fedele, F. & Novo, S. Tako-Tsubo cardiomyopathy and microcirculation. *Journal of Clinical Monitoring and Computing*, Vol.24, No.2, (2010), pp.101–105.

Fineschi, V.; Michalodimitrakis, M.; D'Errico, S.; Neri, M.; Pomara, C.; Riezzo, I. & Turillazzi. E. Insight into stress-induced cardiomyopathy and sudden cardiac death due to stress. A forensic cardio-pathologist point of view. *Forensic Science International*, Vol.194, No. 1-3, (2010), pp.1–8.

Flavahan, NA. A farewell kiss triggers a broken heart? *Circulation Research,* Vol.98, No.9, (2006), pp.1117–1119.

Gallerani, M.; Manfredini, R.; Ricci, L.; Grandi, E.; Cappato, R.; Calö, G.; Pareschi, PL. & Fersini, C. Sudden death from pulmonary thromboembolism: chronobiological aspects. *European Heart Journal,* Vol.13, No. 5, (1992), pp.661-665.

Galiuto, L.; De Caterina, AR.; Porfidia, A.; Paraggio, L.; Barchetta, S.; Locorotondo, G.; Rebuzzi, AG. & Crea, F. Reversible coronary microvascular dysfunction: a common pathogenetic mechanism in Apical Ballooning or Tako-Tsubo Syndrome. *European Heart Journal,* Vol.31, No.11, (2010), pp.1319–1327.

Gavish, D.; Rozenman, Y.; Hafner, R.; Bartov, E. & Ezri, T. Takotsubo cardiomyopathy after general anesthesia for eye surgery. *Anesthesiology,* Vol.105, No.3, (2006), pp.621-623.

Gianni, M.; Dentali, F.; Grandi, AM.; Sumner, G.; Hiralal, R. & Lonn, E. Apical ballooning syndrome or takotsubo cardiomyopathy: a systemic review. *European Heart Journal,* Vol.27, No.13, (2006), pp.1523-1529.

Gibson, CM.; Cannon, CP.; Daley, WL.; Dodge, JT Jr.; Alexander, B Jr.; Marble, SJ.; McCabe, CH.; Raymond, L.; Fortin, T.; Poole, WK. & Braunwald, E. TIMI frame count: a quantitative method of assessing coronary artery flow. *Circulation,* Vol.93, No.5, (1996), pp.879–888.

Hachamovitch, R.; Chang, JD.; Kuntz, RE.; Papageorgiu, P.; Levin, MS. & Goldberger, AL. Recurrent reversible cardiogenic shock triggered by emotional distress with no obstructive coronary disease. *American Heart Journal,* Vol.129, No.5, (1995), pp.1026-1028.

Haghi, D.; , Athanasiadis, A. ; Papavassiliu, T. ; Suselbeck, T.; Fluechter, S.; Mahrholdt, H.; Borggrefe, M. & Sechtem, U. Right ventricular involvement in Takotsubo cardiomyopathy. *European Heart Journal,* Vol.27, No.20, (2006), pp.2433-2439.

Haghi, D.; Fluechter, S.; Suselbeck, T.; Saur, J.; Bheleel, O.; Borggrefe, M. & Papavassiliu, T. Takotsubo cardiomyopathy (acute left ventricular apical ballooning syndrome) occurring in the intensive care unit. *Intensive Care Medecine,* Vol.32, No.7, (2006), pp.1069-1074.

Haghi, D.; Fluechter, S.; Suselbeck, T.; Kaden, JJ.; Borggrefe, M. & Papavassiliu, T. Cardiovascular magnetic resonance findings in typical versus atypical forms of the acute apical ballooning syndrome (Takotsubo cardiomyopathy). *International Journal of Cardiology,* Vol.120, No.2, (2007), pp.205–211.

Haghi, D.; Papavassiliu, T.; Heggemann, F.; Kaden, JJ.; Borggrefe, M. & Suselbeck, T. Incidence and clinical significance of left ventricular thrombus in tako-tsubo cardiomyopathy assessed with echocardiography. *QJM: monthly Journal of the Association of Physicians,* Vol.101, No.5, (2008), pp.381-386.

Hahn, JY.; Gwon, HC.; Park, SW.; Chol, SH.; Chol, JH.; Chol, JO.; Lee, SC.; On, YK.; Kim, JS.; Kim, DK.; Jeon, ES.; Lee, SH.; Hong, KP. & Park, JE. The clinical features of transient left ventricular nonapical ballooning syndrome: comparison with apical ballooning syndrome. *American Heart Journal,* Vol.154, No.6, (2007), pp.1166-1173.

Hawthorne, L. & Lyons, G. Cardiac arrest complicating spinal anaesthesia for cesarean section. *International Journal of Obstetric Anesthesia*, Vol.6, No.2, (1997), pp.126–129

Heubach, JF.; Ravens, U. & Kaumann, AJ. Epinephrine activates both Gs and Gi pathways, but norepinephrine activates only the Gs pathway through human beta2-adrenoceptors overexpressed in mouse heart. *Molecular Pharmacology,* Vol.65, No.5, (2004), pp.1313-1322.

Hinojosa-Laborde, C.; Chapa, I.; Lange, D. & Haywood, JR. Gender differences in sympathetic nervous system regulation. *Clinical and Experimental Pharmacology & Physiology,* Vol.26, No.2, (1999), pp.122-126.

Hoyt, J.; Lerman, A.; Lennon, RJ. ; Rihal, CS. & Prasad, A. Left anterior descending artery length and coronary atherosclerosis in apical ballooning syndrome (Takotsubo/stress induced cardiomyopathy). *International Journal of Cardiology,* Vol.145, No.1, (2010), pp.112-115.

Hurst, RT.; Askew, JW.; Reuss, CS.; Lee, RW.; Sweeney, JP.; Fortuln, FD.; Oh, JK & Tajik, AJ. Transient midventricular ballooning syndrome: a new variant. *Journal of the American College of Cardiology,* Vol.48, No.3, (2006), pp.579-583.

Hurst, RT.; Prasad, A.; Askew, JW.; Sengupta, PP. & Tajik, AJ. Takotsubo Cardiomyopathy: A Unique Cardiomyopathy With Variable Ventricular Morphology. *JACC. Cardiovascular Imaging,* Vol.3, No.6, (2010), pp.641–649.

Ionescu, CN.; Aguilar-Lopez, CA.; Sakr, AE.; Ghantous, AE. & Donohue, TJ. Long-term Outcome of Tako-tsubo Cardiomyopathy. *Heart, Lung and Circulation,* Vol.19, No.10, (2010), pp.601–605.

Itoh, H.; Miyake, Y.; Hioki, I.; Tanaka, S. & Okabe, M. Report of Takotsubo cardiomyopathy occurring during cardiopulmonary bypass. *The Journal of Extra-Corporeal Technology,* Vol.39, No.2, (2007), pp.109-111.

Jabaudon, M.; Bonnin, M.; Bolandard, F.; Chanseaume, S.; Dauphin, C. & Bazin, JE. Takotsubo syndrome during induction of general anesthesia. *Anaesthesia,* Vol.62, No.5, (2007), pp.519-523.

Kawai, S.; Suzuki, H.; Yamaguchi, H.; Tanaka, K.; Sawada, H.; Aizawa, T.; Watanabe, M.; Tamura, T.; Umawatari, K.; Kawata, M.; Nakamura, T.; Yamanaka, O. & Okada, R. Ampulla cardiomyopathy ('takotsubo' cardiomyopathy): reversible left ventricular dysfunction with ST segment elevation. *Japanese Circulation Journal,* Vol.64, No.2, (2000), pp.156–159.

Kaski, JC. Cardiac syndrome X in women: the role of oestrogen deficiency. *Heart,* Vol. 92, No.S3, (2006), pp.5-9.

Kawai, S.; Kitabatake, A.; Tomoike, H. & Takotsubo Cardiomyopathy Group. Guidelines for diagnosis of Takotsubo (ampulla) cardiomyopathy. *Circulation Journal,* Vol.71, No.6, (2007), pp.990–992.

Kim, S.; Yu, A.; Filippone, LA.; Kolansky, DM & Raina, A. Inverted Takotsubo Pattern Cardiomyopathy Secondary to Pheochromocytoma: A Clinical Case and Literature Review. *Clinical Cardiology,* Vol.33, No.4, (2010), pp.200–205.

Kimura, K.; Tanabe-Hayashi, Y.; Noma, S. & Fukuda, K. Rapid formation of left ventricular giant thrombus with Takotsubo cardiomyopathy. *Circulation,*Vol.115, No.23, (2007), pp.620-621.

Klinčeva, M.; Widimský, P.; Pešl, L.; Stásek, J.; Tousek, F.; Vambera, M. & Bílková D. Prevalence of stress-induced myocardial stunning (Tako-Tsubo cardiomyopathy) among patients undergoing emergency coronary angiography for suspected acute myocardial infarction. *International Journal of Cardiology*, Vol.120, No.3, (2007), pp.411–413.

Kolkebeck, TE.; Cotant, CL. & Krasuski, RA. Takotsubo cardiomyopathy: an unusual syndrome mimicking an ST-elevation myocardial infarction. *The American Journal of Emergency Medicine*, Vol.25, No.1, (2007), pp.92-95.

Krishnan, U.; Zacharzewski, A. & Schmitt, M. Nonapical Tako-tsubo Cardiomyopathy Associated with Coronary Slow Flow: A Case Report and Review of the Literature. *Clinical Cardiology*, Vol.32, No.11, (2009), pp.63–66.

Kume, T.; Akasaka, T.; Kawamoto, T.; Yoshitani, H.; Watanabe, N.; Neishi, Y.; Wada, N. &Yoshida, K. Assessment of coronary microcirculation in patients with takotsubo-like left ventricular dysfunction. *Circulation Journal*, Vol.69, No.8, (2005), pp.934–939.

Kurisu, S.; Sato, H.; Kawagoe, T.; Ishihara, M.; Shimatani, Y.; Nishioka, K.; Kono, Y.; Umemura, T. & Nakamura, S. Tako-tsubo-like left ventricular dysfunction with ST-segment elevation: a novel cardiac syndrome mimicking acute myocardial infarction. *American Heart Journal*, Vol.143, No.3, (2002), pp.448–455.

Kurisu, S.; Inoue, I.; Kawagoe, T.; Ishihara, M.; Shimatani, Y.; Nakamura, S.; Yoshida, M.; Mitsuba, N.; Hata, T. & Sato H. Time course of electrocardiographic changes in patients with Tako-Tsubo syndrome: comparison with acute myocardial infarction with minimal enzymatic release. *Circulation Journal*, Vol.68, No.1, (2004), pp.77-81.

Kurowski, V.; Kaiser, A.; von Hof, K.; Killermann, DP.; Mayer, B.; Hartmann, F.; Schunkert, H. & Radke PW. Apical and midventricular transient left ventricular dysfunction syndrome (tako-tsubo cardiomyopathy): frequency, mechanisms, and prognosis. *Chest*, Vol.132, No.3, (2007), pp.809-816.

Lamm, G.; Auer, J. & Eber, B. Atypical form of left ventricular ballooning after a violent attack. *International Journal of Cardiology*; Vol.119, No.3, (2007), pp.395-397.

Lentschener, C.; Vignaux, O.; Spaulding, C.; Bonnichon, P.; Legmann, P. & Ozier, Y. Early postoperative Takotsubo-like left ventricular dysfunction: transient left ventricular apical ballooning syndrome. *Anesthesia and Analgesia*, Vol.103, No.3, (2006), pp.580-582.

Littlejohn, F.; Syed, O.; Ornstein, E.; Connolly, ES. & Heyer, EJ. Takotsubo cardiomyopathy associated with anesthesia: three case reports. *Cases Journal*, Vol.1, No.1, (2008), pp.227.

Liu, S.; Bravo-Fernandez, C.; Riedl, C.; Antapli, M. & Dhamee, MS. Anesthetic management of Takotsubo cardiomyopathy: general versus regional anesthesia. *Journal of Cardiothoracic and Vascular Anesthesia*, Vol.22, No.3, (2008), pp.438-441.

Liu, S. & Saeed Dhamee M. Perioperative transient left ventricular apical ballooning syndrome: Takotsubo cardiomyopathy: a review. *Journal of Clinical Anesthesia*, Vol.22, No.1, (2010), pp.64–70.

Litvinov, IV.; Kotowycz, MA. & Wassmann, S. Iatrogenic epinephrine-induced reverse takotsubo cardiomyopathy: direct evidence supporting the role of catecholamines in the pathophysiology of the ''broken heart syndrome''. *Clinical Research in Cardiology*, Vol.98, No.7, (2009), pp.457–462.

Lyon; AR.; Rees, PS.; Prasad, S.; Poole-Wilson, PA. & Harding, SE. Stress (Takotsubo) cardiomyopathy—a novel pathophysilogical hypothesis to explain catecholamine-induced acute myocardial stunning. *Nature Clinical Practice. Cardiovascular Medicine*, Vol.5, No.1, (2008), pp.22–29.

Manfredini, R.; Citro, R.; Previtali, M.; Vriz, O.; Ciampi, Q.; Pascotto, M.; Tagliamonte, E.; Provenza, G.; Manfredini, F. & Bossone, E. Monday preference in onset of takotsubo cardiomyopathy. *The American Journal of Emergency Medicine*. Vol.28, No, 6, (2010), pp.715–719.

Mansencal, N.; El Mahmoud, R. & Dubourg, O. Occurrence of Tako-Tsubo Cardiomyopathy and Chronobiological Variation. *Journal of the American college of Cardiology*, Vol.55, No.5, (2010), pp.5499–5506.

Mansencal, N.; Abbou, N.; N'Guetta, R.; Pillière, R.; El Mahmoud, R. & Dubourg, O. Apical-sparing variant of Tako-Tsubo cardiomyopathy: Prevalence and characteristics. *Archives of Cardiovascular Disease*. Vol.103, No.2, (2010), pp.75—79

Mariscalco, G.; Cattaneo, P.; Rossi, A.; Baravelli, M.; Piffaretti, G.; Scannapieco, A.; Nassiacos, D. & Sala, A. Tako-tsubo cardiomyopathy complicated by ventricular septal perforation and septal dissection. *Heart and Vessels*, Vol.25, No.1, (2010), pp.73–75.

Maron, BJ.; Towbin, JA.; Thiene, G.; Antzelevitch, C.; Corrado, D.; Arnett, D.; Moss, AJ.; Seidman, CE. & Young, JB. Contemporary definitions and classification of the cardiomyopathies. *Circulation*, Vol.113, No.14, (2006), pp.1807–1816.

Matsuoka, H.; Kawakami, H.; Koyama, Y.; Inoue, K.; Nishimura, K.; Saeki, H. & Ito, T. Tako tsubo cardiomyopathy with a significant pressure gradient in the left ventricle. *Heart and Vessels*, Vol.15, No.4, (2000), pp.203

Matsuoka, K.; Okubo, S.; Fujii, E.; & Uhida, F. Evaluation of the arrhythmogenecity of stress-induced "Takotsubo cardiomyopathy" from the time course of the 12-lead surface electrocardiogram. *The American Journal of Cardiology*, Vol.92, No.2, (2003), pp.230-233.

Mazzarotto, P.; Stecconi, P.; Gemelli, F.; Azzarito, M. & Farnetti, F. A case of ballooning syndrome with atypical anterior localization. *Italian Heart Journal*, Vol.6, No.11, (2005), pp.730–734

Mitchell, JH.; Hadden, TB.; Wilson, JM.; Achari, A.; Muthupillai, R. & Flamm, SD. Clinical features and usefulness of cardiac magnetic resonance imaging in assessing myocardial viability and prognosis in Takotsubo cardiomyopathy (transient left ventricular apical ballooning syndrome). *The American Journal of Cardiology*, Vol.100, No.2, (2007), pp.296–301.

Mizutani, K. & Okada, M. A case of intraoperative repeated coronary artery spasm with ST-segment depression. *Masui*, Vol.51, No.10, (2002), pp.1114-1116.

Montassier, E.; Gueffet, JP.; Trewick, D.; Le Conte, P. & Potel, G. À propos d'un cas de syndrome de Tako-Tsubo ou comment une situation stressante peut vous amener en salle de coronarographie… *Journal Européen des Urgences*, Vol.22, No.4, (2009), pp.114-117.

Movaheda, MR. & Donohueb, D. Review: transient left ventricular apical ballooning, broken heart syndrome, ampulla cardiomyopathy, atypical apical ballooning, or Tako-Tsubo cardiomyopathy. *Cardiovascular Revascularization Medicine*, Vol.8, No.4, (2007), pp. 289–292.

Mudd, JO.; Kapur, NK.; Champion, HC.; Schulman, SP. & Wittstein, IS. Patients with stress-induced (takotsubo) cardiomyopathy have an increased prevalence of mood disorders and antidepressant use compared to patients with acute myocardial infarction. *Journal Cardiac Failure*, Vol.13, No.6, (2007), pp.176.

Muller, O.; Roguelov, C. & Pascale P. A basal variant form of the transient 'midventricular' and 'apical' ballooning syndrome. *QJM: montly journal of the association of physicians*. Vol.100, No.11, (2007), pp.738–739.

Novak, G.; Kross, K.; Follmer, K.; Brofferio, A. & Shirani J. Transient biventricular apical ballooning: a unique presentation of the "broken heart.", *Clinical Cardiology*, Vol.30, No7, (2007), pp.355–358.

Nef, HM.; Möllmann, H.; Sperzel, J.; Weber, M.; Brück, H.; Hamm, CW. & Elsässer A. Temporary third-degree atrioventricular block in a case of apical ballooning syndrome. *International Journal of Cardiology*, Vol.113, No.2, (2006), pp.33–35.

Nef, HM.; Möllmann, H.; Kostin, S.; Troidl, C.; Voss, S.; Weber, M.; Dill, T.; Rolf, A.; Brandt, R.; Hamm, CW. & Elsässer A. Tako-Tsubo cardiomyopathy: intraindividual structural analysis in the acute phase and after functional recovery. *European Heart Journal*, Vol.28, No.20, (2007), pp.2456–2464.

Nef, HM.; Möllmann, H. & Elsässer, A. Tako-tsubo cardiomyopathy (apical ballooning). *Heart*, Vol.93, No.10, (2007), pp.1309–1315.

Nef, HM.; Möllmann, H.; Hilpert, P.; Masseli, F.; Troidl, C.; Rolf, A.; Dill, T.; Skwara, W.; Weber, M.; Hamm, C. & Elsässer, A. Severe mitral regurgitation in Tako-Tsubo cardiomyopathy. *International Journal of Cardiology*, Vol.132, No.2, (2009), pp.77–79.

Nef, HM.; Möllmann, H.; Troidl, C.; Kostin, S.; Voss, S.; Hilpert, P.; Behrens, CB.; Rolf, A.; Rixe, J.; Weber, M.; Hamm, CW. & Elsässer, A. Abnormalities in intracellular Ca2+ regulation contribute to the pathomechanism of Tako-Tsubo cardiomyopathy. *European Heart Journal*, Vol.30, No.17, (2009), pp.2155–2164.

Nef, HM.; Möllmann, H.; Hilpert, P.; Troidl, C.; Voss, S.; Rolf, A.; Behrens, CB.; Weber, M.; Hamm, CW. & Elsässer, A. Activated cell survival cascade protects cardiomyocytes from cell death in Tako-Tsubo cardiomyopathy. *European Journal of Heart Failure*, Vol.11, No.8, (2009), pp.758–764.

Nef, HM.; Möllmann, H.; Akashi, YJ. & Hamm, CW. Mechanisms of stress (Takotsubo) cardiomyopathy. *Nature Reviews. Cardiology*, Vol.7, No.4, (2010), pp.187–193.

Ohara, Y.; Hiasa, Y.; Hosokawa, S.; Tomokane, T.; Yamaguchi, K.; Ogura, R.; Miyajima, H.; Ogata, T.; Yuba, K.; Suzuki, N.; Takahashi, T.; Kishi, K. & Ohtani R. Left ventricular free wall rupture in transient left ventricular apical ballooning. *Circulation Journal*, Vol.69, No.8, (2005), pp.621–623.

Ogura, R.; Hiasa, Y.; Takahashi, T.; Yamaguchi, K.; Fujiwara, K.; Ohara, Y.; Nada, T; Ogata, T.; Kusunoki, K.; Yuba, K.; Hosokawa, S.; Kishi, K. & Ohtani, R. Specific findings of the standard 12-lead ECG in patients with 'Takotsubo' cardiomyopathy: comparison with the findings of acute anterior myocardial infarction. *Circulation Journal*, Vol.67, No.8, (2003), pp.687-90.

Ohtsubo, M.; Sakai, H.; Takano, H.; Kon, H.; Okamoto, K.; Yoshida, N. & Fujita, M. Atypical takotsubo cardiomyopathy with preservation of apical contraction: a case report including pathological findings. *Journal of Cardiology*, Vol.46, No.6, (2005), pp.237–242.

Del Pace, SD.; Parodi, G.; Bellandi, B.; Zampini, L.; Venditti, F.; Ardito, M.; Antoniucci, D. & Gensini GF. Anxiety trait in patients with stress-induced cardiomyopathy: a case–control study. *Clinical Research in Cardiology*, (2011).

Park, JH.; Kang, SJ.; Song, JK.; Kim, HK.; Lim, CM.; Kang, DH. & Koh, Y. Left ventricular apical ballooning due to severe physical stress in patients admitted to the medical ICU. *Chest*, Vol.28, No.1, (2005), pp.296-302.

Parodi, G.; Del Pace, S.; Carrabba, N.; Salvadori, C.; Memisha, G.; Simonetti, I.; Antoniucci, D. & Gensini, GF. Incidence, clinical findings, and outcome of women with left ventricular apical ballooning syndrome. *The American Journal of Cardiology*, Vol.99, No.2, (2007), pp.182–185.

Parodi, G. & Antoniucci, D. Transient left ventricular apical ballooning syndrome after inadvertent epidural administration of potassium chloride. *International Journal of Cardiology*, Vol.124, No.1, (2007), pp.14–15

Pavin, D.; Le Breton, H. & Daubert, C. Human stress cardiomyopathy mimicking acute myocardial syndrome. *Heart*, Vol.78, No.5, (1997), pp.509–511.

Pernicova, I.; Garg, S.; Bourantas, C.; Alamgir, F. & Hoye, A. Takotsubo cardiomyopathy: a review of the literature. *Angiology*, Vol.61, No.2, (2010), pp.166–173.

Pilgrim, TM. & Wyss, TR. Takotsubo cardiomyopathy or transient left ventricular apical ballooning syndrome: A systematic review. *International Journal of Cardiology*, Vol.124, No.3, (2008), pp. 283-292.

Pilliere, R. ; Mansencal, N. ; Digne, F.; Lacombe, P.; Joseph, T.; & Dubourg, O. Prevalence of takotsubo syndrome in a large urban agglomeration. *The American Journal of Cardiology*, Vol.98, No.5, (2006), pp.662—665.

Prasad A. Apical ballooning syndrome: an important differential diagnosis of acute myocardial infarction. *Circulation*, Vol.115, No.5, (2007), pp.56-59.

Prasad, A.; Lerman, A. & Rihal, CS. Apical ballooning syndrome (Tako-Tsubo or stress cardiomyopathy): a mimic of acute myocardial infarction. *American Heart Journal*, Vol.155, No.3, (2008), pp.408—417.

Previtali, M.; Repetto, A. & Scuteri, L. Dobutamine induced severe midventricular obstruction and mitral regurgitation in left ventricular apical ballooning syndrome. *Heart*, Vol.91, No.3, (2005), pp.353.

Rajani, R.; Przedlacka, A.; Saha, M. & de Belder, A. Pancreatitis and the broken heart. *European Journal of Emergency Medicine*, Vol.17, No.1, (2010), pp.27–29.

Ramakrishna, G.; Ravi, BS. & Chandrasekaran, K. Apical ballooning syndrome in a postoperative patient with normal microvascular perfusion by myocardial contrast echocardiography. *Echocardiography*, Vol.22, No.7, (2005), pp.606-610.

Reeder, GS. & Prasad, A. In: *Uptodate*, 1.04.2011. Available from Stress-induced (takotsubo) cardiomyopathy http://www.uptodate.com/contents/stress-induced-takotsubo-cardiomyopathy.

Reuss, CS.; Lester, SJ.; Hurst, RT.; Askew, JW.; Nager, P.; Lusk, J.; Altemose, GT. & Tajik, AJ. Isolated left ventricular basal ballooning phenotype of transient cardiomyopathy in young women. *The American Journal Cardiology*, Vol.99, No.10, (2007), pp.1451–1453.

Rivera, JM.; Locketz, AJ.; Fritz, KD.; Horlocker, TT.; Lewallen, DG.; Prasad, A.; Bresnahan, JF. & Kinney, MO. "Broken heart syndrome" after separation (from OxyContin). *Mayo Clinic Proceedings Mayo Clinic*, Vol.81, No.6, (2006), pp.825- 828.

Rossor, AM.; Pearce, SH. & Adams, PC. Left ventricular apical ballooning (Takotsubo cardiomyopathy) in thyrotoxicosis. *Thyroid*, Vol.17, No.2, (2007), pp.181-182.

Rostoff, P.; Latacz, P.; Piwowarska, W.; Konduracka, E.; Bolech, A. & Zmudka, K. Transient ST-segment elevation in lead aVR associated with tako-tsubo cardiomyopathy. *International Journal of Cardiology*, Vol.134, No.3, (2009), pp.97–110.

Sader, MA. & Celermajer, DS. Endothelial function, vascular reactivity and gender differences in the cardiovascular system. *Cardiovascular Research*, Vol.53, No.3, (2002), pp.597-604.

Sakai, K.; Ochiai, H.; Katayama, N.; Nakamura, K.; Arataki, K.; Kido, T.; Iwamoto, H.; Nakamura, S. & Nakamishi, T. A serious clinical course of a very elderly patient with takotsubo cardiomyopathy. *Heart and Vessels*, Vol. 20, No.2, (2005), pp.77-81

Sato, H.; Tateishi, H. & Uchida, T. Takotsubo-type cardiomyopathy due to multivessel spasm. In: Clinical aspect of myocardial injury: From ischemia to heart failure, Kodama, K.; Haze, K.; Hon, M., *Kagakuhyouronsha*, (1990).

Sato, M.; Fujita, S.; Saito, A.; Ikeda, Y.; Kitazawa, H.; Takahashi, M.; Ishiguro, J.; Okabe, M.; Nakamura, Y.; Nagai, T.; Watanabe, H.; Kodama, M. & Aizawa, Y. Increased incidence of transient left ventricular apical ballooning; (so-called 'Takotsubo' cardiomyopathy) after the mid-Niigata Prefecture earthquake. *Circulation journal*, Vol.70, No.8, (2006), pp.947-953.

Sato, A.; Yagihara, N.; Kodama, M.; Mitsuma, W.; Tachikawa, H.; Ito, M.; Hanawa, H. & Aizawa, Y. Takotsubo cardiomyopathy after delivery in an oestrogen-deficient patient. *International Journal of Cardiology*, (2009).

Sharkey, SW.; Lesser, JR.; Zenovich, AG.; Maron, MS.; Lindberg, J.; Longe, TF. & Maron, BJ. Acute and reversible cardiomyopathy provoked by stress in women from the United States. *Circulation*, Vol.111, No.4, (2005), pp.472-479.

Sharkey, SW.; Lesser, JR.; Maron, MS. & Maron, BJ. Stress cardiomyopathy. *Journal of the American College of Cardiology*, Vol. 49, No8, (2007), pp.921.

Sharkey, SW.; Lesser, JR.; Menon, M.; Parpart, M.; Maron, MS. & Maron, BJ. Spectrum and significance of electrocardiographic patterns, troponin levels, and thrombolysis in myocardial infarction frame count in patients with stress (tako-tsubo) cardiomyopathy and comparison to those in patients with ST-elevation anterior wall myocardial infarction. *The American Journal of Cardiology,* Vol.101, No.12, (2008), pp.1723-1728.

Sharkey, SW.; Windenburg, DC.; Lesser, JR.; Maron, MS.; Hauser, RG.; Lesser, JN.; Haas, TS.; Hodges, JS. & Maron, BJ. Natural history and expansive clinical profile of stress (tako-tsubo) cardiomyopathy. *Journal of the American College of Cardiology,* Vol.55, No.4, (2010), pp.333-341.

Silva, C.; Gonçalves, A.; Almeida, R.; Dias, P.; Araújo, V.; Gavina, C. & Maciel, MJ. Transient left ventricular ballooning syndrome. *European Journal of Internal Medicine.* Vol.20, No.5, (2009), pp.454-456.

Stajer, D.; Mozina, H.; Noc, M. & Rode, P. Correlation between QTcinterval durationandleft ventricular systolic dysfunction in patients with acute myocardial infarction. *Journal of Electrocardiology,* vol.26, No.4, (1993), 333-340.

Strunk, B.; Shaw, RE.; Bull, S.; Adams, J.; Baer, M.; Gershengorn, K.; Kao, A.; Keeffe, B.; Sklar, J.; Sperling, D.; Sperling, R.; Wexman, M. & Young, J. High incidence of focal left ventricular wall motion abnormalities and normal coronary arteries in patients with myocardial infarctions presenting to a community hospital. *Journal of Invasive Cardiolology,* Vol.18, No.8, (2006), pp.376-381.

Suzuki, K.; Osada, N.; Akasi, YJ.; Suzuki, N.; Sakakibara, M.; Miyake, F.; Maki, F. & Takahashi, Y. An atypical case of "Takotsubo cardiomyopathy" during alcohol withdrawal: abnormality in the transient left ventricular wall motion and a remarkable elevation in the ST segment. *Internal Medicine.* Vol.43, No.4, (2004), pp.300-305.

Takayama, N.; Iwase, Y.; Ohtsu, S. & Sakio, H. "Takotsubo" cardiomyopathy developed in the postoperative period in a patient with amyotrophic lateral sclerosis. *Masui,* Vol.53, No.4, (2004), pp.403-406.

Takigawa, T.; Tokioka, H.; Chikai, T.; Fukuschima, T.; Ishizu, T. & Kosogabe, Y. A case of undiagnosed "takotsubo" cardiomyopathy during anesthesia. *Masui,* Vol.52, No.10, pp.1104-1106.

Tamura, A.; Kawano, Y.; Watanabe, T.; Aso, T.; Abe, Y.; Yano, S. & Kadota, JA. Report of 2 cases of transient mid-ventricular ballooning. *International Journal of Cardiology,* Vol.122, No.2, pp.10-12.

Teh, AW.; New, G. & Cooke, J. A Single-centre Report on the Characteristics of Tako-tsubo Syndrome. *Heart, Lung and Circulation,* Vol.19, No.2, (2010), pp.63-70.

Trebouet, E.; Lipp, D.; Dimet, J.; Orion, L. & Fradin, P. Cardiologic emergencies and natural disaster. Prospective study with Xynthia tempest. Annales de Cardiologie et d' Angeiologie. Vol.60, No1, (2011), pp.39-41.

Tsuchihashi, K.; Ueshima, K.; Uchida, T.; Oh-mura, N.; Kimura, K.; Owa, M.; Yoshiyama, M.; Miyazaki, S.; Haze, K.; Ogawa, H.; Honda, T.; Hase, M.; Kai, R. & Morii, I. Transient left ventricular apical ballooning without coronary artery stenosis: a novel heart syndrome mimicking acute myocardial infarction. Angina Pectoris-Myocardial Infarction Investigations in Japan. *Journal of the American College of Cardiology,* Vol.38, No.1, (2001), pp.11-18.

Ueyama, T.; Hano, T.; Kasamatsu, K.; Yamamoto, K.; Tsuruo, Y. & Nishio, I. Estrogen attenuates the emotional stress-induced cardiac response in the animal model of

Tako-tsubo (Ampulla) cardiomyopathy. *The Journal of Cardiovascular Pharmacology,* Vol.42, No.S1, (2003), pp.117-119.

Valbusa, A.; Abbadessa, F.; Giachero, C.; Vischi, M.; Zingarelli, A.; Olivieri, R. & Visconti, LO. Long-term follow-up of Tako-Tsubo-like syndrome: a retrospective study of 22 cases. *The Journal of Cardiovascular Medicine,* Vol.9, No.8, (2008), pp.805—809.

Van de Walle, SO.; Gevaert, SA.; Gheeraert, PJ.; De Pauw, M. & Gillebert, TC. Transient stress-induced cardiomyopathy with an "inverted takotsubo" contractile pattern. *Mayo Clinic Proceedings Mayo Clinic,* Vol.81, No.11, (2006), pp.1499-1502.

Vidi, V.; Rajesh, V.; Singh, PP.; Mukherjee, JT.; Lago, RM.; Venesy, DM.; Waxman, S.; Pyne, CT.; Piemonte, TC.; Gossman DE. & Nesto, RW. Clinical characteristics of tako-tsubo cardiomyopathy. *The American Journal of Cardiology,* Vol.104, No.4, (2009), pp.578 -582.

Villareal, RP.; Achari, A.; Wilansky, S. & Wilson, JM. Anteroapical stunning and left ventricular outflow tract obstruction. *Mayo Clinic Proceedings Mayo Clinic,* Vol.76, No.1, (2001), pp.76:79.

Watanabe, H.; Kodama, M.; Okura, Y.; Aizawa, Y.; Tanabe, N.; Chinushi, M.; Nakamura, Y.; Nagai, T.; Sato, M. & Okabe, M. Impact of earthquakes on takotsubo cardiomyopathy. *Journal of American Medicine Association,* Vol.294, No.3, (2005), pp.305-307.

Winogradow, J.; Geppert, G.; Reinhard, W.; Resch, M.; Radke, PW. & Hengstenberg, C. Tako-tsubo cardiomyopathy after administration of intravenous epinephrine during an anaphylactic reaction. *International Journal of Cardiology.* Vol.147, No.2, (2011), pp.309-311.

Wittstein, IS.; Thiemann, DR.; Lima, JA.; Baughman, KL.; Schulman, SP.; Gerstenblith, G.; Wu, KC.; Rade, JJ.; Bivalacqua, TJ. & Champion, HC. Neurohumoral features of myocardial stunning due to sudden emotional stress. *The New England Journal of Medicine,*Vol.352, No.6, (2005), pp.539—548.

Yanagi, S.; Nagae, K.; Yoshida, K.; Matsumura, Y.; Nagashima, E.; Okada, M.; Ota, T.; Hirota, K. & Yoshikawa, J. Evaluation of coronary flow reverse using Doppler guide wire in patients with ampulla cardiomyopathy: three case reports. *Journal of Cardiology,* Vol.39, No.6, (2002), pp.305-312.

Yasu, T.; Tone, K.; Kubo, N. & Saito, M. Transient mid-ventricular ballooning cardiomyopathy: a new entity of Takotsubo cardiomyopathy. *International Journal Cardiology,* Vol.110, No.1, (2006), pp.100-101.

Yoshida, T.; Hibino, T.; Kako, N.; Murai, S.; Oguri, M.; Kato, K.; Yajima, K.; Ohte, N.; Yokoi, K. & Kimura, G. A pathophysiologic study of tako-tsubo cardiomyopathy with F-18 fluorodeoxyglucose positron emission tomography. *European Heart Journal,* Vol.28, No.21, (2007), pp.2598-2604.

Yunus, A.; Gillis, AM.; Duff, HJ.; Wyse, DG. & Mitchell, LB. Increased precordial QTc dispersion predicts ventricular fibrillation during acute myocardial infarction. *The American Journal of Cardiology,* Vol.78, No.6, (1996), pp.706-708.

Zaroff, JG.; Rordorf, GA.; Ogilvy, CS. & Picard, MH. Regional patterns of left ventricular systolic dysfunction aftersubarachnoid hemorrhage: evidence for neurally mediated cardiac injury. *The Journal of the American Society of Echocardiography*, Vol.13, No.8, (2000), pp.774–779.

Zdanowicz, JA.; Utz, AC.; Bernasconi, I.; Geier, S.; Corti, R. & Beinder, E. "Broken heart" after cesarean delivery. Case report and review of literature. *Archives of Gynecology and Obstetrics*, Vol.283, No.4, (2011), pp.687-694.

7

Role of Percutaneous Cardiopulmonary Support (PCPS) in Patients with Unstable Hemodynamics During the Peri-Coronary-Intervention Period

Ho-Ki Min[1] and Young Tak Lee[2]
[1]*Department of Thoracic and Cardiovascular Surgery, Haeundae Paik Hospital, Inje University College of Medicine, Busan*
[2]*Department of Thoracic and Cardiovascular Surgery, Samsung Medical Center, Sungkyunkwan University School of Medicine, Seoul*
Korea

1. Introduction

Coronary artery disease remains the principal cause of death in developed countries, with acute coronary syndrome (ACS) contributing greatly to cardiovascular morbidity and mortality. Optimal revascularization therapy in these patients is of major importance and remains the basis for favorable outcomes. The intervention-based strategy plays a major role in the management of acute-phase patients because of the cardiovascular benefits demonstrated in numerous studies. In serious cases, ACS can be encountered with life threatening episodes such as cardiogenic shock or cardiac arrest in the peri-intervention period. Compared with the intra-aortic balloon pump (IABP), percutaneous cardiopulmonary support (PCPS) can maintain hemodynamic stability in the abscence of an intrinsic cardiac rhythm or effective cardiac output and can provide excellent mechanical circulatory support in these urgent or emergent situations because it can be implanted and stabilized promptly in many different hospital locations, including the cardiac catheterization laboratory, and if necessary, in the emergency room or intensive care unit. Some reports use PCPS to rescue ACS patients with cardiopulmonary failure (Sung, 2006; Grambow, 1994). Herein, we present our experience with the use of PCPS for initial stabilization in patients with unstable hemodynamics before or after coronary intervention and discuss some of the pertinent issues related to this topic.

2. Extracorporeal membrane oxygenation

2.1 Introduction

Extra corporeal membrane oxygenation (ECMO) techniques became available40 years ago. In 1972, the first veno-arterial ECMO system for humans was used in a patient with acute respiratory distress syndrome (Hill, 1972). The first successful application of neonatal ECMO was performed by Bartlett in 1976 (Bartlett, 1976), and the concept of veno-venous ECMO to eliminate CO_2 was established by Kolobow in 1980 (Kolobow,

1980). In the last decade, enormous advances have been made and ECMO has become more reliable with improved equipment and increased experience, which is reflected in the improved results. ECMO is used for the management of life threatening pulmonary or cardiac failure (or both), when no other form of treatment has been or is likely to be successful. ECMO is generally used as temporary support while awaiting recovery of organs.

ECMO is essentially a modification of the cardiopulmonary bypass circuit, which is used routinely in cardiac surgery. Blood is drained from the venous system peripherally or centrally, oxygenated with carbon dioxide extracted, then returned back to the arterial system peripherally or centrally.

Although ECMO remains a short-term support device, the use of such a circuit for extended periods (days to weeks) has required some modifications. Specially, the circuit is smaller than a standard cardiopulmonary bypass circuit, transportable, and closed to the atmosphere. The cannulae are also specifically designed for ECMO. The duration of support with ECMO has greatly increased with improving oxygenators and medical management, and whereas support was previously on the order of days, patients can now be maintained on ECMO for weeks. In most patients the duration of support required is approximately 1 week. Most commonly, ECMO is used in an emergency or urgent situation after failure of other treatment modalities.

2.2 Indications for ECMO

ECMO is indicated for all the reversible pulmonary or cardiac failures (or both) refractory to conventional therapy. ECMO is usually used for initial stabilization and temporary support while awaiting recovery of organs. However, physicians should keep in mind that the results of ECMO support are consistently related to the indication for institution of such therapy.

With respect to cardiac failure, ECMO has been used successfully to resuscitate patients with cardiac arrest or cardiogenic shock due to acute coronary syndrome, post-cardiotomy cardiac failure, transplant rejection, intractable dysrhythmia, ruptured coronary artery graft, pericardial tamponade, cardiac trauma, sepsis, and myocarditis. ECMO has also been effective in patients with secondary cardiac failure due to respiratory insufficiency, hypothermic arrest from cold-water submersion, and drug overdose. The indications for ECMO in cardiopulmonary resuscitation are summarized in Table 1.

In making the decision to use ECMO, several considerations must be weighed. Most importantly, physicians must consider the possibility of cardiac recovery. If recovery is not expected, consideration must be given to patient eligibility for heart transplantation, other mechanical assist devices to bridge the patient to transplantation, or a definitive mechanical assist device to be inserted as destination therapy. Moreover, patient selection is the most important prognostic indicator. Although some relative contraindications have been proposed, there are few generally accepted absolute contraindications to ECMO. Unwitnessed cardiac arrest, aortic dissection, and terminal illness are considered to be the most important contraindications. The mortality rate after an unwitnessed cardiac arrest approaches 100% and has not changed with the use of ECMO. Early and effective resuscitation can allow for neurologically-intact survivors, but this is less likely to occur in an unwitnessed arrest. Aortic insufficiency is another relative contraindication, particularly if severe. In such situations, aortic valve replacement should be considered. Lesser degrees of aortic insufficiency may be managed with a left ventricular vent. Failure to insert a vent leads to ventricular distension, compromised subendocardial blood flow with an impact on recovery, and the ability to wean from ECMO.

Renal failure, hepatic failure, and significant neurologic disease are relative contraindications to ECMO, depending on the existence of other therapeutic options and the degree of dysfunction (Meurs, 2005).

With respect to respiratory failure, the most common indication is due to adult respiratory distress syndrome (ARDS), pneumonia, trauma, or primary graft failure following lung transplantation. ECMO is also used for neonatal and pediatric respiratory support. The use of ECMO in premature neonates is the mainstay of treatment for immature lungs and insufficient surfactant.

More recently, indications for ECMO have been expanded to pro-procedural supports, such as major airway intervention/surgery and cardiac intervention, including high-risk coronary angioplasty or arrhythmia ablation (Table 1). In a small and retrospective study, Grambow et al. proposed that patients requiring coronary revascularization by angioplasty who have severe left ventricular dysfunction or target vessels supplying greater than 50% of the myocardium are candidates for elective ECMO (Grambow, 1994).

Indications
Resuscitation
Cardiac arrest
Cardiogenic shock
Cardiac trauma
Respiratory insufficiency
Status asthmaticus
Smoke inhalation
Drug overdose
Pulmonary edema
Massive pulmonary embolism
Hypothermia
Procedural support
Angioplasty
Arrhythmia ablation
Pulmonary embolectomy
Coronary artery bypass grafting
Cerebral arteriovenous malformation resection
Donor heart preservation
Abdominal aortic graft replacement
Tracheal reconstruction
Ventricular assist device placement

Table 1. Indications for ECMO

2.3 Mode of ECMO

ECMO can be inserted in a veno-venous (VV) mode, which provides oxygenation and CO_2 removal, and thus is used for pulmonary failure not responding to mechanical ventilation, or can be used in a veno-arterial (VA) mode providing sufficient end-organ perfusion and gas exchange. VA ECMO can be instituted peripherally or centrally.

VV ECMO refers to blood being drained from the venous system and returned to the venous system. This mode only provides respiratory support and is achieved by peripheral cannulation, usually via the femoral or jugular veins. VA ECMO refers to blood being drained from the venous system and returned to the arterial system. The VA ECMO mode provides cardiac and respiratory support, and can be divided into two groups according to vascular access peripherally or centrally.

When using 'central' cannulation, in which the ascending aorta and right atrium are directly cannulated, this is referred to as 'central' ECMO. Central ECMO allows better flow because of better drainage from the right atrium with a bigger cannula and is usually required in patients with a larger body surface area (> 2.0 m^2). The other advantage of central ECMO is that the flow directly from the outflow cannula into the aorta provides antegrade flow to the arch vessels, coronary arteries, and the rest of the body (Fig. 1). However, central ECMO also has its drawbacks. Insertion of central ECMO requires a median sternotomy to allow the cannulation. This is a time-consuming procedure and increases the risk of bleeding from the sternum and also of infection. In contrast to central ECMO, it can be achieved by peripheral vascular access and is called 'peripheral' ECMO or percutaneous cardiopulmonary support (PCPS), in which insertion is more prompt via a bed-side procedure than central ECMO because there is no need for a sternotomy and the risk of

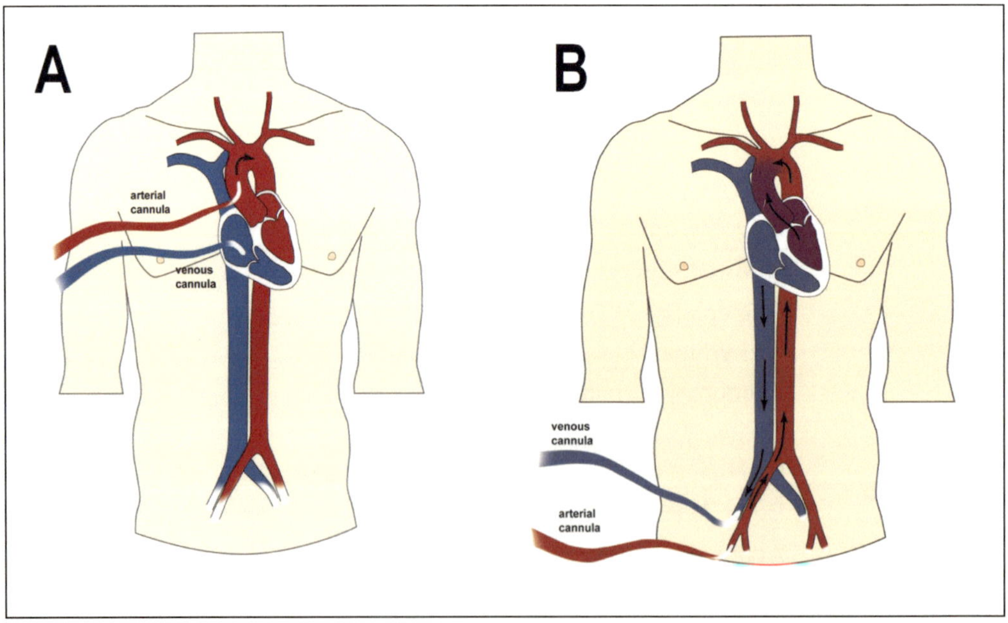

Fig. 1. Mode of ECMO. Panel A represents central ECMO and panel B represents peripheral ECMO.

bleeding is decreased. However, the retrograde aortic flow provided by peripheral ECMO from the femoral artery leads to admixing in the arch (two circulation syndrome). For this reason, monitoring of oxygenation from a right radial arterial line would be prudent. Mechanical ventilation must be continued during ECMO support to maintain oxygen saturation of blood ejected from the left ventricle to at least above 90%. In patients on PCPS, single access cannulae may not be sufficient to achieve satisfactory perfusion and gas exchange. In these patients a second access cannula is inserted via the right internal jugular vein ,so sufficient flow can be achieved.

2.4 Maintenance and Weaning of ECMO

The basic function of VA ECMO in supplying mechanical circulatory support is to drain blood from the venous circulation, oxygenate the blood, and then return the blood to the arterial circulation at physiologic perfusion pressures. Although ECMO efficiently unload the right ventricle, ECMO is not efficient in unloading the left ventricle. Indeed, ECMO increases left ventricular afterload, thus negatively affecting myocardial recovery, even though left ventricular preload is significantly reduced by the diminished return from the lungs. For this reason, attempts to improve left ventricular contractility, reducing left ventricular distension, left ventricular afterload, and clot formation are of utmost importance. Such measures should include inotropic support and may include intra-aortic balloon pumping (IABP), which can decrease left ventricular afterload and therefore reducing wall stress, especially during the critical initial period. Other options include inserting a left ventricular vent to empty the ventricle connecting this line into the venous line of the ECMO circuit, to place an additional drainage catheter in the left atrium that can be placed via the percutaneous route (Aiyagari, 2006), or to perform an atrial septostomy to decompress the left heart (Koenig, 1993).

ECMO flow can be volume-dependent and will drop with hypovolemia, cannula malposition, pneumothorax, and pericardial tamponade, and usually manifests as 'kicking' or 'chatter' of the venous tubing as well as a drop in output. Management includes a volume challenge, and exclusion of intra-abdominal distension or compartment syndrome, cardiac tamponade, or pneumothorax. If a volume challenge does not work, a slight reduction in flow may be helpful or there may be a need to insert another venous cannula. Further, centrifugal pumps in contrast to roller pumps are afterload-dependent, and therefore hypertension is another variable that can reduce flow and should be avoided.

From a respiratory point of view, hypoxia is treated by increasing the flow rate and FiO_2 of the ECMO circuit, not by altering the FiO_2 and PEEP on the ventilator. Attempts to support and rest the lung should be made to wean the FiO_2 on the ventilator and maintain a PEEP level of 8-15 cmH_2O. A protective lung ventilation strategy with low plateau pressures and low tidal volumes should be attempted as well as low respiratory rates, unless attempting to wean off the ECMO circuit. PCO_2 control should be via the ECMO fresh gas flow to the oxygenator, not by altering the respiratory rate on the ventilator.

From a cardiac point of view, the aim should be to minimize the use of inotropes, and thus rest the heart. However, a low-dose inotrope infusion is often maintained to ensure some contractility and adequate emptying of the left ventricle. It is also important to ensure the patient is not hypovolemic.

There are no standardized methods or techniques by which to wean from ECMO. With respect to VV ECMO, weaning and discontinuation are considered when there is evidence of substantial improvement in the underlying disease process and cardiopulmonary function based on radiographs, laboratory parameters, hemodynamic parameters, and gas exchange. While monitoring these parameters, flow through the circuit can gradually be reduced. When a reduction in flow of 75% can be achieved without changes in cardiopulmonary status, membrane gas flow can be stopped. If the patient tolerates those challenges for 12 hours with adequate gas exchange and hemodynamic parameters, VV ECMO can be removed (Gravlee, 2008).

With respect to VA ECMO, weaning and discontinuation are considered when there is evidence of cardiac recovery, including increased blood pressure, return of pulsatility or increased pulsatility on the arterial pressure waveform, and falling central venous and/or pulmonary pressures. Weaning is performed under echocardiographic guidance with regular arterial blood gas and lactate measurements. ECMO flow rates are slowly weaned, while inotropes and ventilator support are adjusted after echocardiography confirms adequate ventricular filling and ejection. Blood gases and serum lactate levels are then assayed to confirm adequate gas exchange and oxygen delivery, respectively. Until a reduction in flow of 75% can be achieved or a flow rate is below 1 - 1.5 liter/min without changes in cardiopulmonary status over 12 - 24 hours, weaning can proceed. If the patient tolerates those challenges for 12 hours with adequate parameters, VA ECMO can be removed.

2.5 Complications of ECMO

Bleeding and hemolysis, multi-organ failure, infection, and equipment failure are the common complications that contribute to morbidity and mortality associated with ECMO in adults. The complications that have been reported to the Extracorporeal Life Support Organization (ELSO) Registry in adult patients treated with ECMO are listed in Table 2, and data on complications and events reported in the ELSO Registry are shown in Table 3 (Meurs, 2005).

The most common complication associated with the use of ECMO is bleeding from cannulation sites, with typical rates ranging 4-14% (Kurusz, 2002). Excessive bleeding is caused by multiple factors. Hepatic congestion and failure, malnutrition, multiple cannulation sites, low-dose anticoagulation with heparin, decreased platelet function, activation of the coagulation cascade secondary to hemolysis, and hyperfibrinolysis from contact with prosthetic surfaces all may contribute to increased bleeding. The use of heparin-coated circuits in addition to the antifibrolytics and vitamin K therapies has contributed to lower bleeding rates. Vena cava tears or rupture with retroperitoneal bleeding, and arterial or aortic injury including dissection and perforation that required surgical exploration and reconstruction have occurred. Other non-cannula-related bleeding complications include pulmonary and gastrointestinal hemorrhage.

Ischemic injury to the brain, kidneys, liver, and other end organs has been attributed to prolonged resuscitation and as well as inadequate pump flow. Recovery from a moderate hypoxic-ischemic insult is possible for most organs; however, neurologic recovery is frequently limited. Emergency ECMO and early coronary perfusion using percutaneous transluminal coronary angioplasty (PTCA) can result in good myocardial recovery. By using mild hypothermia in conjunction with ECMO during PTCA, a 2- to 5-fold increase in the rate of good neurologic recovery was achieved in a series reported by Nagao et al (Nagao, 2000).

Overall infection rates in temporary mechanical circulatory support have been reported to be as high as 30-40% (Patel, 2003). Immobilization, poor nutritional status, and indwelling catheters and tubes are all likely to contribute to the high incidence of infection. Although infrequent now, severe lower limb ischemia leading to amputation has occurred with femoral artery cannulation. Perfusion in the cannulated leg should be monitored closely for evidence of ischemia. Placement of a smaller, additional femoral artery cannula to perfuse the lower limb distal to the ECMO cannula has reduced the risk of this complication. Limb complications have been reported to occur in as many as 25% of patients prior to the use of the distal cannulation technique (Patel, 2003; Schwarz, 2003).

Complications
Cannula related
Perforated femoral or iliac artery
Retroperitoneal bleed
Aortic dissection
Limb ischemia
Poor venous drainage
Failure to cannulate
Hemorrhagic
Bleeding at cannulation site
Bleeding at surgical site
Pulmonary hemorrhage
Gastrointestinal hemorrhage
Cerebrovascular accident
Thromboembolic
Limb ischemia
Pulmonary infarction
Cerebrovascular accident
Insufficient perfusion
Ischemic brain injury
Renal failure
Hepatic failure
Multi-systemic organ dysfunction
Technical
Equipment failure
Hemolysis
Infection
Insufficient ventricular unloading
Ventricular dysfunction and pulmonary edema

Table 2. Complications associated with ECMO

Complications	Pediatric		Adult	
	n	%	n	%
Mechanical				
Air in circuit	21	3.5	4	2.2
Cannula problems	68	11.5	13	7.2
Clots: Bladder	31	5.1		
Bridge	19	3.2	2	1.1
Hemofilter	28	4.6	7	3.9
Oxygenator	60	10	13	7.2
Other	50	8.3	10	5.5
Cracks in pigtail connectors	5	0.8	5	2.8
Heat exchanger malfunction	1	0.2		
Other tubing rupture	4	0.7	2	1.1
Oxygenator failure	52	8.6	39	21.6
Pump malfunction	6	1	1	0.6
Raceway rupture	3	0.5		
Metabolic				
Glucose < 40 mg/dl	14	2.3	1	0.6
Glucose > 240 mg/dl	83	13.8	75	41.4
Hyperbilirubinemia (> 2 direct or > 15 total)	30	5	14	7.7
pH < 7.20	77	12.8	41	22.7
pH > 7.60	25	4.2	14	7.7
Neurologic				
Brain death clinically determined	70	11.6	27	14.9
CNS hemorrhage by US/CT	42	7	1	0.6
CNS infarction by US/CT	43	7.1	24	13.3
Seizures				
Clinically determined	69	11.4	7	3.9
EEG determined	32	5.3	1	0.6
Pulmonary				
Pneumothorax requiring treatment	15	2.5	7	3.9
Pulmonary hemorrhage	55	9.1	11	6.1
Renal				
CAVHD required	41	6.8	39	21.6
Hemofiltration required	170	28.2	22	12.1
Cardiovascular				
Cardiac arrhythmia	110	17.3	44	24.3
CPR required	48	8	12	6.6
Hypertension requiring vasodilators	74	12.3	13	7.2
Inotropes on ECMO	414	68.7	152	84
Myocardial stun by echocardiography	38	6.3	4	2.2
PDA: Bidirectional	2	0.3		
L->R	2	0.3		
R->L	2	0.3		
Tamponade: Blood	35	5.8	21	11.6

Complications	Pediatric		Adult	
	n	%	n	%
Serous	2	0.3		
Hemorrhagic				
Cannulation site bleeding	105	17.4	40	22.1
Disseminated intravascular coagulation	37	6.1	5	2.8
GI hemorrhage	19	3.2	7	3.9
Hemolysis (Hemoglobin > 50 mg/dl)	75	12.4	28	15.5
Surgical site bleeding	101	16.8	53	29.3
Infections				
Culture-proven infection	54	9	28	15.5
White blood cell > 1,500	6	1		

CAVHD = continuous arteriovenous hemodialysis, CNS = central nervous system, CPR = cardiopulmonary resuscitation, CT = computed tomography, EEG = electroencephalogram, GI = gastrointestinal, L->R = left to right shunt, R->L = right to left shunt, US = ultrasound.

Table 3. Complications reported to the ELSO Registry (1994 - July 2005)

In addition, intracardiac thrombus may form within a poorly contracting, nonejecting left ventricle or atrium because little blood reaches the left atrium with good right atrial drainage (Cohn, 2008). Because intracardiac thrombus may induce systemic embolism, thus serial echocardiogram should be followed up for early detection and ECMO patients do require low level heparinization to prevent this complication.

2.6 Outcomes of ECMO

The results of ECMO support are consistently related to the indication for institution of such therapy.

With respect to VV ECMO, Bartlett et al at the University of Michigan were reviewed in 1995 and reported that VV ECMO for respiratory failure provided survival to discharge in 88% of 586 cases of respiratory failure in neonates, 70% for 132 cases of respiratory failure in children and 56% for 146 cases of respiratory failure in adults (Bartlett, 1997). In 2008, the ELSO revealed similar results; specially 972 cases of ECMO support for respiratory failure were reported, of which 53% survived to discharge in the adult population (>18 years). Unfortunately, good quality randomized controlled trials of ECMO outcomes in the adult population are lacking. The incomplete CESAR (Conventional Ventilation or ECMO for Severe Adult Respiratory Failure) was a national randomized controlled trial in the United Kingdom funded by the National Health Service and the Health Technology Assessment Agency; preliminary results were recently released at the 37th Society of Critical Care Medicine Congress in Honolulu in February 2008. The hypothesis was that ECMO will improve survival without severe disability by 6 months post-randomization for patients with severe, but potentially reversible respiratory failure. Severe disability was defined as confined to bed and unable to dress or wash oneself. Suitable patients can be entered from any of the 96 participating hospitals and were randomized to either transfer to Glenfiele hospital for consideration of ECMO or continued conventional management. The conventional group underwent standard clinical practice in the UK. Recruitment was conducted from July 2001 to August 2006. Of the 90 patients assigned to receive ECMO, 22 did not receive ECMO, most often because they improved without it. Patient characteristics were well matched between groups. Of the patients randomly assigned to receive ECMO, 57 of 90 met the primary endpoint of survival or absence of severe disability at 6 months compared with 41 of 87 patients in the conventional ventilation group. This translated to a relative risk in favor of the ECMO group of 0.69 (95% confidence interval, 0.05–0.97; P = 0.03). A significant number of patients had failure of more than 3 organs in both groups (28 in the ECMO group and 27 in the conventional group). The benefit of ECMO was evident, regardless of age, duration of high-pressure ventilation, primary diagnosis at trial entry, and number of organs failing (Peek, 2006; Hitt, 2008).

With respect to VA ECMO, Bartlett et al at the University of Michigan were reviewed in 1995. Their experience with cardiac failure is somewhat smaller with a 33% survival rate in 31 adult patients and 48% survival in 105 pediatric patients (Bartlett, 1997). In 2008, ELSO revealed similar results that 474 patients were supported for cardiac failure of which only 33% survived to discharge. In addition, numerous studies have reported various results according to the disease diagnosis. The data reported to the ELSO registry has shown that myocarditis is associated with a better survival than other diagnosis, with almost three-fifths being successfully weaned from ECMO. Similarly, Acker reported that twenty seven (73.0%) of a group of 37 patients could be weaned from ECMO and 26 patients (70.3%) were discharged from the hospital (Acker, 2001). In this subgroup of patients, ECMO may be used as a bridge to recovery, bridge, or transplantation. Cardiac arrest and shock are the most common indications for ECMO in adults and the benefits of ECMO for cardiac arrest in adults were shown recently (Chen, 2008). Early implementation of ECMO can improve the survival rate to 30-40%, as described in multiple published series and the ELSO registry (Sung, 2006; Meurs, 2005). For acute myocardial infarction, cardiogenic shock is the leading cause of death in hospitalized adults. In these patients, ECMO alone has a limited effect on outcome, but when combined with emergency coronary revascularization by angioplasty, it may improve survival. Also, the concomitant use of an intra-aortic balloon pump with ECMO improves survival in patients with cardiogenic shock. The role of ECMO to provide post-cardiotomy support with severe cardiopulmonary dysfunction after cardiac surgery is well established. Mechanical circulatory support may be required in the post-operative period, either due to the inability to separate from cardiopulmonary bypass, or a progressive low cardiac output syndrome due to a number of factors, such as ventricular dysfunction, pulmonary hypertension, or intractable arrhythmias. The incidence of post-cardiotomy myocardial failure is 2-6% in adult cardiac surgical patients. Rousou et al. reported that 56% of a group of 16 patients survived ongoing post-operative ventricular fibrillation or electromechanical dissociation when ECMO was employed (Rousou, 1994). Similarly, 77% of a group of 13 patients described by Kawahito et al. successfully weaned off ECMO after circulatory collapse from ventricular fibrillation or electromechanical dissociation that was refractory to inotropic agents, IABP, and cardiopulmonary resuscitation (Kawahito, 1994). ECMO has been utilized in the cardiac catheterization laboratory for resuscitation during sudden cardiovascular collapse to provide temporary support for interventional procedures. In a small, retrospective study by Grambow et al., rapid initiation of ECMO (within 20 minutes) resulted in the rescue of patients in cardiogenic shock, but all patients who experienced cardiac arrest died despite ECMO and further interventions. Of those in shocks who were initially salvaged with ECMO, approximately 50% survived for 24 hours but only 25% to hospital discharge. Mortality after 24 hours was attributed to sepsis, multi-organ failure, or congestive heart failure (Grambow, 1994).

3. Our experiences and results

3.1 Study patients

Between May 2005 and December 2010, 402 ECMOs were implanted at the Samsung Medical Center and a retrospective review was performed. Of them, 79 patients were treated with PCPS during peri-intervention period for either refractory cardiac arrest or cardiogenic shock. Patients were considered to have refractory cardiac arrest only if aggressive attempts at resuscitation were unsuccessful in establishing a stable cardiac rhythm. Patients were placed on PCPS for cardiogenic shock if hypotension and peripheral hypoperfusion persist despite aggressive fluid replacement and inotropic support.

3.2 Technique of PCPS

Both femoral areas were draped under sterile conditions if PCPS was indicated. After the intravenous injection of 10 mg/kg of heparin, both the femoral artery and femoral vein were cannulated percutaneously using the Seldinger technique. In some patients, femoral cannulation was completed after an inguinal incision because of difficulties with the percutaneous cannulation. If in the cardiac catheterization, fluoroscopy may be used as well to facilitate guide-wire and cannulae placement. The PCPS could be inserted into all patients for whom it was intended. According to the patient's size, 14 to 21 Fr percutaneous femoral arterial cannulae (DLP; Medtronic Inc, Minneapolis, MN or RMI; Edwards Lifesciences, Irvine, CA) and 17 to 28 Fr percutaneous femoral long venous cannulae (DLP; Medtronic Inc, or RMI; Edwards Lifesciences) were used. In some patients, distal femoral arterial perfusion was performed using a central line catheter (Arrow International, Reading, PA) after distal femoral artery puncture to avoid ischemia of the distal lower leg. The PCPS was then started using the Capiox emergency bypass system (EBS; Terumo Inc, Tokyo, Japan), which comprises a centrifugal pump, a polypropylene hollow fiber membrane oxygenator, and a heparin-coated circuit (Fig 2). The most important benefit of this system is its autopriming, which requires less than five minutes to prime the circuit before use and does not require specially trained personnel. Once the femoral cannulation was established, the PCPS system could be run to stabilize the patient. No hypothermia was applied. If possible, we tried to maintain the hematocrit above 35%, the platelet count above 100,000 per μl and the activated clotting time (ACT) at 150 to 200 seconds to minimize complications of bleeding and thromboembolic complications. After weaning the patients from the PCPS, we surgically removed the femoral artery and venous cannulae and repaired the cannulation sites to avoid ischemic limb complications.

3.3 Results

The clinical characteristics of the patients are listed in Table 4. All patients received VA PCPS and 44 patients (55.7%) had IABP concomitantly, as shown in the Table 4. The data on complications and events are shown in Table 5.

Forty-seven patients (59.5%) were weaned from the PCPS in both groups. Twenty-two patients (48.9%) in the cardiac arrest group could be weaned from the PCPS; the mean duration for PCPS in these patients was 63.1 ± 60.1 (range, 1 to 226; median, 52) hours. Twenty five patients (73.5%) in cardiogenic shock group were weaned from the PCPS; the mean duration for PCPS in these patients was 71.4 ± 66.2 (range, 1 to 306; median, 57) hours. Thirty three patients (41.8%) were discharged from the hospital; fifteen patients (33.3%) were in the cardiac arrest group and eighteen patients (50.0%) were in the cardiogenic shock

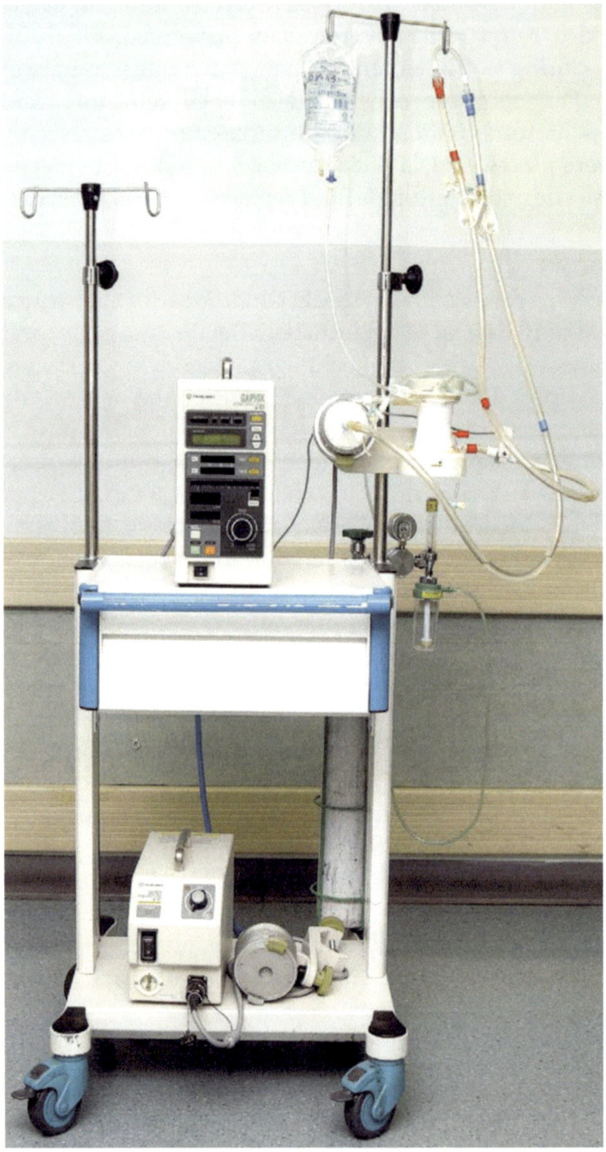

Fig. 2. The percutaneous cardiopulmonary support system used at our institution. It consists of a pump console, flowmeter, back-up console, and a holder for the centrifugal pump and oxygenator module with a drive motor. This system can be transported using a cart or clamped onto the bed. The emergency bypass system circuit, which consists of the centrifugal pump, oxygenator, and tubing, is sterilely packed.

	Refractory cardiac arrest	Cardiogenic shock
Patients	45	34
Age (years)	66.6 ± 12.8	65.5 ± 11.7
Male : Female	35 : 10	26 : 8
Timing of PCPS insertion		
Before PCI	24	14
During PCI	10	3
After PCI	11	17
Location of PCPS insertion		
Catheterization room	17	24
Intensive care unit	8	10
Emergency room	16	
Ward	4	
Concomitant use of IABP	22	22
Duration of PCPS (hours)	63.1 ± 60.1 (1 ~ 226)	71.4 ± 66.2 (1 ~ 306)
Weaning (%)	22 (48.9%)	25 (73.5%)
Survived to discharge (%)	15 (33.3%)	18 (50.0%)

PCI = percutaneous coronary intervention, PCPS = percutaneous cardiopulmonary support, IABP = intra-aortic balloon pump.

Table 4. Clinical characteristics

Complications	No.
Limb ischemia	8
Cannula site bleeding requiring revision	2
Cardiac tamponade requiring pericardiocentesis	2
Pulmonary hemorrhage	1
Hemothorax	1
Pneumothorax	1
Hemopneumothorax	1

Table 5. Complications associated with PCPS

group. There was no statistical difference in weaning from PCPS and survival discharge between the groups.

We divided 79 patients according to the timing of insertion, as follows: group A was instituted before coronary intervention; group B was instituted during intervention; and group C was instituted after intervention. In group A, 25 (65.8%) of 38 patients were weaned from the PCPS and 18 (47.4%) patients survived to discharge; In group B, 8 (61.5%) of 13 patients were weaned from the PCPS and all patients survived to discharge; In group C, 14 (50%) of 28 patients were weaned from the PCPS and 10 (35.7%) patients survived to discharge. There was no statistical difference in weaning from PCPS and survival discharge between the groups.

4. Conclusion

Our results show that PCPS may be a feasible option as a procedural support during coronary intervention. Moreover, we suggest that rescue PCPS combined with early coronary revascularization by angioplasty may improve survival when acute coronary syndrome results in circulatory collapse, and PCPS should be considered in patients with no definite contraindications. However, further evaluation and investigation are needed because the limitations of the study included the absence of a control group for comparison and selection bias.

5. Acknowledgment

The author would like to acknowledge Mrs. Nam Kyung Choi for her dedicated assistance of manuscript editing and English revision.

6. References

Acker MA. (2001). Mechanical Circulatory Support for Patients With Acute-Fulminant Myocarditis. *Ann Thorac Surg*, 71:S73–6. ISSN 0003-4975

Aiyagari RM.; Rocchini AP. Remenapp RT. & Graziano JN. (2006) Decompression of the left atrium during extracorporeal membrane oxygenation using a transseptal cannula incorporated into the circuit. *Crit Care Med*, 34(10):2603-6. ISSN 0090-3493

Bartlett RH.; Gazzaniga AB. Jefferies MR. Huxtable RF. Haiduc NJ. Fong SW. (1976). Extracorporeal membrane oxygenation (ECMO) cardiopulmonary support in infancy. *Trans Am Soc Artif Intern Organs*, 22:80-93.

Bartlett RH. (1997) Extracorporeal life support registry report 1995. *ASAIO J*, 43:104–7, ISSN 1058-2916

Chen YS.; Lin JW. Yu HY. Ko WJ. Jerng JS. Chang WT. Chen WJ. Huang SC. Chi NH. Wang CH. Chen LC. Tsai PR. Wang SS. Hwang JJ. & Lin FY. (2008). Cardiopulmonary resuscitation with assisted extracorporeal life-support versus conventional cardiopulmonary resuscitation in adults with in-hospital cardiac arrest: an observational study and propensity analysis. *Lancet*, 372:554–561. ISSN 0140-6736

Cooper DS. Jacobs JP. Moore L. Stock A. Gaynor JW. Chancy T. Parpard M. Griffin DA. Owens T. Checchia PA. Thiagarajan RR. Spray TL. & Ravishankar C. (2007) Cardiac extracorporeal life support: state of the art in 2007. Cardiol Young, 17 Suppl. 2: 104–115. ISSN 1047-9511

Cohn, LH. (2008). *Cardiac surgery in the adult 3rd edition*, McGraw-Hill Education, http://cardiacsurgery.ctsnetbooks.org/

Ganslmeier P.; Philipp A. Rupprecht L. Diez C, Arlt M. Mueller T. Pfister K. Hilker M. & Schmid C. (2011). Percutaneous cannulation for extracorporeal life support. *Thorac Cardiov Surg*, 59: 103-7. ISSN 0171-6425

Grambow DW.; Deeb GM. Pavlides GS. Margulis A. O'Neill WW. & Bates ER. (1994) Emergent percutaneous cardiopulmonary bypass in patients having cardiovascular collapse in the cardiac catheterization laboratory. *Am J Cardiol*, 73:872-5. ISSN 0002-9149

Gravlee GP.; Davis RF. Stammers AH. & Ungerleider RM. (2008) Cardiopulmonary bypass principles and practice. 3rd edition, Lippincott Williams & Wilkins, ISBN 978-0-7817-6815-3, United States of America

Hitt E. (2008), CESAR trial: extracorporeal membrane oxygenation improves survival in patients with severe respiratory failure. *Medscape Medical News www.medscape.com;* [accessed 21.05.08]

Hill JD.; De Leval MR. Fallat RJ. Bramson ML. Eberhart RC. Schulte HD. Osborn JJ. Barber R. & Gerbode F. (1972) Acute respiratory insufficiency. Treatment with prolonged extracorporeal oxygenation. *J Thorac Cardiovasc Surg*, 64(4):551-62. ISSN 0022-5223

Kawahito K.; Ino T. Adachi H. Ide H. Mizuhara A. & Yamaguchi A. (1994) Heparin coated percutaneous cardiopulmonary support for the treatment of circulatory collapse after cardiac surgery. ASAIO J, 40:972-6. ISSN 1058-2916

Koenig PR.; Ralston MA. Kimball TR. Meyer RA. Daniels SR. & Schwartz DC. (1993). Balloon atrial septostomy for left ventricular decompression in patients receiving extracorporeal membrane oxygenation for myocardial failure. *J Pediatr*, 122:S95-9. ISSN 0022-3476

Kolobow T.; Solca M. Gattinoni L. & Pesenti A. (1981) Adult respiratory distress syndrome (ARDS): why did ECMO fail? *Int J Artif Organs*. 4(2):58-9. ISSN 0391-3988

Kurusz M.; Zwischenberger JB. (2002) Percutaneous cardiopulmonary bypass for cardiac emergencies. *Perfusion*, 17:269-77. ISSN 0267-6591

Meurs KV.; Lally KP. Peek G. & Zwischenberger JB. (2005) ECMO: Extracorporeal cardiopulmonary support in critical care. 3rd edition, ELSO, ISBN 0-9656756-2-9, United States of America

Marasco SF.; Lukas G. McDonald M. McMillan J. & Ihle B. (2008). Review of ECMO (extra corporeal membrane oxygenation) support in critically ill adult patients. *Heart Lung Circ*, 17 Suppl 4:S41-7. ISSN 1443-9506

Nagao K.; Hayashi N. Kanmatsuse K. Arima K, Ohtsuki J, Kikushima K,.& Watanabe I (2000) Cardiopulmonary cerebral resuscitation using emergency cardiopulmonary bypass, coronary reperfusion therapy and mild hypothermia in patients with cardiac arrest outside the hospital. *J Am Coll Cardiol*, Sep;36(3):776-83. ISSN 0735-1097

Patel H.; & Pagani FD. (2003) Extracorporeal mechanical circulatory assist. *Cardiol Clin*. 21(1):29-41. ISSN: 0733-8651

Peek GJ.; Clemens F. Elbourne D. Firmin R. Hardy P. Hibbert C. Killer H. Mugford M. Thalanany M. Tiruvoipati R. Truesdale A. & Wilson A. (2006) CESAR: conventional ventilatory support vs. extracorporeal membrane oxygenation for severe adult respiratory failure. *BMC Health Serv Res*, 23(6):163, http://creativecommons.org/liscences/by/2.0

Rousou JA.; Engelman RM. Flack JE 3rd. Deaton DW. & Owen SG. (1994) Emergency cardiopulmonary bypass in the cardiac surgical unit can be a lifesaving measure in post-operative cardiac arrest. *Circulation*, 90:1280-4. ISSN 0009-7322

Schwarz B.; Mair P. Margreiter J. Pomaroli A. Hoermann C. Bonatti J. & Lindner KH. (2003) Experience with percutaneous venoarterial cardiopulmonary bypass for emergency circulatory support. *Crit Care Med*, 31(3):758-64. ISSN 0090-3493

Sung K. Lee YT. Park PW. Park KH. Jun TG. Yang JH. & Ha YK. (2006) Improved survival after cardiac arrest using emergent autopriming percutaneous cardiopulmonary support. *Ann Thorac Surg*, 82 suppl 2:651-6. ISSN 0003-4975

8

Coronary Angiography Before and After Renal Transplantation

Mihas Kodenchery, Samrat Bhat, Mohamed El-Ghoroury, Hiroshi Yamasaki and Peter A. McCullough[1]
St. John Providence Health System, St. John Hospital and Medical Center, Detroit,
[1]Providence Park Heart Institute, Novi
USA

1. Introduction

Cardiovascular diseases are the leading cause of morbidity and mortality in both dialysis dependent patients and those either waiting for or following up after renal transplantation. Concerns about the risk of contrast-induced acute kidney injury (CI-AKI) associated with coronary angiography in patients with stage 4 or 5 chronic kidney disease (CKD) have sometimes resulted in coronary angiography being delayed until after transplantation. Pretransplant cardiovascular disease is a well established risk factor for post transplant cardiovascular disease and cardiovascular mortality. In addition, post transplant dyslipidemia, [1-3] hypertension, [4-7] allograft dysfunction, delayed or slow graft function[8] and post transplant erythrocytosis [9, 10] are some of the more specific factors that increase cardiovascular risk in renal transplant recipients as compared to the general population. Prompt diagnosis and treatment of cardiovascular disease in CKD and end stage renal disease population prior to transplant is aimed to reduce cardiovascular morbidity and mortality in the perioperative period and beyond. Several studies have demonstrated that left ventricular function and hypertrophy improve after renal transplantation. Ferreira et al prospectively studied 24 patients with end stage renal disease and demonstrated a significant decrease in hypertension, reduction in left ventricular hypertrophy and dilation, and improvement in systolic function after successful renal transplantation.[11] Wali et al followed up 103 renal patients with left ventricular ejection fraction less than 40% with radionuclide ventriculography and renal transplantation and found the mean left ventricular ejection fraction increased from 31.6% to 52.2% at 12 months after transplantation. A longer pre-transplantation interval decreased the likelihood of normalization of ejection fraction. New York Heart Association functional status improved significantly concordant with an improvement of ejection fraction. These studies indicate that renal transplantation should not be withheld for patients with severe cardiac dysfunction as both left ventricular function and survival are expected to improve with renal transplantation.[12]

This chapter will describe the approach to patients with CKD who are being considered for renal transplantation. Careful consideration to the background history, risk of cardiovascular disease, and risk of atherosclerotic events with the transplant operation will be discussed. The risks and benefits of coronary revascularization will be outlined in the context of a patient with very little renal function remaining at the time of evaluation. Finally, we will summarize the major caveats for coronary angiography in patients who have received a kidney transplant and are being evaluated for new symptoms.

2. Preoperative cardiovascular evaluation prior to renal transplantation

Cardiovascular screening is recommended in certain groups of high risk CKD patients prior to transplantation.[13] These include persons with diabetes, men over age 45 years, women over 55 years, previous history of ischemic heart disease, an abnormal electrocardiogram, left ventricular dysfunction, smoking history and duration of dialysis more than 2 years.[14] Controversies exist regarding the ideal screening test for coronary artery disease among exercise stress test, dobutamine stress echocardiogram, and myocardial perfusion studies. Lentine et al in 2008 analyzed the United States Renal Data System on 27,786 eligible patients for renal transplantation and concluded that 46.3% of patients underwent cardiac evaluation prior to transplantation, of whom 9.5% required coronary revascularization. Among patients transplanted without cardiovascular evaluation, the three-year incidence of post transplant acute myocardial infarction was 3% in lower risk group and 10% in higher risk group.[15]

All patients should be assessed for ischemic heart disease before renal transplantation. The minimum workup required includes a history, physical examination, electrocardiogram, and a chest radiograph.[13] Assessment of functional status is critical. In general, if a patient can sustain a moderate or high work rate (> 5 metabolic equivalents of work) without symptoms, then there is a low risk of perioperative myocardial infarction or cardiovascular death. The pretest probability of coronary artery disease plays a major role in determination of cardiac testing. The Canadian society of transplantation recommends noninvasive testing for symptomatic patients or patients with prior history of coronary artery disease, as well as asymptomatic patients with diabetes mellitus or multiple risk factors for coronary artery disease.[17] The choice of noninvasive testing has been a matter of debate with nuclear scintigraphy showing a high negative predictive value and performing well in diabetic patients.[18-21] Marwick et al has shown that the sensitivity of dipyridamole thallium scintigraphy in patients with CKD is lower than that of controls.[22] The speculated reasons for this observation are reduced coronary flow reserve, left ventricular hypertrophy and interstitial cardiac fibrosis. Results with stress echocardiography have been found to be comparable to nuclear imaging, [23, 24] and the expertise of technical and physician personnel often plays the major role in determining which test will be done at each institution. The Society further recommends coronary angiography be performed in patients with a positive noninvasive test or in very high risk patients irrespective of a noninvasive test. De Lima and colleagues have shown that coronary angiography is the best predictor of cardiac events in renal transplant candidates when compared to clinical risk stratification and non invasive testing.[16] Some centers advocate angiography in most transplant candidates with diabetes, while others pursue cardiac catheterization only in candidates with positive screening examination.[25] Low risk patients, asymptomatic patients with a negative noninvasive test result or noncritical disease on angiography on appropriate medical therapy, or who have undergone successful intervention can be considered eligible for transplantation without any further evaluation. Coronary angiography remains the gold standard for evaluation of coronary arteries among patients with positive screening tests or high risk of cardiovascular events. It is complicated by its invasive nature and the risk of contrast nephropathy and cholesterol embolism which will be discussed below.[14] The yield of coronary angiography in this population is high. De Lima et al in 2003 found that about 42% of patients in this group had significant coronary artery stenosis (more than 70% by visual estimation). Significant coronary artery stenosis was also the most significant predictor of cardiac events at 48 months.[16] A suggested approach to preoperative cardiovascular assessment and non invasive stress testing in CKD patients prior to renal transplantation is proposed by Karthikeyan et al in Figure 1.[39] Abnormal results on non invasive stress tests such as coronary CT angiography and myocardial perfusion imaging often need invasive coronary angiography for diagnosis and possible intervention. This will lead to unnecessary delay, contrast and radiation exposure. So initial invasive coronary angiography is preferable in patients with multiple co-morbidities and risk factors and those with intermediate to high pre-test probability for non-invasive stress testing.

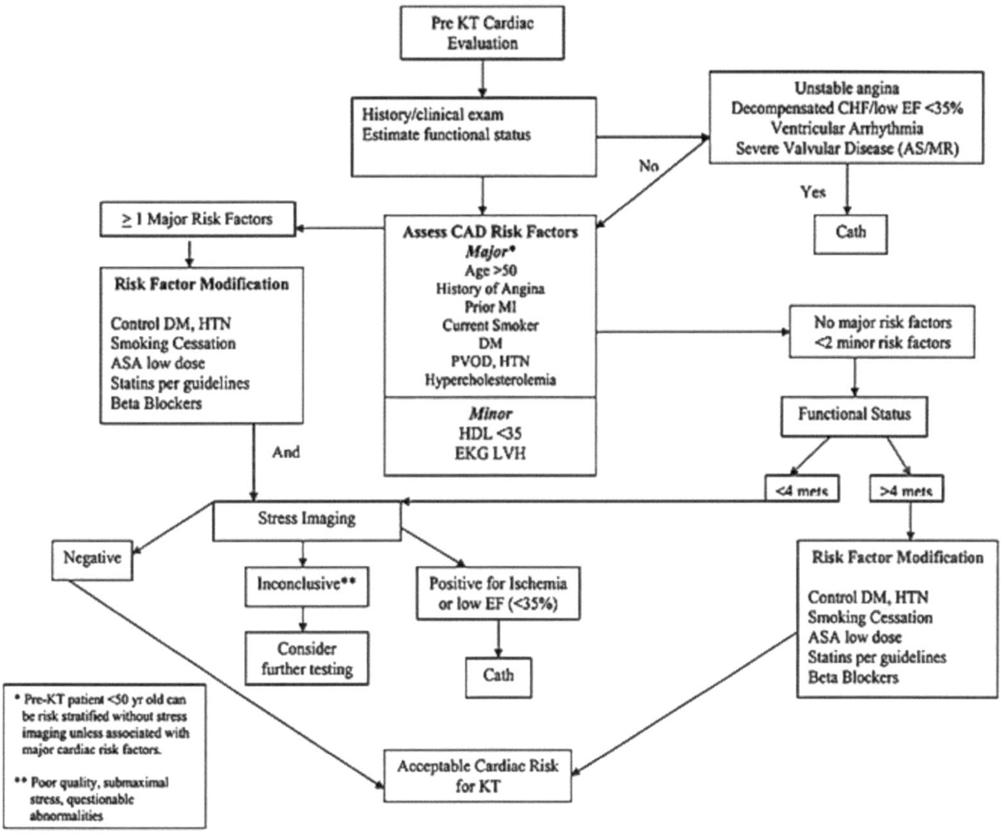

Fig. 1.
Adapted from Cardiology Review (2009); 5: page 183

3. Risk and benefits of coronary angiography in transplant recipients

The major risks of coronary angiography in renal transplant candidates are CI-AKI and cholesterol embolism which may hasten the progression to dialysis. In the general population, the risk of CI-AKI is 3.3 – 14.5%.[26] Risk factors include reduced renal filtration function, older age, diabetes, congestive heart failure and preprocedure myocardial infarction.[27] Acute kidney injury requiring dialysis is rare but may occur in 0.44 to 0.77% of patients. This development is associated with a significant in hospital mortality rate of 35.7 to 39%. The risk of CI-AKI is higher among pretransplant candidates because of their underlying advanced chronic kidney disease and is estimated to be 4-50% with 8-26% eventually requiring dialysis at some point prior to transplantation.[28] Gruberg et al reported that 4.9% of patients with baseline creatinine more that 1.8mg/dl required temporary dialysis after coronary angiography.[29] Cholesterol embolism occurs from disruption of vascular endothelial plaques resulting in release of cholesterol crystals into the blood stream. In severe forms, it may lead to localized inflammation and fibrosis most commonly seen in the skin, digits, kidney and eye. The reported incidence after coronary angiography is as high as 2% and manifests as persistent elevation of creatinine up to 3 weeks after the procedure.[30] The relative contribution of subtle degrees of cholesterol embolism without peripheral signs to AKI is unknown. Further studies are warranted to assess the exact impact of this entity on pretransplant candidates undergoing coronary angiography and evaluate potential measures to reduce their incidence.

4. Safety of coronary angiography in pretransplant candidates

Contrast-induced AKI remains an important and potentially avoidable complication after coronary angiography and coronary and vascular interventions.[40] A direct inverse relationship exists between a patient's estimated glomerular filtration rate (eGFR) and their risk of contrast-induced AKI.[41] In the setting of severely reduced renal filtration, the risk of sustained intrarenal vasoconstriction, tubular and peritubular stasis of contrast agents, cellular toxicity and permanent loss of functioning nephrons are greatly increased.[42] Because coronary events are a major cause of perioperative risk and postoperative morbidity in patients considered for renal transplantation, coronary angiography is frequently performed prior to transplantation, particularly in patients with a history of angina or provocable myocardial ischemia on stress testing.[43] If coronary disease becomes a concern after renal transplantation, the intravascular administration of a contrast agent is associated with a high risk (>15%) of contrast-induced AKI in the transplanted kidney.[44] Thus it is reasonable to consider upfront contrast-induced AKI in the native kidneys before transplantation. Kumar and co-workers reported on the intermediate-term outcomes of 76 predialysis patients with CKD undergoing coronary angiography prior to renal transplantation.[45] The mean eGFR before contrast exposure was 12.5 ± 3.4 ml/min/1.73 m^2 and the mean iodinated contrast load administered was 55.7 ± 50.2 ml. In total, 25 of the 76 patients (32.9%) who had coronary angiography subsequently underwent transplantation; 22 of the patients who underwent transplantation had not received any form of dialysis beforehand. Exposure to contrast media did not seem to hasten progression to end-stage renal disease. The cumulative dialysis-free survival among all 76 patients who had coronary angiography was 89.1% at 6 months post coronary angiography. A number of factors probably worked together to produce these excellent results and a 'safe landing' after coronary angiography. Patients were stable and relatively young (mean age 56.3 years). Other factors that contributed to favorable outcome include discontinuation of all potentially nephrotoxic drugs 24 hours before the angiogram, use of statins, generous hydration prior to procedure, use of N-acetylcysteine and iso-osmolar contrast and the use of biplane angiography.

Statins have pleiotropic effects and their anti-oxidant properties may play a role against the oxidative stress involved in the pathogenesis of contrast induced AKI.[46,47] Hydration prior to administration of contrast may have multiple theoretical benefits for the kidney which include decreased activity of renin angiotensin system, downregulation of tubuloglomerular feedback, augmentation of diuresis and sodium excretion, dilution of contrast media, prevention of renal cortical vasospasm, reduced pre-constriction of vessels, avoidance of tubular obstruction and reduction of endothelin and other renal vasoconstrictors. [48] Reactive oxygen species generated by radiocontrast in the renal tubules and peritubular space are believed to be central in the pathogenesis of CI-AKI. The potential benefit of N-acetylcysteine has been reported in multiple trials including the Acetylcysteine to Prevent Angiography-Related Renal Tissue Injury trial.[49,50] But the recently completed, large Acetylcysteine for Contrast-Induced Nephropathy Trial reported by Berwanger and colleagues has cast a doubt on the effectiveness of this agent to prevent this complication. Iodixanol is an iso-osmolar, non ionic dimer used in coronary angiography. It is associated with a significantly lower incidence of AKI after contrast exposure especially in patients with CKD.[51] Finally, biplane angiography is associated with a reduction in angiographic contrast volume in patients with CKD. [52, 53] Staging complicated intervention can decrease the contrast volume used in a single session and thus decrease the risk of AKI provided a sufficient long interim time period is observed (>10 days). Kumar and colleagues have demonstrated that the prudent use of intravascular iodinated contrast agent and coronary revascularization—with due attention to renal protection—did not hasten the progression to end-stage renal disease. Prevention of contrast-induced AKI is almost certainly a product of multimodality prophylaxis after careful patient selection and pre-, intra-, and post-procedural management.[49] **Table 1** lists caveats concerning nephrotoxic medications and other drugs used in routine management with suggestions to possibly reduce adverse events with coronary angiography.

Medications	**Cardiovascular and Renal Effects**	**Recommendation**
NSAIDs	Inhibition of production of vasodilatory prostaglandins leading to vasoconstriction of afferent arterioles, increased risk of AKI, fluid retention, and the development of heart failure	Discontinue at least 3 days prior to contrast exposure, switch to narcotics or alternative pain treatment
Antihypertensive medications *Special mention ACE inhibitors	Reduce the decline in renal function Can impair tubuloglomerular feedback	Continue Consider holding before angiography
Loop, thiazide, and other diuretics	Volume depletion, electrolyte abnormalities	Hold day of procedure
Aminoglycosides	Interstitial and medullary renal injury	Avoid if possible, close monitoring by levels if no alternative
Vancomycin	Enhance nephrotoxic potential of other nephrotoxic medications, direct chemotoxicity	Continue, closely monitor drug levels

Medications	Cardiovascular and Renal Effects	Recommendation
Amphotericin B	Acute renal vasoconstriction and distal tubular epithelial damage, loss of concentrating ability	Avoid if possible. Intensive monitoring of renal function, hydration and acid base status if no alternative or switch to newer less nephrotoxic agents such as caspofungin
Metformin	Increased risk of lactic acidosis if continued after glomerular filtration rate drops	Hold the day of contrast procedure, and generally recommended for another 10 days
Statins	May be protective against contrast-induced AKI	Continue
Cyclosporine, tacrolimus	Hypertension, dyslipidemia, diabetes mellitus, powerful inhibitor of CYP450 isozyme 3A4 and increases levels of some statins including lovastatin, atorvastatin, and simvastatin	Hold for three days prior to procedure. CCB and ACEI preferred choice for hypertension. To treat dyslipidemia, consider lowering dose, change to tacrolimus, diet control and/or lipid-lowering drugs usually statin with preference to pravastatin or rosuvastatin therapy. Watch for statin induced muscle toxicity/ rhabdomyolysis. Avoid toxic levels of cyclosporine and monitor blood glucose closely. Initiate early therapy for post-transplantation diabetes mellitus.
Sirolimus	Dyslipidemia, no significant impact on hypertension or post-transplant diabetes mellitus. It may interact with drugs metabolized by CYP450 isozyme system.	Treat dyslipidemia with diet control plus lipid-lowering drug therapy usually statins with preference to pravastatin or rosuvastatin. Consider lowering dose and/or change to alternative immune-suppressant drug if resistant dyslipidemia.
Corticosteroids	Hypertension, dyslipidemia, hyperglycemia, diabetes mellitus	Treat hypertension with CCB, ACEI or beta-blockers. Treat dyslipidemia with diet control plus lipid-lowering drug therapy. Monitor blood sugar levels closely and initiate early therapy for post transplantation diabetes mellitus. Use of lower dosing, if possible.
Mycophenolate mofetil and Azathioprine	Both pose low cardiometabolic risks.	Monitoring for hypertension, diabetes mellitus and dyslipidemia when used in conjunction with any of the above mentioned immunosuppressant drugs.

Table 1. Common medications and caveats with respect to coronary angiography in renal transplant candidates or recipients.

5. Coronary revascularization in transplant candidates

Jones et al divided 250 transplant candidates based on coronary angiography into group 1 with less than 50% stenosis, group 2 with more than 50% stenosis in 1 vessel, and group 3 with more than 50% stenosis in 2 or more vessels. Survival was significantly worse in group 3 when compared to groups 1 and 2. However survival was much better in patients who received transplantation in all 3 groups. Therefore severe coronary artery disease should not delay or disqualify a CKD patient from receiving renal transplantation.[31] Coronary intervention in CKD patients is associated with multiple complicated issues that determine the outcome. Dialysis patients with coronary stenosis of more than 70% have a higher risk of cardiac events and death than patients without coronary artery lesions.[14] The Coronary Artery Revascularization Prophylaxis (CARP) trial examined the impact of coronary revascularization in patients requiring major vascular surgery. Revascularization was not associated with any benefit in survival except in patients with left main coronary artery disease. Similarly, the American College of Physicians does not recommend prophylactic revascularization of asymptomatic patients undergoing noncardiac surgery, stressing the fact that asymptomatic low risk pretransplant candidates do not need coronary revascularization for renal transplantation.[32] Kasiske et al suggested that revascularization of significant coronary artery stenosis should occur prior to renal transplantation.[13] The prolonged survival benefit was confined to left main coronary artery stenosis, left main equivalent disease, triple vessel disease with abnormal left ventricular function, and two vessel disease with more than 75% stenosis of the left anterior descending artery. Revascularization is recommended for left main disease and its equivalents and symptomatic patients refractory to medical treatments.[33] Manske et al randomized 26 diabetic pretransplant candidates with significant coronary artery disease into revascularization and medical therapy groups prior to renal transplantation. The outcome of patients managed medically was significantly inferior to those treated by revascularization. Only 2 out of 13 revascularized patients had cardiovascular end points when compared to 10 out of 13 in the medically managed group.[34] Coronary revascularization in renal patients is associated with a three fold increase in mortality when compared to patients not requiring renal replacement therapy.[35] Compared to percutaneous coronary intervention, coronary artery bypass grafting is associated with approximately three time greater short term risk of postoperative hemodialysis dependence among non-hemodialysis dependent CKD patients.[36] Similarly, survival rates are significantly lower in dialysis patients at 2 years when compared to the general population.[35] Percutaneous coronary intervention is shown to have a better in hospital and 30 day survival in dialysis patients when compared to coronary artery bypass surgery. However coronary artery bypass surgery has better long term survival.[37] It also appears that there is a higher rate of restenosis of revascularized vessels in patients with CKD.[38] The use of drug eluting stents may decrease the incidence of restenosis, however these stents mandate the use of aspirin and clopidogrel for at least 1 year as per the present guidelines. Premature discontinuation of an antiplatelet agent is associated with significant risk of stent thrombosis. Thus, the combined use of aspirin and clopidogrel may delay renal transplantation. For that reason, if coronary intervention is contemplated, bare metal stent, balloon angioplasty or bypass grafting should be considered if the anatomy is feasible.[39]

6. Angiography in patients after renal transplantation

Coronary angiography continues to be the gold standard for identifying coronary artery disease even in post transplant patients. Renal transplantation does not protect one from the adverse effect of contrast on the kidney. Transplant recipients are at high risk of CI-AKI due to chronic allograft dysfunction and the high prevalence of diabetes and concomitant use of immunosuppressants like cyclosporine and tacrolimus. Agrawal et al found a 15.4% incidence of contrast induced nephropathy among post transplant patients undergoing coronary angiography. Intravenous hydration, bicarbonate infusion, N-acetylcysteine and the use of iso-osmolar contrast agent show varying efficacy in reducing its incidence.[44] Thus, the renal transplant recipient, appears to be at enhanced risk for CI-AKI compared to patients with similar glomerular filtration and bilateral native kidneys. Renal transplant recipients should be informed of this increased risk and unnecessary or optional contrast exposure should be avoided.

7. Conclusions

There are specific cardiovascular benefits to early renal transplantation in CKD patients including improved left ventricular function, enhanced overall functional capacity and quality of life, and decreased morbidity and mortality. Delay in renal transplantation and longer duration of hemodialysis decreases the likelihood of normalization of cardiac systolic dysfunction after transplantation. CKD patient with cardiac dysfunction should be thoroughly evaluated for underlying ischemia and aggressively treated with anti-anginals, angiotensin converting enzyme inhibitors or angiotensin receptor blockers and beta blockers before, perioperatively, and after renal transplantation. Every effort must be made to promote early renal transplantation when feasible with a living donor.[12] An early cardiovascular assessment, preferably by cautious coronary angiography utilizing the above mentioned renoprotective measures should be performed if indicated, to decrease the cardiovascular event rate associated with transplant surgery. A multidisciplinary approach involving a cardiologist, an interventionist, a nephrologist, a cardiothoracic and transplant surgeon can expedite the process and thus improve post transplant morbidity, mortality, functional capacity and overall quality of life.

8. Abbreviations

KT = Kidney transplantation,
CAD = Coronary artery disease,
CHF = Congestive Heart Failure,
EKG = Electrocardiogram,
EF = Ejection Fraction,
MI = Myocardial infarction,
DM = Diabetes mellitus,
AS = Aortic stenosis,
MR = Mitral regurgitation,
LDL = Low density lipoprotein,
PVOD = Peripheral vascular disease,

CI-AKI = Contrast induced acute kidney injury,
NSAIDs = Non steroidal anti-inflammatory drugs,
AKI = acute kidney injury,
CCB = calcium channel blockers,
ACEI = angiotensin converting enzyme inhibitors,
eGFR = estimated glomerular filtration rate,
MDRD = Modification of Diet in Renal Disease,
AKI = Acute Kidney Injury,
CKD = Chronic Kidney Disease,
ESRD = End Stage Renal Disease

9. References

[1] Kasiske BL, Vazquez MA, Harmon WE, et al. Recommendations for the outpatient surveillance of renal transplant recipients. American Society of Transplantation. *J. Am. Soc. Nephrol.* 2000;11 Suppl 15:S1-86.

[2] Meier-Kriesche H, Baliga R, Kaplan B. Decreased renal function is a strong risk factor for cardiovascular death after renal transplantation. *Transplantation.* 2003;75(8):1291-1295.

[3] Mortazavi M, Tohidi M, Rahbani-Nobar M. Evaluation of serum levels of lipids and lipoproteins in kidney-transplanted patients. *Transplant. Proc.* 2001;33(5):2689-2690.

[4] Pérez Fontán M, Rodríguez-Carmona A, García Falcón T, Fernández Rivera C, Valdés F. Early immunologic and nonimmunologic predictors of arterial hypertension after renal transplantation. *Am. J. Kidney Dis.* 1999;33(1):21-28.

[5] Zeier M, Mandelbaum A, Ritz E. Hypertension in the transplanted patient. *Nephron.* 1998;80(3):257-268.

[6] Kobashigawa JA, Kasiske BL. Hyperlipidemia in solid organ transplantation. *Transplantation.* 1997;63(3):331-338.

[7] Guidi E, Menghetti D, Milani S, et al. Hypertension may be transplanted with the kidney in humans: a long-term historical prospective follow-up of recipients grafted with kidneys coming from donors with or without hypertension in their families. *J. Am. Soc. Nephrol.* 1996;7(8):1131-1138.

[8] First MR, Neylan JF, Rocher LL, Tejani A. Hypertension after renal transplantation. *J. Am. Soc. Nephrol.* 1994;4(8 Suppl):S30-36.

[9] Kasiske BL. Risk factors for accelerated atherosclerosis in renal transplant recipients. *Am. J. Med.* 1988;84(6):985-992.

[10] Wickre CG, Norman DJ, Bennison A, Barry JM, Bennett WM. Postrenal transplant erythrocytosis: a review of 53 patients. *Kidney Int.* 1983;23(5):731-737.

[11] Ferreira SRC, Moisés VA, Tavares A, Pacheco-Silva A. Cardiovascular effects of successful renal transplantation: a 1-year sequential study of left ventricular morphology and function, and 24-hour blood pressure profile. *Transplantation.* 2002;74(11):1580-1587.

[12] Wali RK, Wang GS, Gottlieb SS, et al. Effect of kidney transplantation on left ventricular systolic dysfunction and congestive heart failure in patients with end-stage renal disease. *J. Am. Coll. Cardiol.* 2005;45(7):1051-1060.

[13] Kasiske BL, Cangro CB, Hariharan S, et al. The evaluation of renal transplantation candidates: clinical practice guidelines. *Am. J. Transplant.* 2001;1 Suppl 2:3-95.

[14] Pilmore H. Cardiac assessment for renal transplantation. *Am. J. Transplant.* 2006;6(4):659-665.

[15] Lentine KL, Schnitzler MA, Brennan DC, et al. Cardiac evaluation before kidney transplantation: a practice patterns analysis in Medicare-insured dialysis patients. *Clin J Am Soc Nephrol.* 2008;3(4):1115-1124.

[16] De Lima JJG, Sabbaga E, Vieira MLC, et al. Coronary angiography is the best predictor of events in renal transplant candidates compared with noninvasive testing. *Hypertension.* 2003;42(3):263-268.

[17] Knoll G, Cockfield S, Blydt-Hansen T, et al. Canadian Society of Transplantation: consensus guidelines on eligibility for kidney transplantation. *CMAJ.* 2005;173(10):S1-25.

[18] Patel AD, Abo-Auda WS, Davis JM, et al. Prognostic value of myocardial perfusion imaging in predicting outcome after renal transplantation. *Am. J. Cardiol.* 2003;92(2):146-151.

[19] Feola M, Biggi A, Ribichini F, et al. Predicting cardiac events with Tl201 dipyridamole myocardial scintigraphy in renal transplant recipients. *J. Nephrol.* 2002;15(1):48-53.

[20] Le A, Wilson R, Douek K, et al. Prospective risk stratification in renal transplant candidates for cardiac death. *Am. J. Kidney Dis.* 1994;24(1):65-71.

[21] Derfler K, Kletter K, Balcke P, Heinz G, Dudczak R. Predictive value of thallium-201-dipyridamole myocardial stress scintigraphy in chronic hemodialysis patients and transplant recipients. *Clin. Nephrol.* 1991;36(4):192-202.

[22] Marwick TH, Steinmuller DR, Underwood DA, et al. Ineffectiveness of dipyridamole SPECT thallium imaging as a screening technique for coronary artery disease in patients with end-stage renal failure. *Transplantation.* 1990;49(1):100-103.

[23] West JC, Napoliello DA, Costello JM, et al. Preoperative dobutamine stress echocardiography versus cardiac arteriography for risk assessment prior to renal transplantation. *Transpl. Int.* 2000;13 Suppl 1:S27-30.

[24] Herzog CA, Marwick TH, Pheley AM, et al. Dobutamine stress echocardiography for the detection of significant coronary artery disease in renal transplant candidates. *Am. J. Kidney Dis.* 1999;33(6):1080-1090.

[25] Manske CL, Thomas W, Wang Y, Wilson RF. Screening diabetic transplant candidates for coronary artery disease: identification of a low risk subgroup. *Kidney Int.* 1993;44(3):617-621.

[26] Rihal CS, Textor SC, Grill DE, et al. Incidence and prognostic importance of acute renal failure after percutaneous coronary intervention. *Circulation.* 2002;105(19):2259-2264.

[27] Lindsay J, Apple S, Pinnow EE, et al. Percutaneous coronary intervention-associated nephropathy foreshadows increased risk of late adverse events in patients with normal baseline serum creatinine. *Catheter Cardiovasc Interv.* 2003;59(3):338-343.

[28] Lorenz EC, Stegall MD, Cosio FG, et al. The effect of coronary angiography on renal function in preemptive renal transplant candidates. *Clin Transplant.* 2010. Available at: http://www.ncbi.nlm.nih.gov/pubmed/21050272.

[29] Gruberg L, Dangas G, Mehran R, et al. Clinical outcome following percutaneous coronary interventions in patients with chronic renal failure. *Catheter Cardiovasc Interv.* 2002;55(1):66-72.
[30] Saklayen MG, Gupta S, Suryaprasad A, Azmeh W. Incidence of atheroembolic renal failure after coronary angiography. A prospective study. *Angiology.* 1997;48(7):609-613.
[31] Jones DG, Taylor AM, Enkiri SA, et al. Extent and severity of coronary disease and mortality in patients with end-stage renal failure evaluated for renal transplantation. *Am. J. Transplant.* 2009;9(8):1846-1852.
[32] McFalls EO, Ward HB, Moritz TE, et al. Coronary-artery revascularization before elective major vascular surgery. *N. Engl. J. Med.* 2004;351(27):2795-2804.
[33] Eleven-year survival in the Veterans Administration randomized trial of coronary bypass surgery for stable angina. The Veterans Administration Coronary Artery Bypass Surgery Cooperative Study Group. *N. Engl. J. Med.* 1984;311(21):1333-1339.
[34] Manske CL, Wang Y, Rector T, Wilson RF, White CW. Coronary revascularisation in insulin-dependent diabetic patients with chronic renal failure. *Lancet.* 1992;340(8826):998-1002.
[35] Herzog CA, Ma JZ, Collins AJ. Comparative survival of dialysis patients in the United States after coronary angioplasty, coronary artery stenting, and coronary artery bypass surgery and impact of diabetes. *Circulation.* 2002;106(17):2207-2211.
[36] Ashrith G, Lee V, Elayda MA, Reul RM, Wilson JM. Short- and long-term outcomes of coronary artery bypass grafting or drug-eluting stent implantation for multivessel coronary artery disease in patients with chronic kidney disease. *Am. J. Cardiol.* 2010;106(3):348-353.
[37] Herzog CA, Ma JZ, Collins AJ. Long-term outcome of dialysis patients in the United States with coronary revascularization procedures. *Kidney Int.* 1999;56(1):324-332.
[38] Sadeghi HM, Stone GW, Grines CL, et al. Impact of renal insufficiency in patients undergoing primary angioplasty for acute myocardial infarction. *Circulation.* 2003;108(22):2769-2775.
[39] Karthikeyan V, Ananthasubramaniam K. Coronary risk assessment and management options in chronic kidney disease patients prior to kidney transplantation. *Curr Cardiol Rev.* 2009;5(3):177-186.
[40] McCullough PA. Contrast-induced acute kidney injury. *J. Am. Coll. Cardiol.* 2008;51(15):1419-1428.
[41] McCullough PA, Adam A, Becker CR, et al. Risk prediction of contrast-induced nephropathy. *Am. J. Cardiol.* 2006;98(6A):27K-36K.
[42] McCullough PA. Radiocontrast-induced acute kidney injury. *Nephron Physiol.* 2008; 109(4):p61-72.
[43] Keeley EC, McCullough PA. Coronary revascularization in patients with end-stage renal disease: risks, benefits, and optimal strategies. *Rev Cardiovasc Med.* 2003;4(3):125-130.
[44] Agrawal V, Swami A, Kosuri R, et al. Contrast-induced acute kidney injury in renal transplant recipients after cardiac catheterization. *Clin. Nephrol.* 2009;71(6):687-696.
[45] Kumar N, Dahri L, Brown W, et al. Effect of elective coronary angiography on glomerular filtration rate in patients with advanced chronic kidney disease. *Clin J Am Soc Nephrol.* 2009;4(12):1907-1913.

[46] McCullough PA, Rocher LR. Statin therapy in renal disease: harmful or protective? *Curr. Diab. Rep.* 2007;7(6):467-473.

[47] Katholi RE, Woods WT, Taylor GJ, et al. Oxygen free radicals and contrast nephropathy. *Am. J. Kidney Dis.* 1998;32(1):64-71.

[48] Erley CM. Does hydration prevent radiocontrast-induced acute renal failure? *Nephrol. Dial. Transplant.* 1999;14(5):1064-1066.

[49] Kelly AM, Dwamena B, Cronin P, Bernstein SJ, Carlos RC. Meta-analysis: effectiveness of drugs for preventing contrast-induced nephropathy. *Ann. Intern. Med.* 2008;148(4):284-294.

[50] Diaz-Sandoval LJ, Kosowsky BD, Losordo DW. Acetylcysteine to prevent angiography-related renal tissue injury (the APART trial). *Am. J. Cardiol.* 2002;89(3):356-358.

[51] McCullough PA, Bertrand ME, Brinker JA, Stacul F. A meta-analysis of the renal safety of isosmolar iodixanol compared with low-osmolar contrast media. *J. Am. Coll. Cardiol.* 2006;48(4):692-699.

[52] Goldfarb S, McCullough PA, McDermott J, Gay SB. Contrast-induced acute kidney injury: specialty-specific protocols for interventional radiology, diagnostic computed tomography radiology, and interventional cardiology. *Mayo Clin. Proc.* 2009;84(2):170-179.

[53] Kane GC, Doyle BJ, Lerman A, et al. Ultra-low contrast volumes reduce rates of contrast-induced nephropathy in patients with chronic kidney disease undergoing coronary angiography. *J. Am. Coll. Cardiol.* 2008;51(1):89-90.

9

Coronary Interventions with Mechanical Circulatory Support

Markus Ferrari
University Heart Centre Thuringia, Jena, Germany

1. Introduction

Patients in cardiogenic shock, with severely impaired left ventricular function, or intervention on the last open supplying coronary artery are summarized as so called "high risk coronary interventions" with significant risk of hemodynamic collapse and increased periprocedural mortality rate [1]. Thus, high risk percutaneous coronary interventions (PCI) may require prophylactic or standby hemodynamic mechanical circulatory support. While infusion of inotropic substances further increases myocardial oxygen consumption, other measures of support may be favourable especially in infarct related acute pump failure.

However, in acute cardiogenic shock, mechanical circulatory support may depict the only option to stabilise the patient for intra- or inter-hospital transfer and further diagnostic and therapeutic measures. This chapter summarises different therapeutic options of mechanical circulatory support in high risk PCI patients. Ongoing technical development as well as clinical studies may further elucidate this field of interventional cardiology in the future.

2. Identification of high risk PCI patients and indication for mechanical circulatory support

Cardiogenic shock is defined as reduction of cardiac index to less than 2.2 $l/min/m^2$ and increase in pulmonary capillary wedge pressure above 18 mmHg. Patients present with systolic blood pressure below 100 mmHg, tachycardia of more than 100 bpm, oliguria or anuria, cold and pale extremities, and impairment of cognitive function. The infusion of volume does not result in termination of shock. One-month-mortality rates of cardiogenic shock range between 40% and 80%. Cardiogenic shock can be caused by multiple reasons (table 1). However, acute myocardial infarction (AMI) accounts for more than 80% of cases. Fastest possible coronary revascularisation is recommended in patients suffering from AMI related cardiogenic shock [2].

Some cardiogenic shock patients with ongoing CPR require mechanical circulatory support upfront to make coronary angiography and/or PCI feasible. Besides catecholamine infusion, mechanical circulatory support provides an increase in arterial blood pressure and therefore in organ perfusion resulting in an improvement of organ function. The prognosis of shock patients is determined by the occurrence of a multi organ dysfunction syndrome (MODS) associated with an extremely high mortality. Hemodynamic support should increase arterial blood pressure to values above 70 mmHg for prevention or reversal of beginning MODS.

Myocardial pump failure	- Myocardial ischemia, myocardial infarction - Myocarditis - Dilatated cardiomyopathy - Hypertrophic or restrictive cardiomyopathy - Takotsubo-Syndrome - Cardiotoxic substances (intoxication, cytostatics, drugs) - Cardiodepressive substances (ß-blockers, Ca-antagonists, drugs, antiarrhythmic-, or antidepressive medication)
Rhythm related pump failure	- Supra-ventricular tachycardia or bradycardia - Conductance disorders (AV-block, pre-excitation) - Ventricular tachycardia or bradycardia - Asystoly, electro-mechanical discordance
Mechanical problems	- Valvular heart disease (stenosis, insufficiency) - Mechanical complications of infarction (rupture of papillary muscle, ventricular septum or wall) - Cardiac tamponade - Pericarditis constrictiva - Intra-cavity thrombus - Hypertrophic obstructive cardiomyopathy - Aortic dissection

Table 1. Reasons of acute cardiogenic shock

Three groups of patients requiring mechanical circulatory support in the catheter laboratory can be identified:

1. Acute pump failure or circulatory arrest with cardiogenic shock.
2. Elective high risk PCI patients requiring prophylactic or standby support if the risk for hemodynamic collapse is relatively high.
3. Effective hemodynamic stabilisation for transfer of shock patients to other departments or other heart centres (e.g. cardiac surgery).

While patients in group 1 and 3 can be easily identified by clinical judgement and hemodynamic evaluation, the indication for mechanical support in high risk elective PCI is still based on individual judgement, although scoring systems like Jeopardy Score or Bergelson's Score may help in the clinical process of decision making [3]. While elective circulatory support can be recommended in patients with severely impaired left ventricular ejection fraction, the standby of assist devices is also an option in hemodynamically stable patients.

High risk PCI is defined as PCI of target vessel supplying more than 50% of vital myocardium, or as PCI in unstable patients with an impaired left ventricular ejection fraction below 25% [1]. Several scoring systems may help to identify high risk PCI candidates based on the coronary anatomy. The Jeopardy Score introduced by Califf et al. in 1988 divides coronary circulation in six major areas. In case of occlusion or severe stenosis each segment accounts one point, in case of akinesia in the area only 0.5 points. If this analysis of the coronary tree adds to more than 3 points the patient is endangered for hemodynamic collapse during PCI [4]. However, all scoring systems origin from data bases of the late 80´s and 90´s when direct stenting and rapid exchange coronary devices were not available in the same extend as today. Due to lack of validated scoring systems, the application of surgical scoring systems like STS- or revised Euro-Score may support the process of clinical decision making for use of circulatory support in high risk PCI. Recent studies suggested a benefit of prophylactic circulatory support with the Impella™ in comparison to an intra aortic balloon pump (IABP) in elective high risk patients [5]. However, this study had relatively high 30-day event rates (Impella 15.3%, IABP 21.3%), which requests for further clinical trials. The optimal decision is mostly based on the individual situation of the patient and the experience of the operator.

3. Mechanical circulatory support devices in the catheter laboratory

3.1 Intra aortic balloon pump (IABP)

The concept of intra aortic counter pulsation was already introduced in the 50`s by the Kantrowitz brothers [6]. They showed an improvement in coronary blood flow when offering a delayed blood pressure pulse to the coronary circulation. Further technical developments included electrical stimulation of muscles wrapped around the abdominal aorta until the final design of an intra aortic balloon with a synchronised counter pulsation was introduced in cardiac surgery [7]. In the 70´s, IABP use increased for treatment of acute myocardial infarction and cardiogenic shock. In case of thrombolytic therapy, IABP significantly improved survival as described in the TIMI-18 study [8]. Today, use of IABP in infarct related cardiogenic shock after successful PCI is under controversial discussion [9]. However, IABP is recommended in cardiogenic shock before and after cardiac surgery, and in acute AMI patients before coronary revascularisation to improve hemodynamic situation. An IABP consists of a helium filled balloon in the descending aorta which is inflated and deflated in a counter pulsating way to the contractions of the left ventricle. Coronary and cerebral diastolic perfusion is increased by abrupt inflation in the early diastolic phase, increasing diastolic blood pressure significantly. However, coronary perfusion is only improved in the presence of hemodynamically relevant stenosis. An abrupt evacuation during systole results in reduction of afterload, therefore increasing left ventricular ejection fraction (LVEF) of about 10%. The combination of better diastolic organ perfusion and systolic afterload reduction can improve cardiac output by up to 1 l/min in severe cardiogenic shock. The 7F IABP catheter can be easily inserted in Seldinger's technique via femoral access. Today, the majority of IABP catheters are inserted in a sheathless way. In some cases, subclavian access can also be used for IABP placement.

4. Axial flow pumps

The concept of continuous left ventricular unloading with an axial flow pump was introduced 25 years ago [10]. The first concept was realized with the Hemopump™ which was driven by an external motor sucking blood through a pump cannula from the left ventricle into the ascending aorta with a small impeller in the distal part of the cannula. Further technical developments included the AMED™-System with the impeller in the descending aorta, avoiding any kinking of the drive line [11]. Today, the Impella™-System is well established in clinical routine. It consists of a pump cannula containing a micro motor and an impeller in its distal end. No external motor is necessary to provide flow rates of 2.5 and up to 5 l/min according to the pump sizes. The continuous unloading of the left ventricle establishes continuous flow into the ascending aorta and rhythm independent increase of arterial blood pressure. Especially in acute myocarditis patients, the Impella has several beneficial effects on the myocardium and the whole circulation.

5. Centrifugal pumps

Centrifugal pumps allow high flow rates of more than 5 l/min. While the TandemHeart™ uses a transseptal venous cannula, placed with its tip in the left atrium, other systems drain the blood through a venous cannula from the right atrium. The TandemHeart™ transfers the oxygenated blood from the left atrium through the centrifugal pump into the abdominal aorta without additional oxygenation. In case of dislocation of the pump cannula the patients are endangered of an abrupt deoxygenation.

Centrifugal pumps with an included membrane oxygenator allow biventricular support taking over completely myocardial and pulmonary functions. The blood from right atrium and cava vein is delivered by the centrifugal pump through the oxygenator back into the abdominal aorta with high flow rates after optimal gas exchange. Thus, these portable cardiopulmonary support devices (pCPS) can be also used in complete circulatory arrest. Miniaturized pCPS systems like the Lifebridge™ allow intra- or inter-hospital patient transfer with optimal oxygenation and organ perfusion. Since emergency pCPS can be inserted percutaneously, these devices are also recommended in cardiopulmonary resuscitation when other means fail to re-establish circulation. External cardiac compression devices like the Lucas™ or Autopulse™-System may be helpful to maintain minimal circulation until the cannulas are placed through the femoral vessels by Seldinger's technique. Percutaneous cannulation allows insertion of cannula sizes between 15 and 21 French without interruption of chest compression. Coronary angiography can be performed by contra-lateral approach in Judkin's technique or brachial approach after transfer of the patient to the catheter laboratory.

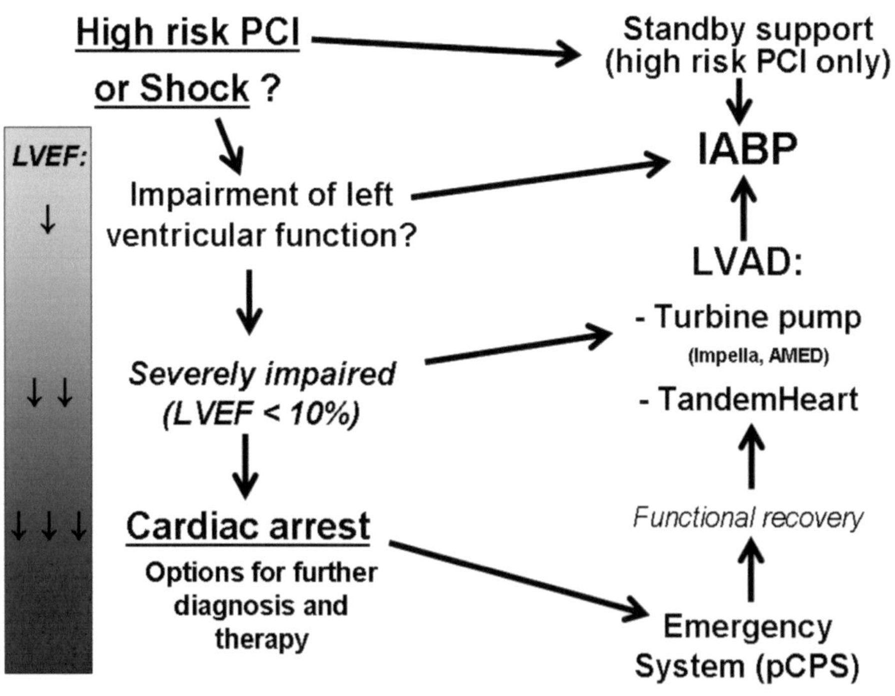

Fig. Options of percutaneous circulatory support in high risk coronary patients (mod. according to [12]).

6. Duration of support and weaning

Mechanical circulatory support may be necessary in cardiogenic shock patients for several days until hemodynamic recovery. In elective high risk PCI, the device can be removed immediately after the intervention. In some cases percutaneous closure devices may be helpful. However, removal of cannulas up to diameters of 20 French is also possible under local compression and application of a compression bandage for 24 hours.

7. Limitations and future perspectives

Mechanical circulatory support in high risk PCI and cardiogenic shock allows hemodynamic stabilization in the acute phase especially during the intervention. Continuous sufficient organ perfusion reduces the rate of shock related MODS. However, foreign surfaces lead to artificial alteration and stimulation of blood cells causing systemic inflammatory response syndrome (SIRS). The time of mechanical circulatory support should be therefore as short as possible. Additional problems are associated with haemolysis and the need for anticoagulation. New coating techniques and optimal design of pump cannulas reduce these clinical problems. Future developments include right heart support devices and foldable systems which can be inserted through minimal diameter peripheral sheaths. After unfolding in the circulation, these devices provide powerful circulatory support [13]. Mechanical support devices are useful tools in a catheter laboratory in close cooperation with cardiac surgery. Some patients with CPR do not recover despite successful coronary revascularisation. Long term circulatory support or heart transplantation may be an option in selected cases [14]. If mechanical complications of myocardial infarction are present in the state of cardiogenic shock, further surgical therapy is recommended, too. The use of circulatory support devices also includes combinations (e.g. CPB and IABP) for a staged weaning process. Future devices may allow the combination of techniques by modification of the cannulas and pump catheters. Immunologic interventions will focus on prevention of SIRS and improved functional recovery of MODS.

8. References

[1] Vogel RA, Shawl F, Tommaso C, et al. Initial report of the National Registry of Elective Cardiopulmonary Bypass Supported Coronary Angioplasty. J Am Coll Cardiol 1990;15:23-29

[2] Hochman JS, Sleeper LA, Webb JG, et al. Early revascularization in acute myocardial infarction complicated by cardiogenic shock. SHOCK Investigators. Should We Emergently Revascularize Occluded Coronaries for Cardiogenic Shock. N Engl J Med 1999;341:625-634

[3] Bergelson BA, Jacobs AK, Cupples LA, et al. Prediction of risk for hemodynamic compromise during percutaneous transluminal coronary angioplasty. Am J Cardiol 1992;70:1540-1545

[4] Califf RM, Phillips HR, 3rd, Hindman MC, et al. Prognostic value of a coronary artery jeopardy score. J Am Coll Cardiol 1985;5:1055-1063

[5] Syed AI, Kakkar A, Torguson R, et al. Prophylactic use of intra-aortic balloon pump for high-risk percutaneous coronary intervention: will the Impella LP 2.5 device show superiority in a clinical randomized study? Cardiovasc Revasc Med 2011;11:91-97

[6] Kantrowitz A. Experimental augmentation of coronary flow by retardation of the arterial pressure pulse. Surgery 1953;34:678-687

[7] Kantrowitz A, Mc KW. The experimental use of the diaphragm as an auxiliary myocardium. Surg Forum 1958;9:266-268

[8] Sanborn TA, Sleeper LA, Bates ER, et al. Impact of thrombolysis, intra-aortic balloon pump counterpulsation, and their combination in cardiogenic shock complicating acute myocardial infarction: a report from the SHOCK Trial Registry. SHould we emergently revascularize Occluded Coronaries for cardiogenic shocK? J Am Coll Cardiol 2000;36:1123-1129

[9] Sjauw KD, Engstrom AE, Vis MM, et al. A systematic review and meta-analysis of intra-aortic balloon pump therapy in ST-elevation myocardial infarction: should we change the guidelines? Eur Heart J 2009;30:459-468

[10] Frazier OH, Wampler RK, Duncan JM, et al. First human use of the Hemopump, a catheter-mounted ventricular assist device. Ann Thorac Surg 1990;49:299-304

[11] Ferrari M, Aboulhosn W, Figulla HR. Successful high-risk coronary angioplasty in a patient with cardiogenic shock under circulatory assist with a 16F axial flow pump. Catheter Cardiovasc Interv 2005;66:557-561

[12] Ferrari M, Figulla HR. Circulatory assist devices in cardiology. Dtsch Med Wochenschr 2005;130:652-656

[13] Thomas JL, Al-Ameri H, Economides C, et al. Use of a percutaneous left ventricular assist device for high-risk cardiac interventions and cardiogenic shock. J Invasive Cardiol 2010;22:360-364

[14] Ferrari M, Hekmat K, Jung C, et al. Better outcome after cardiopulmonary resuscitation using percutaneous emergency circulatory support in non-coronary patients compared to those with myocardial infarction. Acute Card Care 2011;13:30-34

10

Coronary Arteriovenous Fistula

Recep Demirbag
Harran University Medical Faculty, Sanliurfa
Turkey

1. Introduction

Coronary anomalies are defined as rare anatomic patterns and are seen in approximately 1 to 5% of all patients undergoing coronary angiography (Tuncer et al., 2006; Angelini, 1999; Friedman et al., 2007). Classification of anomalies of the coronary arteries is shown in table-1 (Angelini, 2007).

1.	Anomalies of origination and course • Absent left main trunk, • Anomalous location of coronary ostium within aortic root or near proper aortic sinus of Valsalva (for each artery) • Anomalous location of coronary ostium outside normal "coronary" aortic sinuses • Anomalous location of coronary ostium at improper sinus (which may involve joint origination or "single" coronary pattern) • Single coronary artery
2.	Anomalies of intrinsic coronary arterial anatomy • Congenital ostial stenosis or atresia • Coronary ostial dimple • Coronary ectasia or aneurysm • Absent coronary artery • Coronary hypoplasia • Intramural coronary artery (muscular bridge) • Subendocardial coronary course • Coronary crossing • Anomalous origination of posterior descending artery from the anterior descending branch or a septal penetrating branch • Split right or left coronary arteries • Ectopic origination of first septal branch
3.	Anomalies of coronary termination • Inadequate arteriolar/capillary ramifications • Coronary artery fistulas
4.	Anomalous anastomotic vessels

Table 1. Classification of anomalies of the coronary arteries according to Angelini

Coronary artery fistulae (CAF) are classified as abnormalities of termination and are defined as congenital or acquired an abnormal communication between the right or left coronary arterial systems and a cardiac chamber or vessel, having bypassed the myocardial capillary bed (Friedman et al., 2007). They comprise 13% of congenital coronary artery anomalies (Table-2) (Yamanaka et al., 1990).

	No	Incidence (%)	Anomalies (%)
Total coronary arteriograms	126.595		
Total coronary anomalies	1,686	1.33	
Anomalies of origin and distribution	1,461	1.15	87
Coronary artery fistulae	225	0.18	13

Table 2. Isolated congenital coronary artery anomalies (Yamanaka et al. 1990)

The CAFs were first described by Josef Hyrtl in 1851 (Friedman et al., 2007). The incidence of the CAFs is changes according to genetic or ethnic racial factors or either to different geographical regions (Table-3). The true incidence is difficult to evaluate because about most of the cases may be asymptomatic and clinically indictable until an echocardiogram or catheterization is performed. The incidence of CAFs is 0.3–0.8% in patient's undergone diagnostic cardiac catheterizations (Angelini, 1999; Cebi et al., 2008). Echocardiographic studies estimated the incidence of congenital CAFs in children at 0.06 to 0.2% (Sherwood et al., 1999; Hsieh et al., 2002).
Sex predilection is controversial. In a study it is found out that males are more affected than females, with a ratio of 2.3 to 1 (Ata et al., 2009). Another study shows that there is no sex predilection for CAF (Chiu et al., 2008).

Author	Patients	CAFs	Incidence (%)	Population
Gillebert 1986	14,708	20	0.13	Belgian
Yamanaka et al., 1990	126.295	225	0.18	American
Bhandari 1993	4,486	8	0.11	Indian
Cebi 2008	18,272	10	0.05	German
Vavuranakis 1995	33,600	34	0.10	American
Nawa 1996	704	15	2.1	Japanese
Kardos 1997	7,694	5	0.06	Hungarian
Yıldız 2010	12,450	12	0.09	Turkish
Said 2006	30,829	51	0.16	Dutch
Chiu et al. 2008	28.210	125	0.44	Chinese

Table 3. Angiograhic incidence of CAFs in different adult population.

Major sites of origin of the fistulae are from the right coronary artery (40-60%), left anterior descending (30-60%), circumflex and a combination thereof (Gupta-Malhotra, 2010). The CAFs predominantly drain into the right side of the heart (92%) into the right ventricle in 41%, the right atrium in 26%, the coronary sinus in 7%, the pulmonary in 17%, and superior vena cava in 1% of cases (Levin et al., 1978). Its connection between coronary sinus; left atrium, and left ventricle is unusual (Table-4) (Said, 2010).

Termination sites	McNamara 1969 (n=172)	Levin 1978 (n=363)	Hobbs 1982 (n=122)	Kaniya 2002 (n=266)
Right Ventricle	40	41	3	34
Right atrium	35	26	7	18
Pulmonary artery	16	17	66	38
Coronary sinus	-	7	-	-
Left atrium	6	5	7	2
Left ventricle	3	3	17	5
Superior Vena Cava	-	1	-	-
Other sites	-	-	-	3

Table 4. Termination sites of congenital solitary CAFs (%) (Said, 2010)

Approximately 10-30% of patients with CAFs also have another congenital cardiovascular anomaly (Cheung et al., 2001; Holzer et al., 2004). Congenital CAFs may occur as an isolated finding or may appear in the context of other congenital cardiac anomalies or structural heart defects, most frequently in critical pulmonary stenosis or atresia with an intact interventricular septum and in pulmonary artery branch stenosis, tetralogy of Fallot, coarctation of the aorta, hypoplastic left heart syndrome, patent ductus arteriosus, ventricular septal defect, atrial septal defect, and aortic atresia (luo et al., 2006; Ata et al., 2009).

2. Etiology

Exact etiologies of CAFs have not been identified. They are usually occurring congenitally or acquiredly. The congenital causes are responsible for most of them. Congenital fistulous connections between the coronary system and a cardiac chamber appear to represent persistence of embryonic intertrabecular spaces and sinusoids (Lin et al., 2009).

The acquired causes of CAFs include coronary atherosclerosis, Takayasu arteritis, polymyositis, cardiac surgery, percutaneous coronary intervention, septal myectomy, closed-chest ablation of accessory pathway, permanent pacemaker placement, transbronchial lung biopsy, acute myocardial infarction, and after repeated myocardial biopsies in cardiac transplantation (Table-5). The penetrating and nonpenetrating chest trauma may also lead to CAF. Traumatic CAFs are most common between the right coronary artery and the right side of the heart. Although acquired causes are reported to be rare, it is likely that the true incidence is underestimated (Luo et al., 2006).

Seventy-six patients (1985-1995) with 96 CAFs were identified from a review of the literature by Said et al. They reported a congenital origin in 64% of these 76 cases and an acquired cause in 36% (Said et al.,1997).

3. Pathophysiology

Normally, 2 coronary arteries arise from the root of the aorta and taper progressively as they branch to supply the cardiac parenchyma. A fistula exists if a substantive communication arises bypassing the myocardial capillary phase and communicates with a low-pressure cardiac cavity (atria or ventricle) or with a branch of the systemic or pulmonary systems. Anomalies of the coronary arteries can be considered as the result of a rudimentary persistence of an embryologic coronary arterial structure, a failure of normal coronary development, a failure of the normal atrophic process of development, or the misplacement of a connection of an otherwise normal coronary artery. CAFs may appear as a persistence of sinusoidal connections between the lumens of the primitive tubular heart that supply myocardial blood flow in the early embryologic period. The mechanism is related to the diastolic pressure gradient and runoff from the coronary vasculature to a low-pressure receiving cavity. If the fistula is large, the intracoronary diastolic perfusion pressure diminishes progressively. Normal thin-walled vessels exist at the arteriolar level that may drain into the cardiac cavity (arteriosinusoidal vessels) and venous communications (thebesian veins) to the right atrium. These small vessels do not steal significant nutrient flow and do not constitute fistulous connections. Fistulae usually are large (>250 mm) and dilated or ectatic, and they tend to enlarge over time. Often, the limits of what constitutes a fistula and what constitutes a normal vessel are debated (Friedman et al., 2007).

A. Congenital
1. Embryonic
2. Multiple; systemic hemangioma
B. Acquired
1. Closed-chest ablation of accessory pathway
2. Percutaneous coronary balloon angioplasty
3. Hypertrophic cardiomyopathy
4, Right/left ventricular septal myectomy
5. Penetrating and nonpenetrating trauma
6. Acute myocardial infarction
7, Dilated cardiomyopathy
8, Mitral valve surgery
9, "Sign" of mural thrombus
10. Tumor
11. Permanent pacemaker placement
12. Cardiac transplant
13. Endomyocardial biopsy
14. Coronary artery bypass grafting

Table 5. Causes and Associations of Coronary Artery Fistula (Angelini, 1999)

Over time, the coronary artery leading to the fistulous tract progressively dilates, which, in turn, may progress to frank aneurysm formation, intimal ulceration, medial degeneration, intimal rupture, atherosclerotic deposition, calcification, side-branch obstruction, mural thrombosis, and, rarely, rupture (Gupta-Malhotra, 2010). The histopathologic findings which are reported in the literature are myocardial hypertrophy with focal fibrosis, dilatation of the involved vessel, and mural thinning of the fistula wall with fresh thrombosis and concomitant atherosclerosis (Zenooz et al., 2009)

CAFs were classified into 2 types according to different patterns of morphology and pathology: type I was a solitary coronary to cardiac chamber or great vessel fistula, whereas type II comprised coronary artery left ventricle (LV) multiple microfistulas. Type I CAFs were also classified into 2 different sizes: macro (diameter ≥1.5 mm (Figure-1) and small (diameter <1.5 mm) (Chiu et al., 2008).

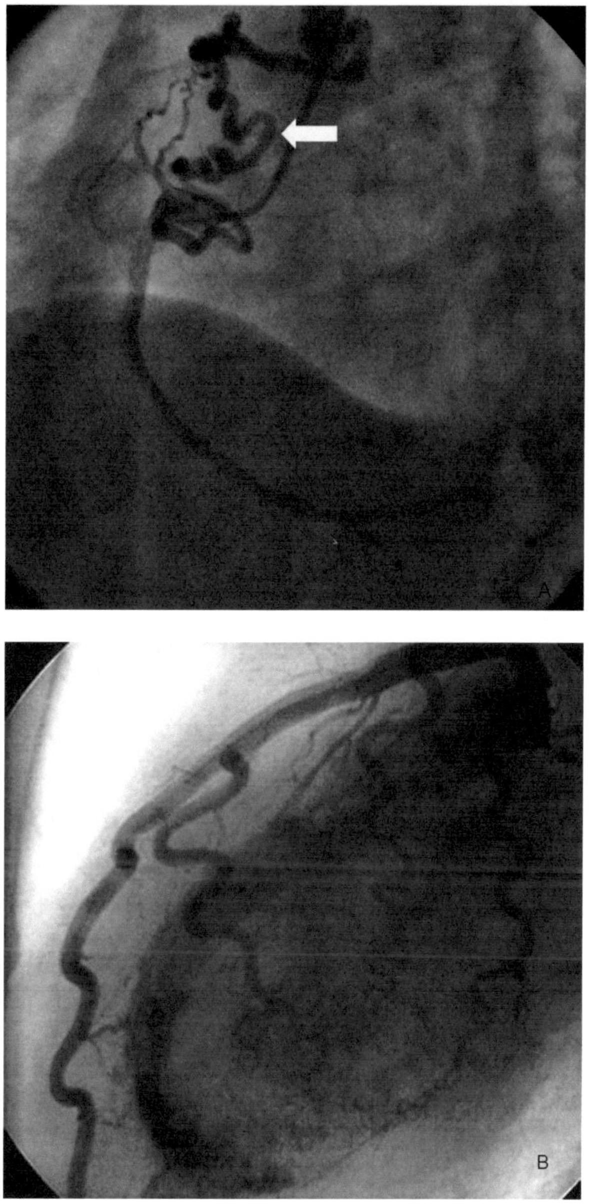

Fig. 1. A. Coronary angiography in the left anterior oblique view (60 degree) shows a large tortuous coronary fistula (thick white arrows) from the proximal right coronary artery (RCA) to the main pulmonary artery (Chiu et al., 2008).
B. Angiogram (left lateral projection) shows the multiple fistulae originating from the left coronary system (Kose et al., 2005)

Origin, termination and pathway of CAFs are explained by Said et al (Said et al.,2006). He reported that recognized for the origin and termination each, two morphological types: single or multiple channels and for the pathways three different types: tortuous/multiple, tortuous/single and straight/single channels with or without aneurysmal formation or dilatation of the fistula-related artery (Figure-2). Fistulas with single communications are much more higher compared with multiple fistulas (Kose & G. Heper, 2005).

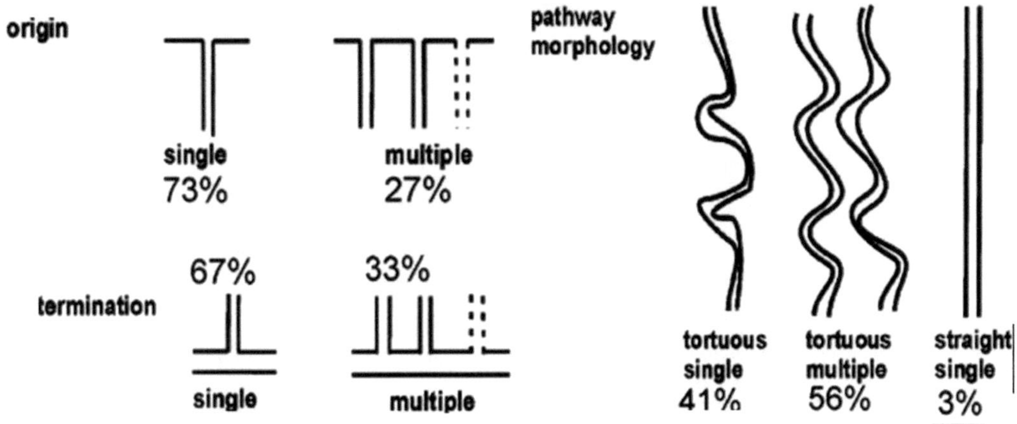

Fig. 2. An art drawing illustrating origin, pathways and ending of CAFs (Said 2006)

The mechanism of myocardial ischemia or heart failure induced by CAFs is thought to be the result of a shunting and steal phenomenon of normal coronary flow, flow-mediated inflammatory vascular changes, vascular trauma or dissection, coronary compression, abnormal myocardial perfusion pressure due to intravascular stenoses or to abnormal drainage compartments, micro- or macro-vascular venous thrombosis, and micro- or macrovascular arterial thrombosis (Chiu et al., 2008; Valente et al., 2010; Gowda et al., 2006). Mechanisms of coronary thrombosis in CAF include abnormal flow patterns associated with vascular ectasia, coronary tortuosity, abrupt changes in vessel caliber, and abnormal vascular connections; potential for congenitally intrinsic local or circulating changes in the clotting or fibrinolytic cascade; and effects of direct vascular trauma (Fahey et al., 2008)

The coronary arterial fistula can be direct in its course and connection, or it can take a convoluted and worm-like path to its site of drainage. Occasionally, the fistulous connections can become aneurysmal. The involved coronary artery is typically dilated when the distal fistula is large, as there is preferential flow, or "steal", from the coronary arterial system into the lower resistance chamber or vessel. The steal phenomenon associated with CAF is classificated by two types. One type is the *persistent steal* caused by the existence of large fistulous tracts. The other type, *episodic steal,* is caused by physiologic factors which can be seen in small and multiple CAF (Angelini, 2002b)

When the fistula drains into the right side of the heart, the volume load is increased in this side as well as in the pulmonary vascular bed, the left atrium and the left ventricle. When the fistula drains into the left atrium or the left ventricle, although there is volume overloading of these chambers, there is no increase in the pulmonary blood flow. A left-to-right shunt exists in over 90% of cases. The size of the shunt is determined by the size of the fistula and the pressure difference between the coronary artery and the chamber into which the fistula drains. However, the shunt ratio is generally small regardless of age; in many cases, a shunt is not detectable. Large shunts are particularly prevalent when the fistula terminates in the atrial chambers (Nakayama et al.,2010). If a large left-to-right shunt exists,

CAFs are complicated as pulmonary hypertension and congestive heart failure; others include rupture or thrombosis of the fistula or associated arterial aneurysm or coronary steal phenomena (Qureshi, 2006; Friedman et al., 2007).

4. Clinical features

The clinical presentation of coronary artery fistulas is mainly dependent on the severity of the left-to-right shunt. The majority of adult patients with CAFs are usually asymptomatic. However, their natural history can be variable and they may cause symptoms in some patients at any age. The type of fistula, shunt volume, site of the shunt, and the presence of other cardiac conditions are associated with the clinical findings of CAF. While small coronary artery fistulae are usually asymptomatic due to small shunt flow, large coronary artery fistulae are mostly symptomatic causing cardiac heart failure, pulmonary arterial hypertension, myocardial infarction, arrhythmias, endocarditis, or rupture (Dursun et al., 2009). The symptoms of CAFs in adult patients usually begin in the 5th or 6th decade (Qureshi, 2006). A smaller percentage of pediatric patients tend to be asymptomatic, unlike adults. It is mentioned in an article that most patients with these fistulas younger than 20 years were asymptomatic compared with patients older than 20 years (Liberthson et al., 1979). It is very rare to diagnose a CAF in the neonate (Zenooz et al., 2010).

Dyspnea on exertion is the most common symptom of CAFs. The other symptoms of CAFs are angina, fatigue, palpitations and paroxysmal nocturnal dyspnea. Angina pectoris may be rarely seen in patients without arteriosclerotic coronary artery disease. Patients with angina pectoris are mostly older than 40 years old and they have coexistent coronary artery stenosis and/or have large or multiple fistulas. Rarely, the presenting feature can be pericardial effusion or sudden death (Chiue et al., 2008; Gowda et al., 2006).

It is commonly believed that the lesion is incidentally detected on routine examination or is an incidental finding during coronary angiogram (Juraschek et al., 2011). The most common clinical presentation of CAF is a continuous heart murmur. CAFs are usually suspected when a murmur is detected in asymptomatic individuals. The prevalence of a continuous murmur varies in different reports depending on the population studied. The location on the chest wall where the murmur is the loudest depends on where the fistula enters the heart. It was reported that a continuous murmur was found in 3-9 % in patients with CAFs (luo et al., 2006). The characteristic of murmur is a soft, at a grade of 2/6-4/6, continuous murmur that tends to be crescendo- decrescendo in both systole and diastole but louder in diastole. The murmur is often confused with other conditions, such as patent ductus arteriosus, arteriovenous shunts. pulmonary arteriovenous fistula, ruptured sinus of Valsalva aneurysm, aortopulmonary window, prolapse of the right aortic cusp with a supracristal ventricular septal defect, internal mammary artery to pulmonary artery fistula, and systemic arteriovenous fistula. It is to be underlined that in these conditions, continuous murmurs reach their peak intensity at the time of the second heart sound. CAFs should be considered in many symptomatic or asymptomatic patients with cardiac murmurs (Ata et al., 2009).

5. Diagnostic methods

Most frequently used diagnostic methods are: usually include physical examination, electrocardiography, chest X-ray, echocardiography, multidetector computed tomography and angiocardiography. The other technical methods are rarely used in the diagnosis of CAF. Cardiac enzyme and brain natriuretic peptid levels may be elevated in patients with CAF. The screening and the treatment guideline suggested by Angelini is shown in Figure-3 (Angelini, 2002b).

Although the electrocardiogram shows the left ventricular volume overload and occasionally ischaemic changes, it is usually unhelpful in CAFs. Generally, the chest x-ray is normal, but occasionally moderate cardiomegaly may be present when there is a large left-to-right shunt (Qureshi, 2006). The treadmill evaluation of coronary function is largely negated by the consistently high incidence of false-positive and false-negative results. This is why the treadmill is not to be used frequently and reliably. Myocardial perfusion scintgraphic studies may be used to assess myocardial ischaemia before and after treatment of CAFs. Magnetic resonance imaging may also help in confirming the diagnosis, as the proximal coronary arteries or even the whole length of the fistula vessel may be seen. Intravascular Doppler ultrasonography provides further insight into the pathophysiology of CAFs.

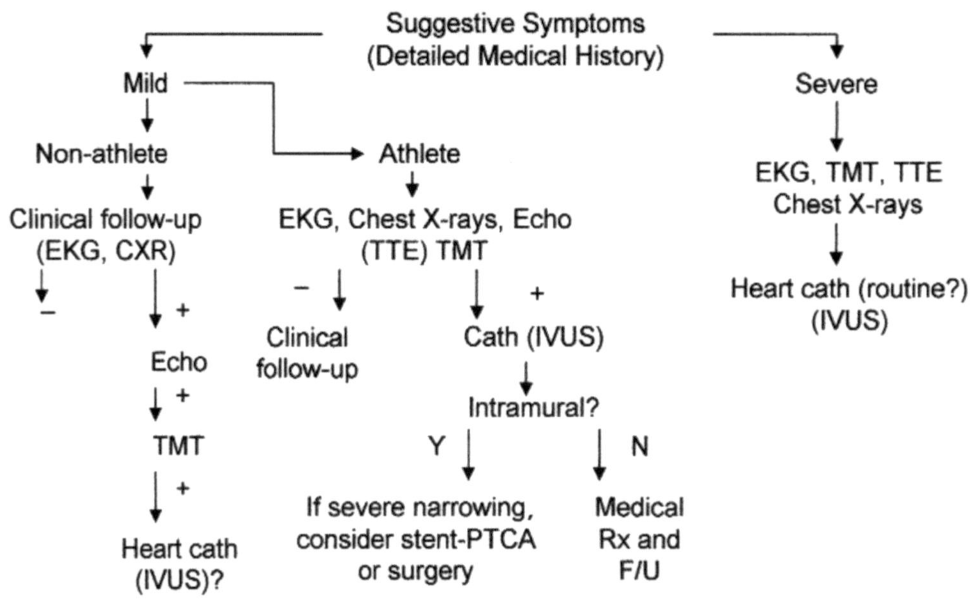

Fig. 3. Proposed diagnostic protocol for adult patients who are at risk for coronary artery anomalies.
– = negative test result; + = positive test result; CXR = chest x-ray; echo = echocardiogram; EKG = electrocardiogram; F/U = follow-up; IVUS = intravascular ultrasound; N = no; PTCA = percutaneous transluminal coronary angioplasty; Rx = treatment; TMT = treadmill test; TTE = transthoracic echocardiogram; Y = yes (Angelini, 2002b)

5.1 Angiography

Coronary angiography is the main diagnostic technique for the precise diagnosis of the CAFs, and its dynamic implication, cannot be ascertained entirely from non-invasive modalities. Cardiac catheterisation and angiography have been used as a method of technique evaluation of CAFs. The catheterization provides the hemodynamic evaluation of the CAFs. Cardiac catheterization remains the modality of choice for defining coronary artery patterns of structure and flow. Most frequently, intracardiac pressures are normal and shunt flow is modest. Aortography or selective coronary arteriography also provide the most detailed anatomy of the fistula, in particular, the size, the origin, the course, presence of any stenosis and the drainage site (Figure-4). In addition, therapeutic embolization using occlusive coils or devices may be performed via catheterization (Krishnamoorth et al., 2004).

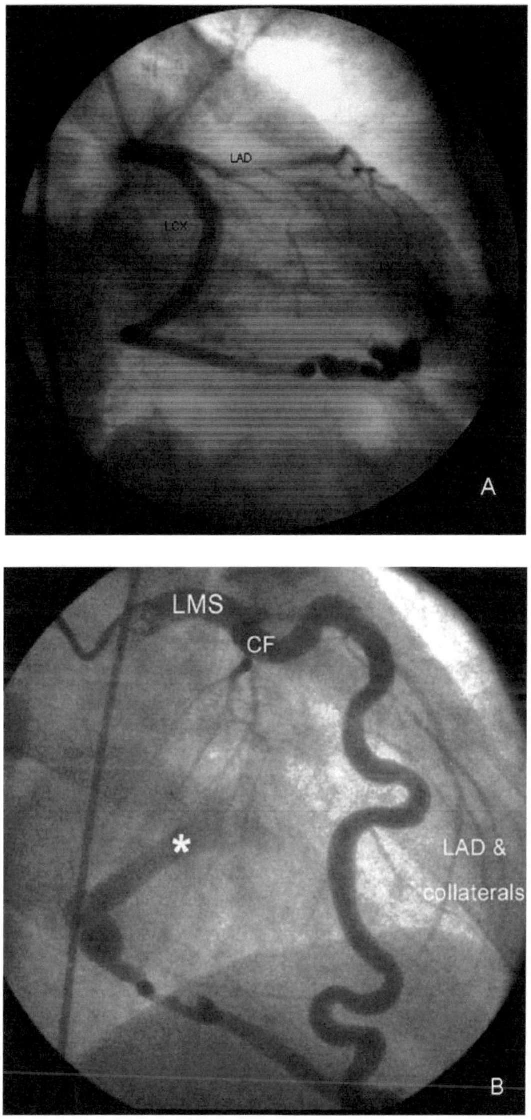

Fig. 4. A. Selective injection shows the fistula from the left circumflex coronary artery to the left ventricle (Dursun et al, 2009).
B. The coronary fistula from the left main coronary artery to the right ventricle, and the coronary steal with rudimentary distal coronary arteries (Marijon et al., 2007).
CF; coronary fistula, LAD; left anterior descending coronary artery, LCX; left circumflex coronary artery, LMS; left main coronary artery, LV; left ventricle.

Coronary angiography still remains the gold standard for imaging the coronary arteries, but sometimes origin and relation of CAFs to adjacent cardiac structures may be ambiguous. It is difficult to measure and observe abnormal tortuous blood vessels with coronary angiography in one section, under such conditions non-invasive methods such as transthoracic and transoesophageal echocardiography, magnetic resonance imaging and contrast enhanced multislice tomography can be used as adjunct to coronary angiography.

5.2 Echocardiography

Echocardiography is helpful in diagnosing most fistulae. Two-dimensional echocardiograms may reveal left atrial and left ventricular enlargement as a consequence of significant shunt flow or decreased regional or global dysfunction as a consequence of myocardial ischemia. A markedly enlarged coronary artery can usually be detected with echocardiography. Echocardiography is not suitable for the evaluation of the functional status of CAFs (Angelini, 2002b).

A coronary artery fistula should be suspected when two dimensional imaging of the main coronary arteries in the parasternal-short axis view shows one coronary artery dilated while the other coronary artery is of normal size. Multiple two-dimensional echocardiographic planes were used in coursing the dilated left coronary artery in the parasternal short-axis plane. But position of the probe, cardiac motion and curvilinear nature of the vessel may limit visualization. High-volume flow may be detected by color-flow imaging at the origin or along the length of the vessel (Figure-5). Carefully seek the site of drainage; often, it is evident as a disturbed flow signal, most frequently within the right ventricle. Recently, some authors have recommended the transesophagial echocardiography for the diagnosis of fistulas because of its better resolution. Transesophageal echocardiogram may be also useful in delineating the origin, course, and drainage of a fistula (Juraschek et al., 2011).

Widespread use of echocardiography coupled with increased awareness and availability of surgical and transcatheter repair of congenital lesions have led to greater potential to perform intervention on CAFs (Valente et al., 2010).

5.3 Multidetector computed tomography

Although echocardiography is often used to detect CAFs, detailed evaluation may be difficult in some patients. Overweight patients present a particular difficulty because of their insufficient acoustic window for echocardiography. In this latter group, Multidetector Computed Tomography (MDCT) may allow excellent adjunctive anatomical delineation, notably of the origin intervening anatomy and distal entry sites of CAFs with high resolution (Lee et al., 2007).

Distal vessel entry depiction by MDCT allows an assessment for the presence or absence of obstruction, which determines the likelihood of a coronary artery steal presentation (Figure-6 and -7). A contrast opacification into the receiving chamber/vessel is useful in confirming the CAFs entry site and patency of the shunt (Dodd et al., 2008)

Cardiac catheterization is the best diagnostic method for identification of CAFs, but it is invasive and has got roughly 1.5% morbidity, 0.15% mortality risk (Lee et al., 2007). Therefore, in patients where echocardiography and angiography are unable to provide adequate anatomical and physiological information, MDCT may provide additional precise details of CAFs, enabling more optimal therapeutic planning (Dodd et al., 2008). Many studies suggest that MDCT has a potential in thoracic imaging, involving not only evaluation of the coronary arteries but other thoracic vessels and coronary-extracoronary communications.

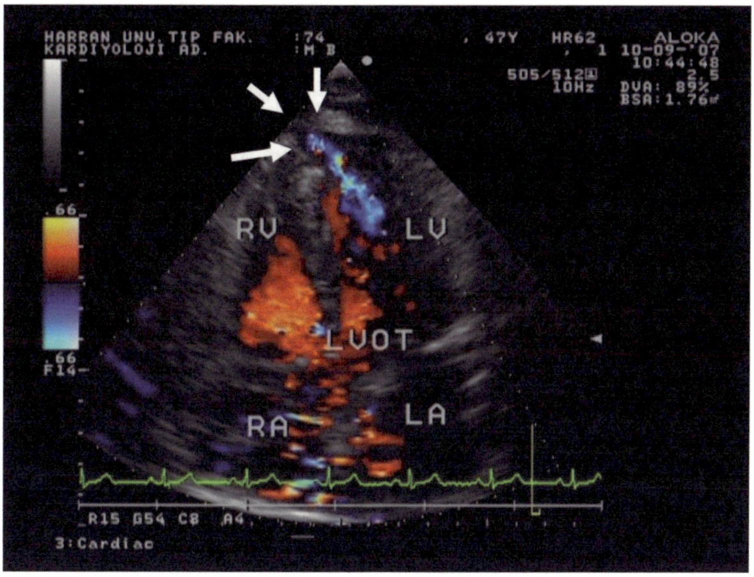

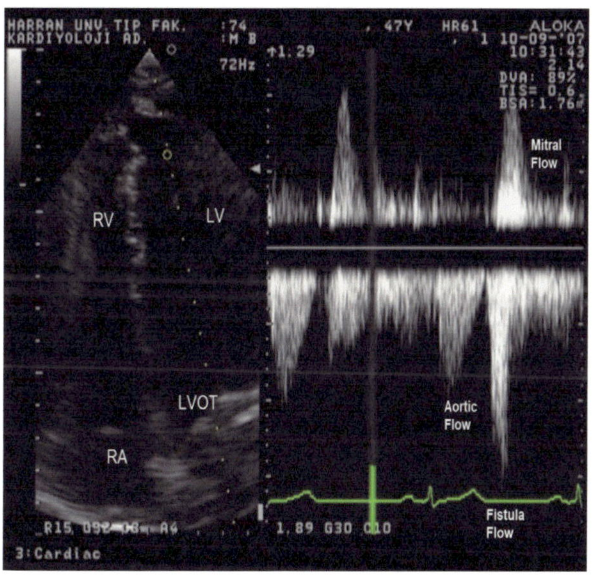

Fig. 5. Colour Doppler and continuo Doppler show fistula form coronary artery to left ventricle. Colour Doppler and continuo Doppler at apical four-chamber view from a transthoracic echocardiogram shows drainage of fistula into the left ventricle apex in diastolic period. IVS; inter-ventricular septum, LV; Left ventricle, LVOT; left ventricular outflow tract, RV; Right ventricle, RA; Right atrium.

The MCDT takes far less time than catheter angiography and requires less skill to carry out. Catheter-related risks, including bleeding at puncture site, haematoma formation, occurrence of arteriovenous fistula etc., are completely eliminated. It also eliminates the more serious complications of catheter angiography like coronary artery dissection, stroke and a small but definite incidence of mortality. The procedure is carried out as an outpatient procedure, and hence, hospitalization is not needed. Thus, MDCT is considered as a good alternative to echocardiography and coronary angiography. The major limitation of MDCT is radiation exposure, which can be substantially lowered by techniques such as automatic tube current modulation and shielding (Zenooz et al., 2009: Srinivasan, 2008).

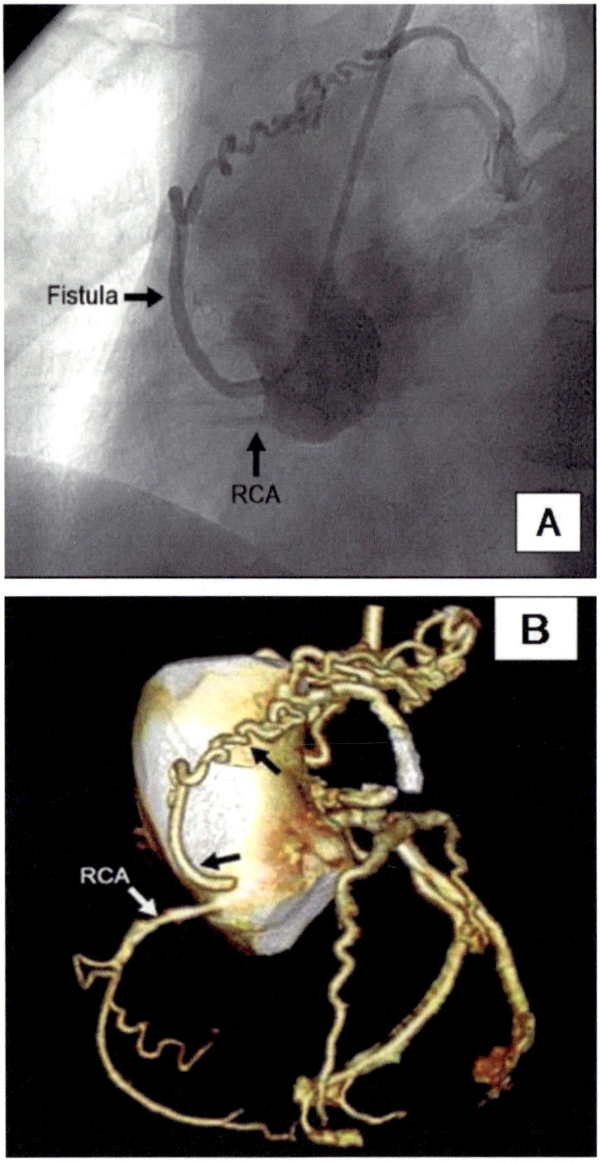

Fig. 6. A: Left anterior oblique view showing the fistula originating from the right sinus of Valsalva and draining into the pulmonary artery.
B: Computed tomographic coronary angiography. Fistula (black arrows) from the circumflex coronary artery to the pulmonary artery. B: Fistula (black arrows) from the right sinus of Valsalva to the pulmonary artery (Acar at al., 2010)
CX – left circumflex artery; LAD – left anterior descending artery; RCA – right coronary artery.

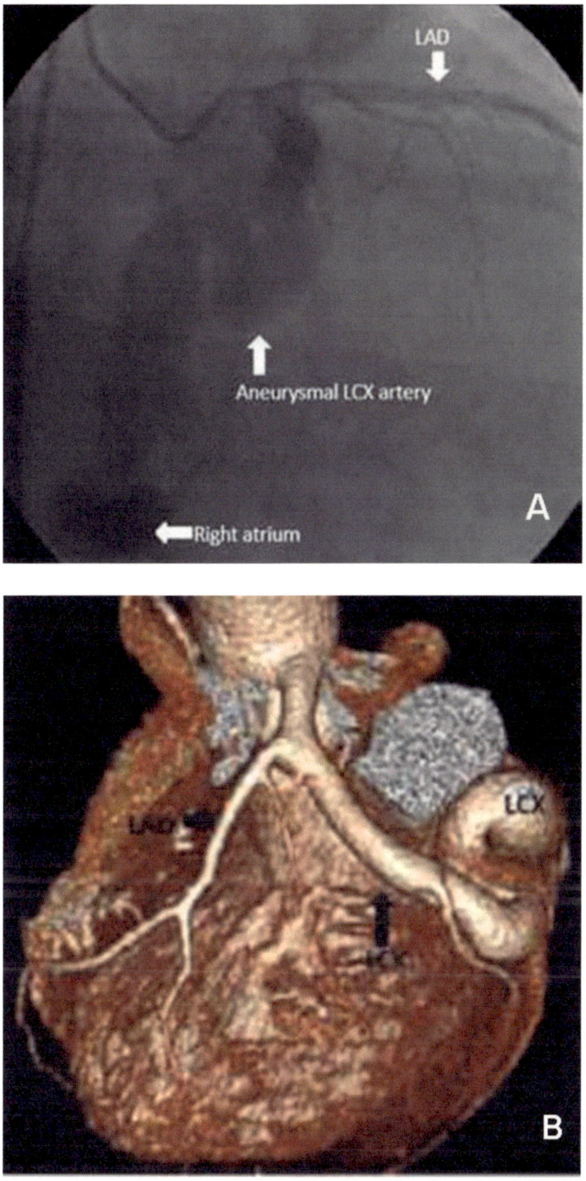

Fig. 7. (A) Coronary angiogram showing a tortuous aneurysmal circumflex artery opacifying the right atrium. (B) Multislice cardiac-gated computed tomography scans showing the left anterior descending artery and a giant circumflex aneurysm with a very tortuous course terminating in a large fistulous connection into the coronary sinus (Pala et al, 2011). LAD: Left anterior descending artery; LCx: Left circumflex artery.

6. Treatment of CAF

The management strategy of patients with CAFs depends on the size of the fistula, presence of symptoms, the anatomy of the fistula, the patient's age and whether the patient has other associated cardiovascular disorders (Lin et al., 2009). Spontaneous closure is rare but may occur in small fistulae. Spontaneous closure is likely to occur in infants younger than 2 years if the CAFs drains into the right heart, especially the right ventricle (Wong et al., 2000). Small fistulous connections in the asymptomatic patients need to be monitored. The majority of small, asymptomatic CAFs in adults do not need surgical or coronary intervention and medical treatment (Angelini et al, 2002b). In borderline situations, close echocardiographic or angiographic follow-up imaging identifying the enlargement of feeding vessel in asymptomatic patients provide significant information. Larger fistulae progressively enlarge over time, and complications, such as congestive heart failure, myocardial infarction, arrhythmias, infectious endocarditis, aneurysm formation, rupture, and death, are more likely to arise in older patients. These complications may be avoided by early closure of the fistula.

Most symptomatic patients with CAFs are treated by closure with transcatheter or surgical ligation. Transcatheter embolization is adviced to all large fistulae but the small fistulous connections. Patients with multiple openings, or significantly aneurysmal dilatation may not be optimal candidates for transcatheter closure. These CAFs are not suitable for the transcatheter approach and preferably are to be addressed surgically.

The preferred method of approach for any patient depends on the anatomy of the fistula, the presence or absence of associated defects and the experience of the interventional cardiologists and surgeons. For the treatment of traumatic CAFs and iatrogenic CAFs, early operative intervention needs to be preferred. Patients which are managed conservatively may develop life-threatening complications. Aneurysmal degeneration, which can lead to mural thrombosis, rupture, or side-branch obstruction, is needed to be treated. For asymptomatic patients, indications for surgery are similar to those diseases which have left to right shunts (e.g., $Qp/Qs>1.5$ or right ventricular volume overload).

6.1 Transcatheter treatment

Transcatheter closure of CAFs avoids the need for surgical intervention, cardiopulmonary bypass, and median sternotomy. In 1983, Reidy and his colleagues first successfully performed transcatheter closure of CAFs (Reidy et al., 1983). Since then, transcatheter closure of CAFs has been reported with satisfactory results, and this is now considered the treatment of choice for this anomaly.

The main indications for embolization are proximal location of the fistulous vessel, single drain site, extraanatomic termination of the fistula away from the normal coronary arteries, older patient age, and the absence of concomitant cardiac disorders requiring surgical intervention (Zenooz et al., 2009). The main technical limitations of embolization consist of extreme vessel tortuosity, small diameter of the coronary artery and presence of multiple drainage sites or coronary branches at the site of optimal device position.

6.1.1 Devices

The choice of device and technique depends on the anatomic characteristics of the CAFs which include tortuosity, the presence of high flow in the fistula, aneurismal dilation of the feeding vessel and the point of the intended occlusion. Other important determinants comprise the age and the size of the patient, the catheter size that can be used in the patient, the size of the vessel to be occluded and the tortuosity of the catheter course to reach the intended point of occlusion (Qureshi, 2006).

Various occlusion devices are available for the closure of the CAFs. These are Gianturco and polyester-covered stainless steel coils, detachable balloons, umbrella devices, covered stent polyvinyl alcohol particles, glue and a combination of these instruments (Tacoy et al., 2009; Zhu et al., 2010).
The above mentioned coils are used primarily in smaller CAFs (Figure-8). Their advantages are smaller sheath and catheter delivery sizes, and their cost. Multiple coil placements may be necessary for closing of the severe, tortuous, high-flow fistula. Mechanical detachable coils are used in patients with high-flow velocity coronary fistulae and these play an important role in avoiding coil migration and these are safe in coil embolization (Naber et al., 2004). Electrically detachable coils are particularly safe with minimal risk of migration due to high-flow velocity (Okamoto et al., 2006).

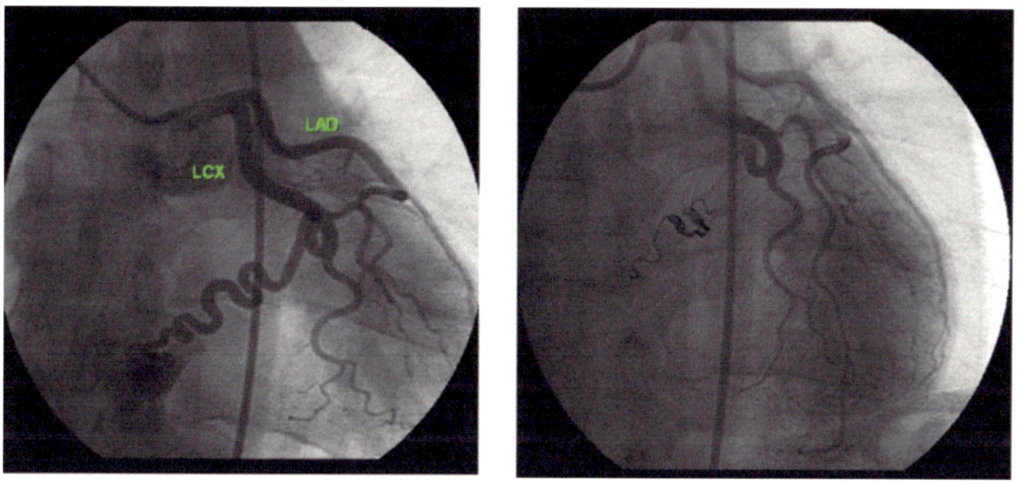

Fig. 8. (A) Selective coronary angiography of the left coronary artery reveals the severe tortuous fistula arising from the distal portion of circumflex artery and draining into the coronary sinus. (B) Complete occlusion following transvenous placement of Guglielmi detachable coils (Tacoy et al., 2009).

The Amplatzer duct occluder is an ideal device for CAFs closure provided the drainage is large enough to allow the passage of the long sheath. This device can be deployed antegradely or retrogradely, and usually use of a single device is enough for complete closure. Another useful device for CAFs closure is the Amplatzer vascular plug. It has wide range of device sizes and can be delivered through a 5–8 French standard coronary guiding catheter. Compared with umbrella devices, the plug affords greater opportunity to close the tortuous fistulae as it can be delivered through a flexible guiding catheter. Detachable coils can also be delivered through a guiding catheter, however, it seems that the plug has advantages over the detachable coil in ease of delivery and incidence of residual flow (Zhu et al, 2010). Double umbrella devices allow more precise positioning and are used in larger fistulae with coronary branches close to the occlusion site (Figure-9) (Armsby et al., 2002).

6.1.2 Technique

The transcatheter approach is a fairly complicated intervention and requires an experienced operator and interventional specialist with expertise in both coronary arteriography and

embolization techniques. A wide range of equipment should be available to deal with all the fistulas, as well as possible complications of the techniques.
Access is usually needed in both the femoral arteries and one femoral vein and sheaths are inserted initially. Afterwards, heparin needs to be administered (100 units/kg). After hemodynamic data is obtained, aortic root angiography and selective coronary angiography are performed in order to demonstrate the anatomy of the fistula, its drainage site, and in order to identify distal coronary branches (Zhu et al, 2010). Coronary angiograms are analyzed using different systems and the diameter of the fistula is measured. Approach to closure is determined by the number and the location of drainage sites, the location of the proximal coronary branches, and the ability to cannulate the distal part of the fistula. Device deployment is performed either antegrade (via the femoral vein) or retrograde (via the femoral artery). Antegrade deployment avoids potential damage to the femoral artery, and allows the use of larger catheters and affords a straighter catheter course. Retrograde deployment is to be attempted if there is a difficulty in establishing an arteriovenous wire loop through the fistula.

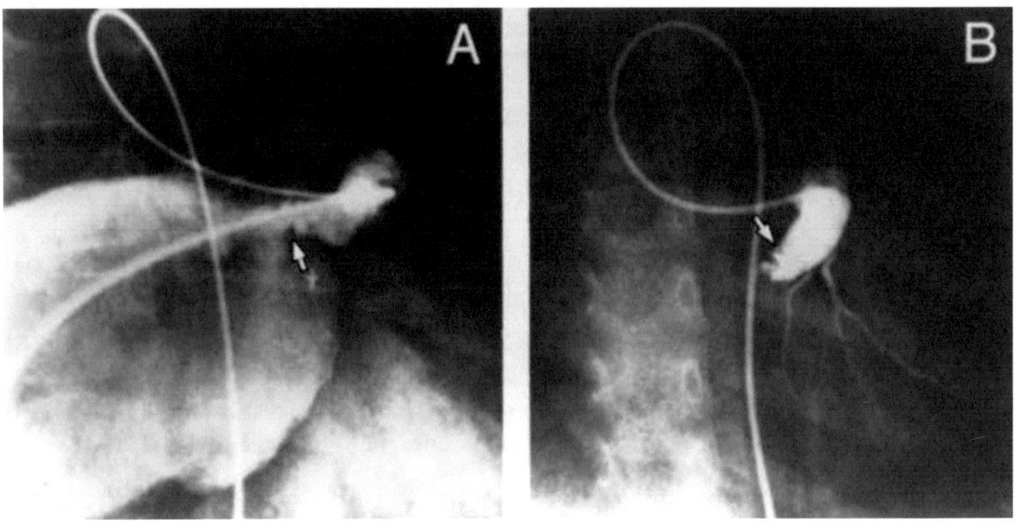

Fig. 9. Coronary artery fistula from left coronary artery to left atrium. (A) Arteriovenous wire loop enabling passage of venous catheter across the atrial septum into the fistula drainage site (**arrow**). (B) Angiogram following transvenous deployment of a 12-mm Rashkind device (**arrow**), showing coronary artery fistula occlusion and coronary artery side branches that were not evident in angiograms performed without balloon occlusion (Armsby et al., 2002).

A Berman or Swan-Ganz type of balloon catheter is passed and the balloon inflated with contrast in order to temporarily occlude the vessel. The purpose of this is to test for ischaemia. In the absence of ischaemic changes, the site, where the balloon has been kept inflated or its beyond, is an acceptable site for occlusion of the fistula (Qureshi, 2006). Afterwards, a guiding coronary catheter is positioned in the artery. With the standard guidewire advanced into the fistula, the guiding catheter may be passed to the point of intended occlusion and then, either Gianturco or Cook-PDA coils can be deployed through this catheter to achieve occlusion. The coil should be up to 30% larger than the vessel to be occluded at the point of occlusion to avoid inadvertent embolisation of the coil. Once the first coil is in correct position, different sizes of coils can be deployed subsequently to form a tight nest (Qureshi, 2006).

Amplatzer occluder type of devices is suitable to the fistula which can be reached via the right side of the heart (Zhou et al, 2006). The fistula vessel should be large, have easy and straight access from the right heart, if needed with the help of an arteriovenous guidewire circuit, and allow a guiding sheath to be passed into the vessel for the occlusion device. In these, either femoral venous or internal jugular venous access is used. Detachable balloons are rarely used nowadays. They can be floated out with the arterial flow and achieve immediate occlusion and then the balloon is detached. They are complex to use and require large introducer catheters (6–8 Fr). Early deflation and premature detachment of these balloons incur further problems, which have made most operators avoid of using them (Qureshi, 2006). Selective coronary angiography in multiple projections is essential before, during and after coil implantation (Olgunturk et al., 2006).

The advantages of the transcatheter closure of CAFs are: shorter hospital stays, less myocardial damage, less invasion, and fewer complications compared with conventional open surgery possible for the patients. Successful occlusion of the CAFs at catheterization was reported in >83-95% of patients. In the remaining patients, they are to be managed conservatively or with surgery (Nakayama et al., 2010).

The procedural complications include transient ischemic changes, unretrieved device embolization, fistula dissection, transient T-wave changes, transient bundle branch block, myocardial infarction, and transient atrial arrhythmia and death. All these complications are rare, apart from inadvertent coil migration, which may occur as a result of high flow in the large fistulas or with undersized coils. Even if the coils do migrate, they can be retrieved with snares (Qureshi, 2006). Catheter-based closure of CAFs has a better clinical outcome and the operative mortality is 1.4% 0% in current transcatheter closure (Olivotti et al, 2008; Armsby et al., 2002; Qureshi, 2006). Intimal dissection of the coronary artery, thrombosis or pericardial effusion may also occur. However, morbidity and mortality rates generally are considered to be low. The pericardial effusion may be associated with increased hydrostatic pressure of pericardial vessels, pericardial inflammation or it is similar to the postpericardiotomy syndrome after open heart surgery. After pericardial tap and anti-inflammatory agents with aspirin, the effusion disappears gradually (Fue et al., 1997).

In order to reduce complications during the procedure, several procedural and clinical details mandate special attention. First, precise identification of the distal coronary branches is difficult before the fistula is closed due to fast blood flow through the fistula vessel. Thus, the optimal site for device placement is the fistula drainage. However, even after the device is placed at the fistula drainage, it does not mean that a small area of myocardial infarction would not occur. Therefore, it is necessary to monitor ST-T changes for 24 to 48 hours after CAFs closure. Secondly, the sizing of the device is difficult due to variation of the fistula morphology. Undersizing of the device may lead to complications such as residual shunt and device migration, especially when the patient is a child (Zhu et al., 2010).

6.2 Surgical treatment

The first surgical treatment of CAFs was performed by Bjork and Crafoord in 1947 (Ata et al. 2009). The indications for surgery include a large CAF characterized by high fistula flow, multiple communications, very tortuous pathways, multiple terminations, significant aneurysmal formation, simultaneous distal bypass, or presence of large vascular branches that can be accidentally embolized (Zenooz et al, 2009). If the placement of the occlusion device is considered to be difficult due to aneurysmatic change and tortuous vessel, or if it occludes a coronary artery branch, operation is needed. In addition, it has been reported that surgery should be carried out earlier for a low surgical risk patient, considering future CAF-related problems, even if the patient does not have symptoms (McMahon et al., 2001).

6.2.1 Techniques

Surgical repair usually is approached via a median sternotomy and cardiopulmonary bypass. Identify the feeding vessel and delineate its course and site of insertion. Identify the site of presumed fistulous drainage prior to institution of the cardiopulmonary bypass. A typical procedure includes opening the chamber into which the fistula drains, identifying the fistula, and then closes it either by external ligation or by internal patching of the orifices (Liberthson et al., 1979).

If the fistula enters the ventricle or if the feeding vessel is large, the coronary artery is opened, and the opening to the fistula is closed with a running suture. The arteriotomy is closed. Large aneurysms may require excision. Rarely, when the fistula is an end artery, it may be ligated with or without bypass.

Some authors have reported successful surgical occlusion of CAFs on beating heart without cardiopulmonary bypass. Ligation of the CAFs may be performed on the outside of the beating heart when it is easily accessible. But some recommend exploration of the pulmonary artery with the use of cardiopulmonary bypass especially in patients who have CAFs in combination with a vascular malformation (Ata et al., 2009).

Complete occlusion of the fistula may be achieved in >95% of cases after surgery. Complications of surgery include myocardial ischemia and/or infarction (reported in 3% of patients) and recurrence of the fistula (4% of patients). The reason for the recurrence includes the fact that there may be multiple fistulas present which are difficult to deal with by surgery.

6.3 Follow-up after transcatheter and surgical closure

The outcome of transcatheter occlusion is as good as that of surgical correction. Patients which are closed by using transcatheter techniques need to be closely followed up for complications such as residual shunts, new fistula formation, formation of thrombus, coronary aneurysma and coronary artery stenosis. Clinical experiences show that the short-, middle- and long-term outcome of transcatheter closure of CAFs has been satisfactory. Residual or recurrent shunts after transcatheter closure have been reported in 10–20% of patients and these may require further procedures to achieve complete occlusion (Liang et al, 2010; Zhu et al, 2010). A study shows that an incidence of major complications which occurs late after closure of CAFs with transcatheter and surgical interventions is 15% (Valente et al, 2010). Mortality related to surgical closure or transcatheter closure of isolated CAFs is low (<1%) (Qureshi, 2006; Urrutia-S et al., 1983).

All patients should be controlled on the following day after a chest radiograph, electrocardiogram, and Doppler echocardiography study and the physical status, electrocardiogram, and Doppler echocardiography need to be followed regularly every 3–6 months during the first year and annually thereafter. Close long-term follow-up with coronary angiography and myocardial scintigraphy after transcatheter or surgical closure of CAFs is very important in order to be able to recognize possible recanalization and complications (Luo et al., 2006; Angelini, 2002b). The late complications are presence of myocardial infarction, coronary thrombosis, ventricular tachycardia, or heart failure. The etiology of the late complications is associated with angiographic and clinical features of CAFs. The drainage of the CAFs into the coronary sinus may lead to late complications of CAFs. Clinical predictors associated with adverse outcomes include older age, tobacco use, diabetes, systemic hypertension, and hyperlipidemia (Valente et al., 2010).

6.4 Medical treatment

Medical treatment is the most common choice for the mild symptoms. (Sam et al., 2006). Patients who are conservatorly treated should be followed up closely for appearance of symptoms. Most of the adult patients who are asymptomatic remain free of symptoms for long periods (Gowda et al., 2006).

Medical management of patients with angina due to CAFs is similar to management of angina in the absence of CAFs. Beta-blockers or calcium channel blockers are usually recommended in angina related diseases. Nitrates must be used cautiously, as they can cause dilation of the fistula and they decrease the end-diastolic pressure of the recipient ventricle, both of which can lead to increased shunt flow and coronary "steal".

Medical management after complete CAFs occlusion remains controversial in the literature. Most studies do not suggest antiaggregan and anticoagulation treatment. However, in view of the persistence of the fistulous cul-de-sac, coronary artery dilation, and potential for thrombus formation (which may lead to myocardial infarction), aspirin is indicated. For severe coronary artery dilatation (>10 mm), some authors advocate anticoagulation with warfarin. Patients treated surgically and with transcatheter techniques should receive maintenance doses of antiplatelet agents and, perhaps, an anticoagulant regime for the first 6 months postoperatively, until the operative surface has endothelizated.

CAFs that drain into the coronary sinus are particularly at high risk of long-term morbidities after CAFs closure, and strategies, including long-term anticoagulation, should be considered in these patients (Valente et al., 2008).

Patients remain at risk for development of endocarditis until the flow is stopped and should receive antibiotic prophylaxis for any dental, gastrointestinal tract, and urologic procedures. Therefore, prophylaxis for bacterial endocarditis is recommended in all CAF patients and in patients after complete fistula occlusion for at least 1 year.

Since advanced age and modifiable coronary risk factors, such as hyperlipidemia, systemic hypertension, diabetes, and tobacco use, are associated with increased risk of CAFs complications, control of these factors is needed.

7. Conclusion

With increased experience and improved devices and techniques, transcatheter closer techniques of CAFs are emerging as a successful therapeutic strategy. The safe and effective results of both surgical closure and transcatheter closer support the current convention of elective closure of clinically significant CAFs in childhood. The preferred method of approach for any individual will depend on the anatomy of the fistula, the presence or the absence of the associated defects and the experience of the interventional cardiologists and surgeons.

Coronary artery fistulas can be safely and effectively closed using transcatheter techniques. Anatomical variations and different sizes of coronary artery fistulas necessitate availability of different sizes and types of devices at the time of catheterization for successful closure.

Recent results of both transcatheter and surgical approaches indicate a good prognosis. Life expectancy is considered normal. Patients need to be closely followed up for complication such as residual shunts, new fistula formation and coronary artery stenosis.

8. Acknowledgment

I am particularly grateful to Assoc. Prof. Recep Cigdem, Paolo Angelini, MD, Salah Said, MD, Gulten Tacoy, MD, and others who gave permission to use their materials.

9. References

Acar, G. et al. (2010). Bilateral coronary artery fistula originating from the right sinus of Valsalva and left circumflex artery,and draining into the pulmonary artery. *Hellenic J Cardiol.*Vol.51, No.5, pp.458-459, ISSN: 1109-9666

Angelini, P.; Villason, S.; Chan, A.V. & Diez, J.G. (1999). Normal and anomalous coronary arteries in humans. In: Angelini P, ed. *Coronary Artery Anomalies.* pp. 27-150. Lippincott Williams & Wilkins ISBN 978-0781710183, Philadelphia.

Angelini, P. et al. (2002a). Coronary anomalies: incidence, pathophysiology, and clinical relevance. *Circulation,* Vol. 105, No.20, pp.2449-2454, ISSN: 0009-7322

Angelini, P. (2002b). Coronary Artery Anomalies—Current Clinical Issues Definitions, Classification, Incidence, Clinical Relevance, and Treatment Guidelines. *Tex Heart Inst J,* Vol.29, No.4, pp.271-278, ISSN:0730-2347

Angelini, P. (2007). Coronary artery anomalies: an entity in search of an identity. *Circulation,* Vol.115, No.10, pp.1296-1305, ISSN: 0009-7322

Armsby, L.R. et al. (2002). Management of coronary artery fistulae. Patient selection and results of transcatheter closure. *J Am Coll Cardiol.* Vol.39, No.6, pp.1026-1032, ISSN: 0735-1097

Ata, Y. et al. (2009). Coronary arteriovenous fistulas in the adults: natural history and management strategies. *J Cardiothorac Surg.* Vol.6, no.4, pp.62, ISSN: 1749-8090

Bhandari, S. et al. (1993). Coronary artery fistulae without audible murmur in adults. *Cardiovasc Interven Radiol,* Vol:16, No.4, pp.219-223, ISSN: 7415-5101

Cebi, N. et al. (2008). Heuer H. Congenital coronary artery fistulas in adults: concomitant pathologies and treatment. *Int J Cardiovasc Imaging.* Vol.24, No.4, pp.349-355, ISSN: 1569-5794

Chiu C.Z. et al. (2008). Angiographic and Clinical Manifestations of Coronary Fistulas in Chinese People 15-Year Experience. *Circ J,* Vol. 72, No.8, pp.1242-1248, ISSN: 1346-9843

Cheung, D.L., et al. (2001). Coronary artery fistulas: long-term results of surgical correction. *Ann Thorac Surg,* Vol.71, No.1, pp.190-195, ISSN; ISSN; 1552-6259

Davis, J.T, et al. (1994). Coronary artery fistula in the pediatric age group: a 19-year institutional experience. *Ann Thorac Surg,* Vol.58, No.3, pp.760-763, ISSN; 1552-6259

Dodd, J.D., et al. (2008. Evaluation of efficacy of 64-slice multidetector computed tomography in patients with congenital coronary fistulas. *J Comput Assist Tomogr.* Vol.32, No.2, pp.265-270, ISSN: 0363-8715

Dursun, A, et al. (2009). Diagnosis of the left circumflex coronary artery fistula drainage into the left ventricle by echocardiographic color Doppler flow imaging. *Int J Cardiol,* Vol.134, No.3, pp. e85–e86, ISSN: 0167-5273

Fahey, J.T. & Asnes, J. (2008). Coronary recanalization due to presumed thrombosis following surgical ligation of a large right coronary artery to right ventricle fistula. *Congenit Heart Dis,* Vol.3, No.4, pp.295-298, ISSN: 1747-0803

Friedman, A.H. et al. (2007). Identification, imaging, functional assessment and management of congenital coronary arterial abnormalities in children. *Cardiol Young*. Vol.17, No.Suppl. 2, pp.56–67, ISSN 1047-9511

Fu, Y.C. et al (1997). Transcatheter embolization of coronary artery fistula: a case report. *Zhonghua Yi Xue Za Zhi (Taipei),* Vol.59, No.3, pp.194-198, ISSN: 0578-1337

Gillebert, C. Et al. (1986). Coronary artery fistulas in an adult population. Eur Heart J, Vol.7, No.5, pp.437-443, ISSN: 1522-9645

Gowda, R.M. et al. (2006). Coronary artery fistulas: clinical and therapeutic considerations, *Int J Cardiol.* Vol.107, No.1, pp.7–10, ISSN: 0167-5273

Gupta-Malhotra, M. (Jan 12, 2010). Coronary artery fistula. In: *Pediatrics Cardiac Disease and Critical Care Medicine,* http://emedicine.medscape.com/article/895749-overview?src=emailthis

Holzer, R. et al. (2004). Review of an institutional experience of coronary arterial fistulas in childhood set in context of review of the literature. *Cardiol Young,* Vol.14, No.4, pp.380-385, ISSN: 1047-9511

Hobbs, R.E. et al. (1982). Coronary artery fistulae: a 10-year review. *Cleve Clin Q,* Vol. 49, No.4, pp.191-197, ISSN: 0009-8787

Hsieh, K.S. et al. (2002). Coronary artery fistulas in neonates, infants, and children: Clinical findings and outcome. *Pediatr Cardiol,* Vol.23, No.4, pp.415-419, ISSN: 1432-1971

Juraschek, S.P. et al. (2011). Heart failure with transient left bundle branch block in the setting of left coronary fistula. *Cardiol Res Pract.* Vol. 2011, No.786287, pp.1-3, ISSN: 2090-0597

Iglesias, J.F. et al. (2010. Transcatheter coil embolization of multiple bilateral congenital coronary artery fistulae. *J Invasive Cardiol,* Vol.22, No.3, pp.142-145, ISSN: 1042-3931

Kardos, A. et al. (1997). Epidemiology of congenital coronary artery anomalies: a coronary arteriography study on a central European population. *Cathet Cardiovasc Diagn,* Vol.42, No.3, pp.270-275, ISSN: 0098-6569

Kamiya, H. et al. (2002). Surgical treatment of congenital coronary artery fistulas: 27 years' experience and a review of the literature. *J Card Surg,* Vol.17, No.2, pp.173-177, ISSN: 0886-0440

Kose, S. & Heper, G. (2005). Increased myocardial ischemia during nitrate therapy: caused by multiple coronary artery-left ventricle fistulae? *Tex Heart Inst J,* Vol.32, No.1, pp.50-52, ISSN: 0730-2347

Krishnamoorthy, K.M., et al. (2004). Transesophagial echocardiography for the diagnosis of coronary arteriovenous fistula. *Int J Cardiol,*Vol.96, No.2, pp. 281– 283, ISSN: 0167-5273

Wong, K. et al. (2000). Coronary arterial fistula in childhood. *Cardiol Young,* Vol.10, No.1, pp.15- 20, ISSN: 1467-1107

Lee, C.M. et al. (2007). Identification of a Coronary-to-Bronchial-Artery Communication With MDCT Shows the Diagnostic Potential of This New Technology Case Report and Review. *J Thorac Imaging,* Vol.22, No.3, pp.274–276, ISSN: 0883-5993

Levin, D.C. et al. (1978). Hemodynamically significant primary anomalies of the coronary arteries: angiographic aspects. *Circulation,* Vol.58, No.1, pp.25 - 34, ISSN: 0009-7322

Liberthson, R.R. et al. (1979). Congenital coronary arteriovenous fistula. Report of 13 patients, review of the literature and delineation of management. *Circulation.* Vol.59, No.5, pp.849-854, ISSN: 0009-7322

Lin, C.T. & Lin, T. K. (2009). The Current Status of Coronary Artery Fistula. *J Intern Med Taiwan,* Vol.20, No.6, pp.484-489, ISSN: 1016-7390

Luo, L. et al. (2006). Coronary arterial fistulas. *Am J Med Sci,*Vol.332, No.2, pp.79–84, ISSN: 1538-2990

Marijon, E. et al. (2007). Coronary fistula as an unusual cause of angina in a middle-aged man. *Pediatr Cardiol,* Vol.209, No.5, pp.993-994. ISSN: 0172-0643

McMahon, C.J. et al. (2001). Coronary artery fistula: management and intermediate-term outcome after transcatheter coil occlusion. *Tex Heart Inst J,* Vol.28, No.1, pp.21–25, ISSN: 0730-2347

McNamara, J.J. & Gross, R.E. (1969). Congenital coronary artery fistula. *Surgery;* Vol.65, No.1, pp.59-69, ISSN: 0039-6060.

Naber, C.K. et al. (2004). Percutaneous coil embolization of a large, congenital coronary—pulmonary fistula using hydrophiliccoated detachable platinum coils. *Herz,* Vol.29, No.2, pp.218-219, ISSN: 1615-6692

Nakayama, Y. et al. (2010). Surgical repair of complicated coronary arteriovenous fistula and coronary artery aneurysm in an elderly patient after 26 years of conservative therapy. *Heart Vessels,* Vol.26, No.1 pp. 111-116, ISSN: 1615-2573

Nawa, S. Et al. (1996). Clinical and angiographic analysis of congenital coronary artery fistulae in adulthood. Is there any new trend? *Jpn Heart J,* Vol.37, No.1, pp.95-104, ISSN: 0021-4868

Okamoto, M. et al. (2006). Successful coil embolization with assistance of coronary stenting in an adult patient

with a huge coronary arterial—right atrial fistula. *Intern Med,* Vol.45, No.14, pp.865-870. ISSN: 1445-5994

Olgunturk, R. et al. (2006). Transcatheter closure of a rare form of coronary arteriovenous fistula (circumflex artery to coronary sinus). *Int J Cardiol,* Vol.113, No.2, pp.261–263, ISSN: 0167-5273

Olivotti, L. et al. (2008). Percutaneous closure of a giant coronary arteriovenous fistula using free embolization coils in an adult patient. *J Cardiovasc Med (Hagerstown),*Vol.9, No.7, pp.733-736. ISSN: 1558-2035

Pala, S. et al. (2011). Noninvasive evaluation of a giant circumflex coronary artery aneurysm fistulized into the coronary sinus by multislice computed tomography. *Arch Turk Soc Cardiol,* Vol.39, No.1, pp. 39:88

Qureshi, S.A. (2006), Coronary arterial fistulas. *Orphanet J Rare Dis*, Vol.1, No.51, pp.1-6, ISSN: 1750-1172

Qureshi, S.A. et al. (1996). Use of interlocking detachable coils in embolization of coronary arteriovenous fistulas. *Am J Cardiol*, Vol.78, No.1, pp:110-113, ISSN: 1879-1913

Gowda, R.M. et al. (2006). Coronary artery fistulas: Clinical and therapeutic considerations. *Int J Cardiol,* Vol.107, No.1, pp.7–10, ISSN: 0167-5273

Reidy, J.F. et al. (1983). Thranscatheter occlusion of coronary to bronchial anastomosis by deta balloon combined

with coronary angioplasty at same procedure. *Br Heart J,* Vol.49, No.3, pp.284–287, ISSN: 0007-0769

Said, S.A.M. & Wert, T. (2006). Dutc survey of congenital coronary artery fistulas in adults: Coronary artery-left ventricular multiple micro-fistulas multi-center observational survey in the Netherlands. *Int J Cardiol,* Vol.110, No.1, pp.33-39, ISSN: 0167-5273

Said, S.A.M. (2010). Congenital solitary coronary artery fistulas characterized by their drainage sites. *World J Cardiol.* Vol.2, No.1, pp. 6-12, ISSN: 1949-8462

Shewood, M.C. et al. (1999). Prognostic significance of clinically silent coronary artery fistulas. *Am J Cardiol*, Vol.83, No.3, pp.407-411, ISSN: 0002-9149

Srinivasan, K.G. (2008). Congenital coronary artery anomalies: diagnosis with 64 slice multidetector row computed tomography coronary angiography: a single-centre study. *J Med Imaging Radiat Oncol.* Vol.52, No.2, pp.148-154, ISSN: 1754-9485

Tacoy, G. et al. (2009). Congenitally severe tortuous circumflex artery fistula draining into the coronary sinus: Transcatheter closure with Guglielmi detachable coils via different delivery system. *J Cardio*, Vol.54, No.2, pp.317-321, ISSN: 1876-4738

Urrutia-S, C.O. et al. (1983). Surgical management of 56 patients with congenital coronary artery fistulas. *Ann Thorac Surg,* Vol.35, No.3, pp.300-307, ISSN: 1552-6259

XU Liang, X.U. et al. (2010). Transcatheter closure of coronary artery fistula in children. *Chin Med J,* Vol.123, No.7, pp.822-826, ISSN: 0366-6999

Valente, A.M. et al. (2010). Predictors of Long-Term Adverse Outcomes in Patients With Congenital Coronary Artery Fistulae. *Circ Cardiovasc Interv.* No.3, No.2, pp.134-139, ISSN: 1941-7632

Vavuranakis, M. et al. (1995). Coronary artery fistulas in adults: incidence, angiographic characteristics, natural history. *Cathet Cardiovasc Diag,* Vol.35, No.2, pp.116-120, ISSN: 0098-6569

Yamanaka, 0. Hobbs, R.E. (1990). Coronary artery anomalies in 126,595 patients undergoing coronary arteriography. *Cathet Curdiovasc Diugn*, Vol.21, No.1, pp.28-40, ISSN: 0098-6569

Yildiz, A., et al. (2010). Prevalence of coronary artery anomalies in 12,457 adult patients who underwent coronary angiography. *Clin Cardiol*, Vol.33, No.12, pp.60-64, ISSN: 0160-9289

Zenooz, N.A. et al. (2009). Coronary Artery Fistulas: CT Findings. *RadioGraphics*, Vol.29, No.3, pp.781–789, ISSN: 1527-1323

Zhou, T. et al. (2006). Transcatheter closure of a giant coronary artery fistula with patent duct occluder. *Chin Med J (Engl),* Vol.119, No.9, pp.779-781, ISSN: 0366-6999

Zhu, X.Y. et al. (2010). Transcatheter Closure of Congenital Coronary Artery Fistulae: Immediate and Long-Term Follow-Up Results. *Clin Cardiol,* Vol.32, No.9, pp.506–512, ISSN: 1932-8737

11

Association Between Fatty Liver and Cardiovascular Disease: Mechanism and Clinical Implications

Nseir W.[1,3] and Assy N.[2,3]
[1]*Departments of Internal Medicine, Holy Family Hospital, Nazareth,*
[2]*Liver Unit, Ziv Medical Center, Safed*
[3]*Faculty of Medicine, Technion, Haifa,*
Israel

1. Introduction

NAFLD is associated with major cardiovascular risk factors including type 2 diabetes mellitus (T2DM), obesity, dyslipidemia, hypertension and insulin resistance and constitutes a new component of the metabolic syndrome (MetS) [1-2].The association of MetS and NAFLD is so strong that NAFLD is considered as the hepatic manifestation of MetS [3]. The clinical implication of NAFLD and nonalcoholic steatohepatitis (NASH) are mainly derived from their common occurrence in the general population (15%-30%) and their potential to contribute to CAD, extra hepatic cancer, diabetes, and progression to fibrosis (30%-40%), cirrhosis (20%-30%) and hepatocellular carcinoma [4-5]. Although the mechanisms underlying liver disease progression remain unclear, insulin resistance and obesity-related inflammation, obesity related ectopic fat and lipotoxicity play a key role, along with possible genetic, dietary and life style factors [6].

Most studies show that MetS is associated with a two-fold increase in CAD risk and a 5-fold increased risk for incidences of T2DM [7-12]. The importance of NAFLD component within the MetS is now increasingly recognized, and this has stimulated an interest in the possible relationship between NAFLD and cardiovascular disease (CVD). This review focuses on the relationship between NAFLD and CAD, the Biological mechanisms linking NAFLD and CAD and a proposed new treatment approach for patients with NAFLD.

2. The relationship between NAFLD and CAD

Prevalence: NAFLD affects 15-30% of the general population [13]. The prevalence is also high in overweight and obese children [14]. Factors contributing to NAFLD include sedentary life style, and increased consumption of foods with high fat and high fructose corn syrup content (soft drinks). Steatosis is associated with an increased prevalence and incidence of CAD and cardiovascular mortality. [15- 16].

Clinical studies: Targher et al showed a significant increase of carotid intima-media thickness (IMT) in the presence of NAFLD [17]. Brea et al showed that patients with NAFLD had increased intima-media thickness (IMT), independently by the MetS [18]. Lin et al showed that patients with NAFLD were more likely to have CAD compared to patients without NAFLD, independent of obesity and other risk factors [19]. Villanova et al showed that NAFLD patients have a significant decrease in brachial artery flow- mediated vasodilatation, which correlates with the extent of liver disease. Furthermore, the 10-year probability of coronary heart disease (as calculated according to the Framingham risk score) was moderately increased in NAFLD patients, and particularly in patients with NASH [20]. This study and others provide evidence of severe endothelial dysfunction and increased risk of cardiovascular events in NAFLD [21]. Targher et al showed an increased prevalence of CAD in patients with T2DM and NAFLD as compared with diabetic patients without NAFLD [22] and that the severity of liver histology among NAFLD patients is strongly associated with early carotid atherosclerosis, independent of classical risk factors, insulin resistance, and the presence of MetS [23]. Akabame et al showed that NAFLD is a novel risk factor for vulnerable plaques, using a multislice computed tomography (MSCT) [24]. Recently, we showed that patients with NAFLD, even without MetS, have more vulnerable coronary soft plaques than healthy controls. [25] (Figure 1). Pacifico et al demonstrated that obese children with NAFLD have a marked increase in carotid IMT in comparison with control healthy children, and that the carotid IMT was higher for obese children with NAFLD than obese children without liver involvement but with similar body mass index (BMI) [26].

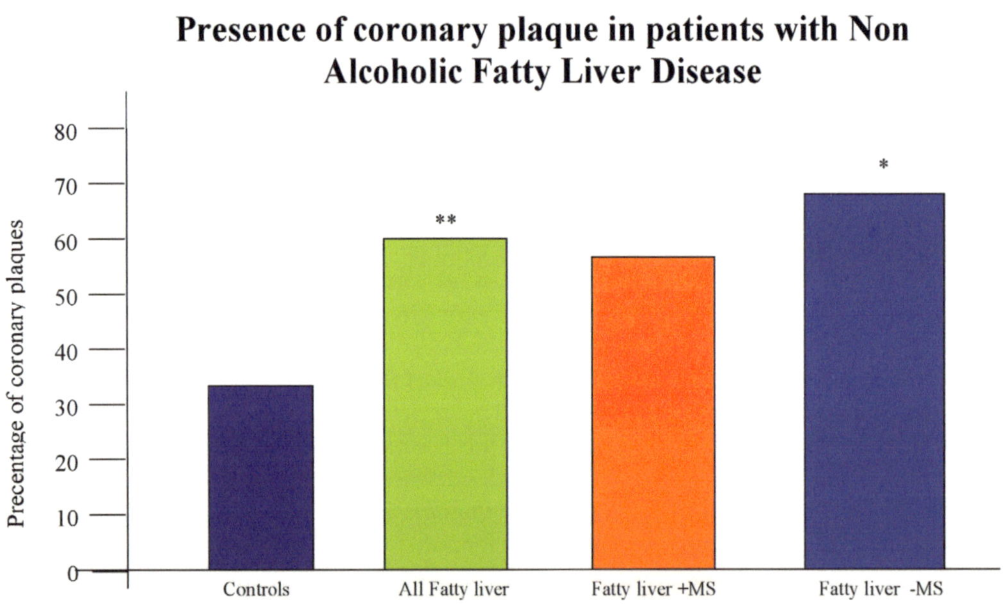

Graph of coronary plaque in NAFLD patients with or without metabolic syndrome (MS) and in controls *$P<0.07$; fatty liver without metabolic syndrome versus fatty liver with metabolic syndrome. **$P<0.001$;all fatty liver versus controls.(reference 25)

Fig. 1. Presence of coronary plaque in patients with Non Alcoholic Fatty Liver Disease

3. Cause of death in patients with NAFLD

The mortality rate among patients with NAFLD followed for 8 years was higher than in the general population, [27]. In another study consisting of biopsy-proven, NAFLD patients who were followed for 18 years, CVD was among the common causes of death after all of the cancers combined [28]. In the Valpolicella Heart Diabetes Study, Targher et al showed that NAFLD patients have been associated with an increased incidence of major CVD events after excluding classical risk factors, diabetes duration, glycemic control, medication use, and components of the metabolic syndrome [29-30]. Dunn et al showed that NAFLD patients had significantly increased all-cause mortality and cardiovascular mortality, especially in the 45-54 years age group [31]. A strong association between mildly elevated serum liver enzymes as a surrogate marker of NAFLD and increased risk for CVD mortality and morbidity was reported in several population-based cohort studies [21, 32, 33]. A Swedish study consisting of 129 patients with NAFLD showed that patients with NASH had higher incidences of cardiovascular mortality compared to the reference population [34]. Recently, other studies with 28 years follow up showed that CAD was the leading cause of death in patients with NAFLD, followed by hepatic and extra hepatic malignancy and finally by cirrhosis and its complications [35, 36, Table 1].

Cause of death	Number of patients	%
CAD	15	35.0
Extra hepatic cancer	12	28.0
Liver cancer, cirrhosis	8	18.6
Diabetes mellitus	3	7.0
Poisoning	3	6.8
Intestinal Perforation	1	2.3
Alcohol abuse	1	2.3

Table 1. Causes of Death in 143 patients with NAFLD (death= 43)

4. Classical and emerging risk factors for atherosclerosis

The new risk factors for CAD include markers for inflammation (e.g. CRP, lipoprotein A), homocystine, markers of fibrinolytic and homeostatic function (e.g. fibrinogen, tissue plasminogen activator, and plasminogen activator inhibitor-1). These markers are also associated with NAFLD [37-41]. The classic common risk factors for NAFLD and CAD are age and gender [42, 43], physical inactivity [44- 47], T2 DM [48-52], hyperlipidemia [53- 56], obesity [57-63], and hypertension [64- 66]. These risk factors are well known and beyond the scope of this review.

5. Mechanisms linking NAFLD and CAD

The biological mechanisms potentially responsible for accelerated atherogenesis in NAFLD patients may either have origin in the liver or have the liver as the target of systemic abnormalities. Here we will discuss the biological mechanisms linking NAFLD and CAD, the novel risk factors for CAD, and the common pathways of both diseases (Figure 2)

A) Oxidative stress

Oxidative stress plays an important role in the progression from simple steatosis to steatohepatitis [67]. The role of oxidative stress is supported by different animal models of

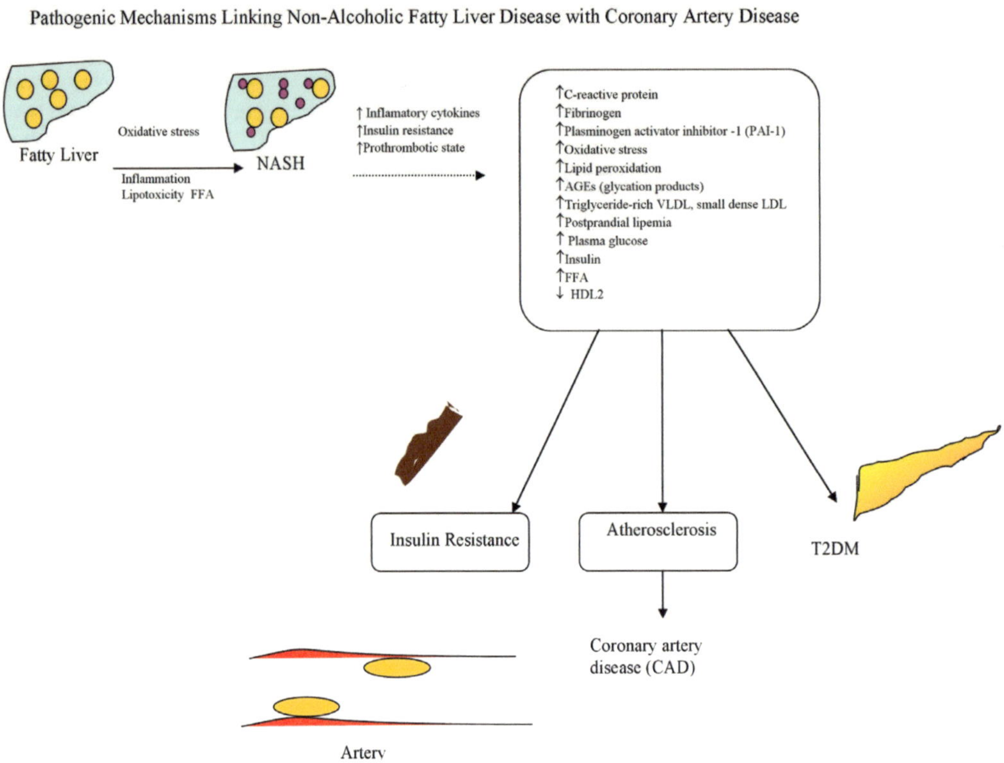

Fig. 2. Biological mechanism of accelerated atherosclerosis in patients with NAFLD. Fat accumulation in the liver induces hyperglycemia, sub clinical inflammation, atherogenic dylipidemia, lipotoxicity, and the secretion of cytokines. Thereby inducing insulin resistance, atherosclerosis, and diabetes mellitus. All contributes to coronary artery diseases.

NASH which show either increased reactive oxygen species (ROS) formation or evidence of extensive lipid peroxidation [68,69]. The association between oxidative stress and NAFLD in humans is supported by the immunohistochemical detection of lipid peroxidation products and 8-hydroxy-deoxyguanosine in the plasma and liver biopsies from patients with NAFLD [70, 71]. The earliest events in the pathogenesis of atherosclerosis are thought to be changes in endothelial functions, in turn triggered by oxidative modification of low-density lipoproteins (LDL), leading to the formation of oxidized LDL in the subintimal space [72]. The expression of chemotactic factors such as monocyte chemotactic protein-1
(MCP-1) is enhanced by oxidative stress and oxidized LDL Endothelial expression of vascular cell adhesion molecule-1 (VCAM-1), which is regulated through a redox-sensitive mechanism, promotes the adhesion of monocytes to the endothelium. The release of macrophage colony-stimulating factor (M-CSF) is also stimulated by modified LDL. Expression of these factors results in the attraction and adhesion of monocytes to the arterial wall and the promotion of their differentiation into tissue macrophages. Exposure to the superoxide ion, a ROS, activates the nuclear factor kappa-B (NF-kappa B) regulatory complex and triggers the transcription of several atherosclerosis-related genes (VCAM-1, MCP-1, tumor necrosis factor (TNF), matrix metalloproteinase (MMP)-9 and procoagulant

tissue factor). This series of events leads to the accumulation of macrophages in the arterial wall, which then avidly incorporate oxidized LDL to form foam cells. Oxidized LDL, in turn, stimulates the release of interleukin-1 from macrophages. The activity of MMPs is also regulated by oxidative stress and appears to be closely linked to smooth muscle cell activation and migration. MMPs have also been implicated in the physiopathology of plaque rupture. Furthermore, ROS can lead to platelet activation and thrombus formation. Therefore, oxidative stress appears to be important in both the early and later stages of the atherosclerotic process [73, 74].

B) Insulin resistance

NAFLD is strongly associated with hepatic and adipose tissue insulin resistance (IR), as well as reduced whole-body insulin sensitivity [75]. Previous studies have documented a reduction of 45-50% in glucose disposal, and an impaired ability of insulin to suppress endogenous glucose production (hepatic IR) in subjects with NAFLD [76]. The spectrum of metabolic disturbances associated with IR extends beyond hyperglycemia and includes dyslipidemia, obesity, hypercoagulability, and inflammation. In long-term follow-up of patients with T2DM, IR was independently predictive of CAD, with a 1-unit increase in IR assessed by the homeostasis model assessment (HOMA) associated with a 5.4% increased risk for CAD [77]. Increased levels of fatty acids, (NEFA), lipotoxicity and disturbances in adipokine secretion, are believed to be related to insulin resistance. Increased levels of NEFA might affect the endothelial nitric oxide production, thereby impairing endothelium-dependent vasodilatation. They may increase myocardial oxygen requirements and, therefore. ischemia. Recent evidence in older men with CAD has shown that NEFAs are independently associated with cardiovascular mortality [78]. The Insulin Resistance and Atherosclerosis Study (IRAS) also confirmed the relation between IR and atherosclerosis in the carotid artery [79]. Overall, growing evidence suggests that hepatic insulin resistance is sufficient to induce several components of the metabolic syndrome and promote progression to cardiovascular disease

C) Sub clinical inflammation

Targher et al showed that in healthy non-smoking volunteers, plasma CRP, fibrinogen, von Willebrand factor (v-WF) and plasminogen activator inhibitor-1 (PAI-1) activity levels were markedly higher in subjects with hepatic steatosis than in those without, even after controlling for other confounders such as age, BMI, blood pressure, insulin resistance and triglyceride levels [80]. Recently, Il-6 and CRP have been shown to correlate with higher degrees of fibrosis and inflammation (i.e. NASH) in patients with NAFLD [81]. Thus, NAFLD/NASH should be considered a chronic inflammatory condition. Recent advances in basic science have established a fundamental role for inflammation in mediating all stages of atherosclerosis from initiation through progression and, ultimately, the thrombotic complications of atherosclerosis.

Prospective epidemiological studies have found increased vascular risk in association with increased inflammatory markers such as, IL-6, TNF-α, CRP and fibrinogen [82-85]. Elevated values of circulating inflammatory markers commonly accompany acute coronary syndrome (ACS). Such elevations correlate with in-hospital and short-term prognosis [85, 86].Chronic subclinical inflammation is a common finding in NAFLD and in atherosclerosis. Moreover, chronic sub clinical inflammation is strongly involved in IR and MetS, as mainly demonstrated by mechanistic studies in animal models [87]. Ectopic fat deposition in visceral adipose depots, heart and other depots increases the expression of visceral

proinflammatory mediators such as monocyte chemotactic protein-1 and IL-6, leading to local macrophage infiltration and associated systemic chronic inflammation [88].
Hepatic steatosis is associated with increased production of pro-inflammatory cytokines by hepatocytes and non-parenchymal cells, including Kupffer cells and hepatic stellate cells. Increased intra-hepatic cytokine expression results from local NF-kB activation, mediated by hepatocellular damage and fat-derived factors, and is likely to play a major role in NAFLD progression and CVD pathogenesis [81, 88-90].
An atherogenic role of liver inflammation is supported by the observation that CAD risk is greater in NASH than in simple hepatic steatosis [27, 28].
D) Adiponectin
Liver fat accumulation, NEFAs, adiponectin, low-grade inflammation in the context of insulin resistance patient with fatty liver, might explain the development of endothelial dysfunction and early cardiovascular disease. Mature adipocytes act as an active endocrine and paracrine organ, secreting an increasing number of growth factors that participate in diverse metabolic processes, particularly IR. Patients with NAFLD exhibit reduced levels of adiponectin, which are inversely correlated with the severity of NAFLD histology [91-93]. The reduced production of adiponectin associated with obesity may contribute to the progression of NAFLD [89]. Adiponectin increases the expression of messenger RNA and protein production of tissue inhibitor of metalloproteinase in macrophages through the induction of IL-10 synthesis and selectively suppresses endothelial cell apoptosis [94, 95]. This suggests that adiponectin protects plaque rupture by the inhibition of matrix metalloproteinase function. Endothelium-dependent vasoreactivity is impaired in people with hypoadiponectinaemia, which might be at least one cause of hypertension in visceral obesity [96]. The protein inhibits the expression of adhesion molecules, such as vascular cell adhesion molecule-1 (VCAM-1), ICAM-1 and E-selectin, through the inhibition of NF-κB activation; it also suppresses foam-cell formation. From this, it is clear that adipokines are capable of contributing to remodeling of the myocardial extracellulat matrix [96]
E) Myocardial Lipotoxicity
Increasing plasma free fatty acids for few hours causes endothelial dysfunction and induces the production of systemic inflammation, and pro coagulants in vitro, in animal models and in humans. Of interest, free fatty acid impairs nitric oxide production by endothelial cells through the activation of an IKKb- mediated response. For instance, subjects with either glucose intolerance or T2DM have a significant increase in myocardial triglyceride content. There is a significant correlation between the development of fatty liver and abnormalities in left ventricular energy metabolism. [97]. In Diabetic patients with NAFLD, fatty liver and elevated aminotransferases coexist with myocardial insulin resistance and coronary dysfunction [97]
F) Atherogenic dyslipidemia
Liver fat accumulation originate from peripheral fats stored in adipose tissue that flow to the liver via the plasma nonesterified fatty acid (NEFA, 60%) pool, fatty acids newly made within the liver through de novo lipogenesis (DNL, 30%), and from dietary fatty acid uptake (10%). The fat of lipids entering the liver may be secreted as very low-density lipoprotein (VLDL) triglycerides, oxidized or stored. The major component of dyslipidemia in NAFLD patients is an elevation of serum triglycerides (TG) which comes mainly from increased concentration of VLDL. In addition to increased synthesis of VLDL, there is also decreased clearance of triacylglycerol-rich lipoprotein (TRLs) induced by a decrease in lipoprotein lipase activity [98]. Other components of dyslipidemia, such as formation of small dens low-density lipoprotein (LDL), are closely associated with IR and hypertriglyceridemia [99].

VLDL1 triglyceride is a major predictor of LDL size. It seems that stimulated hepatic lipase activity favors the formation of small dense LDL particles. The increased activity of hepatic lipase in IR conditions such as in NAFLD and obesity produces smaller HDL particles, leading to increased HDL elimination [100]. In addition, increased levels of VLDL1 alter the composition of HDL, leading finally to an increased catabolism of these particles, which explains the inverse correlation of HDL and liver fat [101]. In summary, patients with NAFLD have increased levels of VLDL, TG, and small dense LDL particles and decreased levels of HDL. The presence of small dense LDL particles is associated with increased CVD risk [102]. Small dense LDL particles can move through endothelial fenestrations, entering the subendothelial space where inflammation and transformation into plaque can occur, and leading finally to coronary artery diseases [103]. Further, alterations in smooth muscle ion channels, Ca^{2+} handling, and cell signaling may be important mechanisms leading to coronary micro vascular dysfunction [103].

G) Postprandial lipemia

Exaggerated postprandial lipemia is an established CVD risk in T2DM [104]. Studies comparing the postprandial response of TG and FFA to a fat rich meal in nondiabetic subjects with biopsy proven NASH to control subjects showed that patients with NASH had significantly higher postprandial TG levels than healthy control subjects [105]. Other studies support a close relationship between dietary habits, postprandial lipemia and CAD [106]. The atherosclerotic risk of postprandial hyperlipidemia is derived from an increase of remnant lipoproteins (RLPs) [107]. In patients with IR, an increase of postprandial RLP values usually occurs and becomes a coronary risk factor. The RLP is easily taken into the macrophage in the arterial wall via the apolipoprotein B48 receptor, promoting foam cell formation of macrophages and performing the atherosclerotic lesion as is oxidized LDL [108]. Stanhope et al showed that consumption of fructose-sweetened but not glucose-sweetened beverages for 10 weeks increases de novo lipid synthesis and the 24-hour postprandial TG including increased levels of apoB, LDL, oxidized LDL, RLP triglyceride, and the apoB / apoA1 ratio (all biomarkers of increased for CAD) [109].

Dietary habits and genetic determinants, including microsomal transfer protein (MTP) polymorphisms, may promote NASH and atherogenesis via hypoadiponectinaemia [110,111]. Recently, Musso et al reported that the risk of adiponectin single-nucleotide polymorphisms (SNPs) 45TT and 276 GT are significantly more prevalent in NAFLD than in the general population and are associated with the severity of liver disease. In addition, an association with an atherogenic postprandial lipoprotein profile in NASH was detected independently of fasting adipokine and lipid levels [112].

H) Pro-coagulation and hypofibrinolysis

The prothrombotic state in the atherosclerosis process encompasses platelets hyperaggregability, hypercoagulability and hyperfibrinolysis. Markers of fibrinolytic and hemostatic function (e.g. fibrinogen, tissue plasminogen activator, and plasminogen activator inhibitor 1-antigens), are strongly associated with NAFLD. Plasminogen activator inhibitor-1(PAI-1) is expressed in visceral adipose tissue. It is mainly expressed in stromal cells including monocytes, smooth muscle cells and pre-adipocytes [113]. Plasma PAI-1 levels are more closely related to fat accumulation and PAI-1 expression in the liver than in adipose tissue, suggesting that, among insulin-resistant individuals, the fatty liver is an important site of PAI-1 production [114]. We showed also that there is an association between the thrombotic risk factors and the extent of fibrosis in patients with NAFLD [40]. This confirms the central role of the liver in these processes. Fibrinogen, von

Willebrand factor (vWF) and PAI-1 are also considered markers of the acute-phase reaction of inflammation and thrombosis, and has been closely linked to CAD and diabetes mellitus [115]. CRP increases PAI-1 expression and activity in human aortic endothelial cells [116].

6. Clinical implications

It is evident that patients with NASH are more prone to develop CAD (Increase mortality by 86%) than patients with simple steatosis (increase mortality by 55%, 117); however, it has not been clear until now whether the treatment of NAFLD patients will prevent CAD development. We suggest adding a new modality of approaching patients with NAFLD. Once the diagnosis of NAFLD was made, the first step will be a lifestyle intervention using a combination of diet, active walking, and behavior modification [118], with a goal of >10% weight reduction [119]. Mediterranean diet derived mainly from olive oil (rich in omega-9) is recommended [120,121]. We advise to reduce or discontinue the consumption of fast foods and regular soft drinks, which contain fructose [122]. Recently Dunn et al showed that modest wine drinking (20-30 gram/daily) offers protection against suspected NAFLD [123].The second step is to assess the risk of hepatic fibrosis: There are two modalities of assessment of fibrosis in NAFLD: The noninvasive methods of fibrosis include BARD score or Angulo score [124,125]. The invasive methods (liver biopsy) remains the only reliable means to determine prognosis based on the severity of fibrosis.

The third step will include the assessment of cardiovascular risk stratification: We suggest the use of the Framingham score with effort test and/or measurements of the carotids arteries (IMT) as well as biomarkers of inflammation (CRP, fibrinogen), oxidative stress, (MDA, Paraoxonase), Insulin Resistance, (HOMA), lipotoxicity (TG, HDL, LDL, TC), OGTT, and microalbumin/creatinin ratio [126].

The fourth step includes the assessment of malignancy: For patients older than > 45. Colonoscopy, mammography, chest X-ray, gynecology consultation, and tumor markers (CEA, AFP, PSA, and CA19-9, and CA125, stool blood) are recommended since malignancy is the second most common cause of death in patients with NAFLD [127]. The final step is to initiate an appropriate therapy according to the comorbidities, and the clinical status of each patient. A combination therapy is favored.

A) Patients with metabolic syndrome

The most effective antidiabetic agent is metformin especially in obese T2DM or pioglitazone in non-obese patients [128,129]. We advice to delay early insulin therapy because it may increase fibrosis and weight [130]. Whether insulin increases the risk of HCC or not is still under debate. Exenatide induces significant weight loss, which may lead to an insulin-sensitizing effect [131]. Gliptins are a group of drugs, which increase incretin levels by inhibiting the enzyme DPP-4. These agents are relatively new and, as for the GLP-1 analogues, improve insulin resistance in prediabetic individuals and patients with T2DM after weight loss [132]. Lipid-lower agents are mandatory treatment in diabetic patients with NAFLD, statins and fibrates for dyslipidemic and diabetic patients [133-135] are recommended. Renin-angiotensin system (RAS) inhibitors or alpha-blockers for hypertensive patients [136,137]. However, these types of medicines are not approved solely for fatty liver. Low dose aspirin is reasonable for patients with 10 years cardiovascular disease risk >10% and no risk factors for bleeding.

B) Patients without metabolic syndrome

Best evidence for metformin or pioglitazone for 1-2 year in treating NAFLD patients without MetS. However, routine prescription of this drug (pioglitazone) needs further clarification. Vitamin E (400 IU/day) and omega-3 may be recommended [138,139]. However, vitamin E is not approved yet and high dosage may increase all cause mortality (140). Ursodeoxycholic acid has no benefit for NASH patients as compared to placebo (141). Statins for dyslipidemic patients. Aspirin to prevent CAD according to Framingham score (142). Diagnosis of NAFLD may be a clear indication for diabetes screening, and cardiovascular risk screening and should be performed with the use of existing risk calculators and should be guided by established cardiovascular risk factors.

a. For patients with metabolic syndrome: tailored therapy
   - Metformin/ Pioglitazon/Insulin for T2DM.
   - However, routine prescription needs further clarification
   - Statins /Fibrates for atherogenic dyslipidemia
   - Renin angiontensin system inhibitors/ α- blockers for hypertension
b. For patients without metabolic syndrome:
   - Best evidence for metformin/ pioglitazone or vitamin E.
   - However, high dose vitamin E (>400 IU/day) may increase mortality
   - Currently, high dose ursodeoxycholic acid has no benefit for NASH patients
   - Omega-3 and vitamin D (2000 IU/day) may be beneficial.
c. For the future:
   - Promising agents awaiting randomized controlled trials (Fatostatin,
   - (Aramchol, DPP-4 inhibitors, GLP-1 agonists and combination therapy)

Table 2. Pharmacologic treatment of patients with NAFLD

7. Conclusion

NAFLD is a growing public health problem worldwide. The clinical impact of NAFLD on CAD risk deserves particular attention in view of the implications for screening and surveillance strategies in the growing number of NAFLD patients. NAFLD is associated with increased biomarkers level of chronic inflammation and atherosclerosis. Pharmacotherapy should be given for patients at high risk for complications (NASH, T2DM, obesity, atherogenic dyslipidemia). However, it is not currently known whether improving NAFLD will prevent the development and progression of CAD. Moreover, the prognostic value of NAFLD in CAD risk stratification has yet to be determined. NAFLD patients should be candidate not only for aggressive treatment of their liver disease , but also for aggressive treatment of underlying CAD risk factors, because many patients with NAFLD will have major CAD events and die prior to the development of advanced liver disease.

8. References

[1] Angulo P. Nonalcoholic fatty liver disease. N Engl J Med 2002; 346: 1221-1231.
[2] Targher G, Arcaro G. Non-alcoholic fatty liver disease and increased risk of cardiovascular disease. Atherosclerosis 2007; 191:2:235-240.

[3] Marchesini G, Bugianesi E, Forlani G, Cerrelli F, Lenzi M, Manini R, et al. Nonalcoholic fatty liver, steatohepatitis, and the metabolic syndrome. Hepatology 2003;4: 917-923.

[4] Younossi Z, Diehl AM, Ong JP. Nonalcoholic fatty liver disease: an agenda for clinical research. Hepatology 2002; 35:746-52.

[5] Bruke A, Lucey MR. Non-alcoholic fatty liver disease, non-alcoholic steatohepatitis and orthotopic liver transplantation. Am J Transplant 2004;5: 686-693.

[6] Petersen KF, Dufour S, Hariri A, Nelson-Williams C, Foo JN, Zhang XM, et al. Apolipoprotein C3 gene variants in nonalcoholic fatty liver disease. N Engl J Med 2010; 362:1082-1089.

[7] Gami AS, Witt BJ, Howard DE, Erwin PJ, Gami LA, Somers VK, et al. Metabolic syndrome and risk of incident cardiovascular events and death: a systemic review and meta-analysis of longitudinal studies. J Am Coll Cardiol 2007; 30:4:403-414.

[8] Ford ES, Schulze MB, Pischon T, Bergmann MM, Joost HG, Boeing H. Metabolic syndrome and risk of incident diabetes: findings from the European Prospective Investigation into Cancer and Nutrition-Potsdam Study. Cardiovasc Diabetol 2008; 7:35.

[9] Ford ES, Li C, Sattar N. Metabolic syndrome and incident diabetes: current state of the evidence. Diabetes Care 2008;9:1898-904.

[10] Lakka HM, Laaksonen DE, Lakka TA, Niskanen LK, Kumpusalo E, Tuomilehto J, et al. The metabolic syndrome and total and cardiovascular disease mortality in middle-aged men. JAMA 2002;21:2709-2716.

[11] Isomaa B, Almgren P, Tuomi T, Forsén B, Lahti K, Nissén M, et al. Cardiovascular morbidity and mortality associated with the metabolic syndrome. Diabetes Care 2001; 24:683-689.

[12] Malik S, Wong ND, Franklin SS, Kamath TV, L'Italien GJ, Pio JR, et al. Impact of the metabolic syndrome on mortality from coronary heart disease, cardiovascular disease, and all causes in United States adults. Circulation 2004;10:1245-1250.

[13] Browning JD, Szczepaniak LS, Dobbins R, Nuremberg P, Horton JD, Cohen JC, et al. Prevalence of hepatic steatosis in an urban population in the United States: impact of ethnicity. Hepatology 2004; 40:1387-1395.

[14] Sagi R, Reif S, Neuman G, Webb M, Phillip M, Shalitin S. Nonalcoholic fatty liver disease in overweight children and adolescents. Acta Paediatr 2007; 96:1209-1213.

[15] Hamaguchi M, Kojima T, Takeda N, Nagata C, Takeda J, Sarui H, et al. Nonalcoholic fatty liver disease is a novel predictor of cardiovascular disease. World J Gastroenterol 2007;13:1579-1584.

[16] Abid A, Taha O, Nseir W, Farah R, Grosovski M, Assy N. Soft drink consumption is associated with fatty liver disease independent of metabolic syndrome. J Hepatol 2009; 51:918-924.

[17] Targher G, Bertolini L, Padovani R, Zenari L, Zoppini G, Falezza G. Relation of nonalcoholic hepatic steatosis to early carotid atherosclerosis in healthy men: role of visceral fat accumulation. Diabetes Care 2004;10:2498-2500.

[18] Brea A, Mosquera D, Martin E, Arizti A, Cordero JL, Ros E. Nonalcoholic fatty liver disease is associated with carotid atherosclerosis: a case-control study. Arterioscler Thromb Vasc Biol 2005; 5:1040-1050.

[19] Lin YC, Lo HM, Chen JD. Sonographic fatty liver, overweight and ischemic heart disease. World J Gastroenterol 2005;11:4838-4842.
[20] Villanova N, Moscatiello S, Ramilli S, Bugianesi E, Magalotii D, Vanni E, et al. Endothelial dysfunction and cardiovascular risk profile in nonalcoholic fatty liver disease. Hepatology 2005; 2:473-480.
[21] Schindhelm RK, Diamant M, Bakker SJ, van Dijk RA, Scheffer PG, Teerlink T, et al. Liver alanine aminotransferase, insulin resistance and endothelial dysfunction in normotriglyceridaemic subjects with type 2 diabetes mellitus. Eur J Clin Invest 2005;6:369-374.
[22] Targher G, Bertolini L, Padovani R, Poli F, Scala L, Tessari R, et al. Increased prevalence of cardiovascular disease in Type 2 diabetic patients with non-alcoholic fatty liver disease. Diabet Med 2006; 23:403-409.
[23] Targher G, Bertolini L, Padovani R, Rodella S, Zoppini G, Zenari L, et al. Relation between carotid artery wall thickness and liver histology in subjects with nonalcoholic fatty liver disease. Diabetes Care 2006; 29:1325-1330.
[24] Akabame S, Hamaguchi M, Tomiyasu K, Tanaka M, Kobayashi- Takenaka Y, Nakano K, et al. Evaluation of vulnerable coronary plaques and non-alcoholic fatty liver disease (NAFLD) by 64-detector multislice computed tomography (MSCT). Circ J 2008;72:618-625.
[25] Assy N, Djibre A, Farah R, Grosovski M, Marmor A. Presence of coronary plaques in patients with nonalcoholic fatty liver disease. Radiology 2010; 254:393-400.
[26] Pacifico L, Cantisani V, Ricci P, Osborn JF, Schiavo E, Ferrara E, et al. Nonalcoholic fatty liver disease and carotid atherosclerosis in children. Paediatr Res 2008; 63:423-427.
[27] Adams LA, Lymp JF, St Sauver J, Sanderson SO, Lindor KD, Feldstein A, et al. The natural history of nonalcoholic fatty liver disease: a population-based cohort study. Gastroenterology 2005;1:113-121.
[28] Matteoni CA, Younossi ZM, Gramlich T, Boparai N, Liu YC, McCullough AJ. Nonalcoholic fatty liver disease: a spectrum of clinical and pathological severity. Gastroenterology 1999; 6:1413-1419.
[29] Targher G, Bertolini L, Poli F, Rodella S, Scala L, Tessari R, et al. Nonalcoholic fatty liver disease and risk of future cardiovascular events among type 2 diabetic patients. Diabetes 2005; 54:3541-3546.
[30] Targher G, Bertolini L, Rodella S, Tessari R, Zenari L, Lippi G, et al. Nonalcoholic fatty liver disease is independently associated with an increased incidence of cardiovascular events in type 2 diabetic patients. Diabetes Care 2007; 8:2119-2121.
[31] Dunn W, Xu R, Wingard DL, Rogers C, Angulo P, Younossi ZM, et al. Suspected nonalcoholic fatty liver disease and mortality risk in a population-based cohort study. Am J Gastroenterol 2008;9:2263-2271.
[32] Ruttmann E, Brant LJ, Concin H, Diem G, Rapp K, Ulmer H. Gamma-glutamyltransferase as a risk factor for cardiovascular disease mortality: an epidemiological investigation in a cohort of 163,944 Austrian adults. Circulation 2005;14:2130-2137.
[33] Lee DS, Evans JC, Robins SJ, Wilson PW, Albano I, Fox CS, et al. Gamma glutamyl transferase and metabolic syndrome, cardiovascular disease, and mortality risk: the Framingham Heart Study. Arterioscler Thromb Vasc Biol 2007;1:127-133.

[34] Ekstedt M, Franzen LE, Mathiesen UL, Thorelius L, Holmqvist M, Bodemar G, et al. Long-term follow-up of patients with NAFLD and elevated liver enzymes. Hepatology 2006; 40: 865-873.
[35] Ong JP, Pitts A, Younossi ZM. Increased overall mortality and liver-related mortality in non-alcoholic fatty liver disease. J Hepatol 2008; 49:608-612.
[36] Soderberg C, Stal P, Askling J, Glaumann H, Lindberg G, Marmur J,et al. Decreased survival of subjects with elevated liver function tests during a 28-year follow-up. Hepatology 2010;2:595-602.
[37] Park SH, Kim BI, Yun JW, Kim JW, Park DI, Cho YK, et al. Insulin resistance and C-reactive protein as independent risk factors for non-alcoholic fatty liver disease in non-obese Asian men. J Gastroenterol Hepatol 2004; 6:694-698.
[38] Lee S, Jin Kim Y, Yong Jeon T, Hoi Kim H, Woo OH S, Park Y, et al. Obesity is the only independent factor associated with ultrasound-diagnosed non-alcoholic fatty disease: a cross-sectional case-control study. Scand J Gastroenterol 2006; 51:566-572.
[39] Hirsch S, Poniachick J, Avendano M, Csendes A, Burdiles P, Smok G, et al. Serum folate and homocysteine levels in obese females with non-alcoholic fatty liver. Nutrition 2005; 2: 137-141.
[40] Assy N, Bekirov I, Mejritsky Y, Solomon L, Szvalb S, Hussein O. Association between thrombotic risk factors and extent of fibrosis in patients with non-alcoholic fatty liver diseases. World J Gastroenterol 2005;37:5834-5839.
[41] Sookoian S, Castano GO, Burgueno AL, Rosselli MS, Gianotti TF, Mallardi P, et al. Circulating levels and hepatic expression of molecular mediators of atherosclerosis in nonalcoholic fatty liver disease. Atherosclerosis 2010; 2:585-591.
[42] Ruhl CE, Everhart JE. Epidemiology of nonalcoholic fatty liver. Clin Liver Dis 2004;3:501-519.
[43] Carulli L, Lonardo A, Lombardini S, Marchesini G, Loria P. Gender, fatty liver and GGT. Hepatology 2006; 44:278-279.
[44] Powell KE, Thompson PD, Caspersen CJ, Kendrick JS. Physical activity and the incidence of coronary heart disease. Annu Rev Public Health 1987; 8:253-287.
[45] Hsieh SD, Yoshinaga H, Muto T, Sakurai Y. Regular physical activity and coronary risk factors in Japanese men. Circulation 1998; 97: 661-665.
[46] Church TS, Kuk JL, Ross R, Priest EL, Biltoft E, Blair SN. Association of cardiorespiratory fitness, body mass index, and waist circumference to nonalcoholic fatty liver disease. Gastroenterology 2006;7:2023-2030.
[47] Zelber-Sagi S, Nitzan- Kaliski D, Goldsmith R, Webb M, Zvibel I, Goldiner I, et al. Role of leisure-time physical activity in alcoholic fatty liver disease: a population-based study. Hepatology 2008;48:1791-1798.
[48] Stamler J, Vaccaro O, Neaton JD, Wentworth D. Diabetes, other risk factors, and 12-yr cardiovascular mortality for men screened in the Multiple Risk Factor Intervention Trial. Diabetes Care 1993; 16:434-444.
[49] Adlerberth AM, Rosengren A, Wilhelmsen L. Diabetes and long-term risk of mortality from coronary and other causes in middle-aged Swedish men. A general population study. Diabetes Care 1998; 21:539-545.
[50] De Marco R, Locatelli F, Zoppini G, Verlato G, Bonora E, Muggeo M. Cause-specific mortality in type 2 diabetes. The Verona Diabetes Study. Diabetes Care 1999; 22:756-761.

[51] Marchesini G, Marzocchi R, Agostini F, Bugianesi E: Nonalcoholic fatty liver disease and metabolic syndrome.Curr Opin Lipidol 2005;16:421-427.
[52] Hanley AJ, Williams K, Festa A, Wagenknecht LE, D'Agostino RB Jr, Kempf J, et al. Insulin resistance atherosclerosis study. Diabetes 2004; 53:2623-2632.
[53] Stamler J, Wentworth D, Neaton JD. Is relationship between serum cholesterol and risk of premature death from coronary heart continues and graded? Findings in 356,222 primary screenees of the Multiple Risk Factor Intervention Trial (MRFIT). JAMA 1986; 256:2823-2828.
[54] Assy N, Kaita K, Mymin D, Levy C, Rosser B, Minuk G. Fatty infiltration of liver in hyperlipidemic patients. Dig Dis Sci 2000; 45:1929-1934.
[55] Clark JM, Diehl AM. Nonalcoholic fatty liver disease: an underrecognized cause of cryptogenic cirrhosis. JAMA 2003; 289:3000-3004.
[56] Radu C, Grigoriscu M, Crisan D, Lupsor M, Constantin D, Dina L. Prevalence and associated risk factors of non-alcoholic fatty liver disease in hospitalized patients. J Gastrointestin Liver Dis 2008; 17:255-260.
[57] Rabkin SW, Mathewson FA, Hsu PH. Relation of body weight to development of ischemic heart disease in a cohort of young North American men after a 26 year of observation period: the Manitoba study. Am J Cardiol 1977;39:452-458.
[58] Hubert HB, Feinleib M, McNamara PM, Castelli WP. Obesity as an independent risk factor for cardiovascular disease: a 26-year follow-up of participants in the Framingham Heart Study. Circulation 1983; 67: 968-977.
[59] Ruhl CE, Everhart JE. Determination of the association of overweight with elevated serum alanine aminotransferase activity in the United States. Gastroenterology 2003; 124:71-79.
[60] Marcos A, Fisher RA, Ham JM, Olzinski AT, Shiffman ML, Sanyal AJ, Luketic VA, et al. Selection and outcome of living donors for adult-to-adult right lobe transplantation. Transplantation 2000; 69:2410-2415.
[61] Hilden M, Christoffersen P, Juhl E, Dalgaard JB. Liver histology in a 'normal' population- examination of 503 consecutive fatal traffic casualties. Scand J Gastroenterol 1977; 12:593-597.
[62] Lee RG. Nonalcoholic steatohepatitis a study of 49 patients. Hum Pathol 1989; 20: 594-598.
[63] Gholam PM, Kotler DP, Flancbaum LJ. Liver pathology in morbidity obese patients undergoing Roux-en-Y gastric bypass surgery. Obes Surg 2000; 12:49-51.
[64] Neal B, MacMahon S, Chapman N. Effects of ACE inhibitors, calcium antagonists, and other blood pressure-lowering drugs. Lancet 2000; 356:1955-1964.
[65] Donati G, Stagni B, Piscaglia F, Venturoli N, Morselli-Labate AM, Rasciti L, et al. Increased prevalence of fatty liver in arterial hypertensive patients with normal liver enzymes: role of insulin resistance. Gut 2004; 53:1020-1023.
[66] Yokohama S, Yoneda M, Haneda M, Okamoto S, Okada M, Aso K, et al. Therapeutic efficacy of an angiotensin II receptor antagonist in patients with nonalcoholic steatohepatitis. Hepatology 2004; 40:1222-1225.
[67] Day CP. Non-alcoholic steatohepatitis (NASH): where are we now and where are we going? Gut 2002:50:585-588.
[68] Yang S, Zhu H, Gabrielson K, Trush MA, Diehl AM. Mitochondrial adaptation to obesity-related oxidant stress. Arch Biochem Biophys 2000; 378:259-268.

[69] Leclercq IA, Farrel GC, Field J, Bell DR, Gonzalez FJ, Robertson GR. CYP2E1 and CYP4A as microsomal catalysts of lipid peroxides in murine nonalcoholic steatohepatitis. J Clin Invest 2000;105:1067-1075.

[70] Seki S, Kitada T, Yamada T, Sakaguchi H, Nakatani K, Wakasa K. In situ detection of lipid peroxidation and oxidative DNA damage in non-alcoholic fatty liver disease. J Hepatol 2002; 37:56-62.

[71] Chalasani N, Deeg MA, Crabb DW. Systemic levels of lipid peroxidation and its metabolic and dietary correlates in patients with nonalcoholic steatohepatitis. Am J Gastroenterol 2004; 99:1497-1502.

[72] Berliner JA, Navab M, Fogelman AM, Frank JS, Demer LL, Edwards PA, et al. Atherosclerosis: basic mechanisms. Oxidation, inflammation, and genetics. Circulation 1995;91:2488-2496.

[73] Nishio E, Watanabe Y. The involvement of reactive oxygen species and arachidonic acid in alpha 1-adrenoceptor-ibduced smooth muscle cell proliferation and migration. Br J Pharmacol 1997;121:665-70.

[74] Schulz E, Anter E, Keaney JF. Oxidative stress, antioxidants, and endothelial function. Curr Med Chem 2004; 11:1093-1104.

[75] Bugianesi E, McCullough AJ, Marchesini G. Insulin resistance: a metabolic pathway to chronic liver disease. Hepatology 2005; 42:987-1000.

[76] Seppala-Lindroos A, Vehkavaara S, Hakkinen AM, Goto T, Westerbacka J, Sovijarvi A, et al. Fat accumulation in the liver is associated with defects in insulin suppression of glucose production and serum free fatty acids independent of obesity in normal men. J Clin Endocrinol Metab 2002; 87:3023-3028.

[77] Bonora E, Formentini G, Calcaterra F, Lombardi S, Marini F, Zenari L, et al. HOMA-estimated insulin resistance is an independent predictor of cardiovascular disease in type 2 diabetic subjects: prospective data from the Verona Diabetes Complications Study. Diabetes Care 2002; 25:1135-1141.

[78] Pilz S, Scharnagl H, Tiran B, Seelhorst U, Wellnitz B, Boehm BO, et al. Free fatty acids are independently associated with all-cause and cardiovascular mortality in subjects with coronary artery disease. J Clin Endocrinol Metab 2006 ;91:2542-2547.

[79] Howard G, O'Leary DH, Zaccaro D, Haffner S, Rewers M, Hamman R, et al. Insulin sensivity and atherosclerosis: the Insulin Resistance Atherosclerosis Study (IRAS) Investigators. Circulation 1996; 93:1809-1817.

[80] Targher G, Bertolini L, Scala L, Zoppini G, Zenari L, Falezza G. Non-alcoholic hepatic steatosis and its relation to increased plasma biomarkers of inflammation and endothelial dysfunction in non-diabetic men. Role of visceral adipose tissue. Diabet Med 2005; 22:1354-1358.

[81] Wieckowska A, Papouchado BG, Li Z, Lopez R, Zein NN, Feldstein AE. Increased hepatic and circulating interleukin-6 levels in human nonalcoholic steatohepatitis. Am J Gastroenterol 2008;103:1372-1379.

[82] Ridker PM, Rifai N, Pfeffer M, Sacks F, Lepage S, Braunwald E. Elevation of tumor necrosis factor-alpha and increased risk of recurrent coronary events after myocardial infarction. Circulation 2000; 101:2149-2153.

[83] Ridker PM, Rifai N, Stampfer MJ, Hennekens CH. Plasma concentration of interleukin-6 and the risk of future myocardial infarction among apparently healthy men. Circulation 2000; 101:1767-1772.

[84] Ridker PM, Hennekens CH, Buring JE, Rifai N. C-reactive protein and other markers of inflammation in the prediction of cardiovascular disease in women. N Eng J Med 2000; 342:836-843.
[85] Toss H, Lindahl B, Siegbahn A, Wallentin L. Prognostic influence of increased fibrinogen and C-reactive protein levels in unstable coronary artery disease. FRISC Study Group. Fragmin during Instability in Coronary Artery Disease. Circulation 1997; 96:4204-4210.
[86] Rebuzzi AG, Quaranta G, Liuzzo G, Caligiuri G, Lanza GA, Gallimore JR, et al. Incremental prognosis value of serum levels of troponin T and C-reactive protein on admission in patients with unstable angina pectoris. Am J Cardiol 1998; 82:715-719.
[87] Shoelson SE, Lee J, Goldfine AB. Inflammation and insulin resistance. J Clin Invest 2006; 116:1793-1801.
[88] Van Gaal LF, Mertens IL, De Block CE. Mechanisms linking obesity with cardiovascular disease. Nature 2006; 444:875-880.
[89] Day CP. From fat to inflammation. Gastroenterology 2006; 130: 207-210.
[90] Marra F, Gastaldelli A. Svegliati Baroni G, Tell C, Tiribelli C. Molecular basis and mechanisms of progression of non-alcoholic steatohepatitis. Trends Mol Med 2008;14:72-81.
[91] Libby P. Inflammation in atherosclerosis. Nature 2002; 420:868-874.
[92] Ridker PM, Danielson E, Fonseca FA, Genest J, Gotto AM Jr, Kastelein JJ, et al. JUPITER Study Group. Rosuvastatin to prevent vascular events in men and women with elevated C-reactive protein. N Engl J Med 2008; 359:2195-2207.
[93] Hui JM, Hodge A, Farrell GC, Kench JG, Kriketos A, George J. Beyond insulin resistance in NASH: TNF-alpha or adiponectin? Hepatology 2004;40:46-54.
[94] Kumada M, Kihara S, Ouchi N, Kobayashi H, Okamoto Y, Ohashi K, et al. Adiponectin specifically increased tissue inhibitor of metalloproteinase-1 through interleukin-10 expression in human macrophages. Circulation 2004; 109:2046-2049.
[95] Kobayashi H, Ouchi N, Kihara S, Walsh K, Kumada M, Abe Y, et al. Selective suppression of endothelial cell apoptosis by the high molecular weight form of adiponectin. Circ Res 2004; 94:e27-31.
[96] Schram K, Sweeney G. Implications of myocardial matrix remodeling by adipokines in obesity-related heart failure. Trends Cardiovasc Med. 2008 ;18:199-205.
[97] Lautamäki R, Borra R, Iozzo P, Komu M, Lehtimäki T, Salmi M, Jalkanen S, Airaksinen KE, Knuuti J, Parkkola R, Nuutila P. Liver steatosis coexists with myocardial insulin resistance and coronary dysfunction in patients with type 2 diabetes. Am J Physiol Endocrinol Metab. 2006 ;291:E282-90.
[98] Taskinen MR. Lipoprotein lipase in diabetes. Diabetes Metab Rev 1987;3:551-570.
[99] Verges B. New insight into the pathophysiology of lipid abnormalities in type 2 diabetes. Diabetes Metab 2005;31:429-439.
[100] Frenais R, Nazih H, Ouguerram K, Maugeais C, Zair Y, Bard JM, et al. In vivo evidence for the role of lipoprotein lipase activity in the regulation of Apolipoprotein AI metabolism: a kinetic study in control subjects and patients with type II diabetes mellitus. J Clin Endocrinol Metab 2001; 86:1962-1967.

[101] Adiels M, Taskinen MR, Packard C, Caslake MJ, Soro-Paavonen A, Westerbacka J, et al. Overproduction of large VLDL particles is driven by increased liver fat content in man. Diabetologia 2006;49:755-765.
[102] Gardner CD, Fortmann SP, Krauss RM. Association of small low-density lipoprotein particles with the incidence of coronary artery disease in men and women. J Am Med Assoc 1996;276:875-881.
[103] [103] Kwiterovich PO. Clinical relevance of the biochemical, metabolic, and genetic factors that influence low-density lipoprotein heterogeneity. Am J Cardiol 2002; 90:30i-47i.
[104] Adiels M, Olofsson SO, Taskinen MR, Boren J. Diabetic dyslipidemia. Curr Opin Lipidol 2006; 17:238-246.
[105] Cassader M, Gambino R, Musso G, Depetris N, Mecca F, Cavallo-Perin P, ey al. Postprandial triglyceride-rich lipoprotein metabolism and insulin sensitivity in nonalcoholic steatohepatitis patients. Lipids 2001; 36;1117-1124.
[106] Roche HM, Gibney MJ. The impact of postprandial lipemia in accelerating atherothrombosis. J Cardiovasc.Risk 2000; 7:317-324.
[107] Tanaka A. Postprandial hyperlipidemia and atherosclerosis. J Atheroscler Thromb 2004;11:322-329.
[108] Brown ML, Ramprassad MP, Umeda PK, Tanaka A, Kobayashi Y, Watanabe T, et al. A macrophage receptor for apolipoprotein B48: cloning, expression, and atherosclerosis. Proc Natl Acad Sci USA 2000; 97:7488-7493.
[109] Stanhope KL, Schwarz JM, Keim NL, Griffen SC, Bremer AA, Graham JL, et al. Consuming fructose-sweetened, not glucose- sweetened, beverages increases visceral adiposity and lipids and decreases insulin sensivity in overweight / obese humans. J Clin Invest 2009;119:1322-1334.
[110] Musso G, Gambino R, Durazzo M, Biroli G, Carello M, Faga E, et al. Adipokines in NASH: postprandial lipid metabolism as a link between adiponectin and liver disease. Hepatology 2005; 42:1175-1183.
[111] Musso G, Gambino R, De Michieli F, Cassader M, Rizzetto M, Durazzo M, et al. Dietary habits and their relations to insulin resistance and postprandial lipemia in nonalcoholic steatohepatitis. Hepatology 2003; 37:909-916.
[112] Musso G, Gambino R, De Michieli F, Durazzo M, Pagano G, Cassader M. Adiponectin gene polymorphisms modulate acute adiponectin responses to dietary fat: Possible pathogenetic role in NASH. Hepatology 2008; 47:1167-1177.
[113] Bastelica D, Morange P, Berthet B, Borghi H, Lacroix O, Grino M, et al. Stromal cells are the main plasminogen activator inhibitor-1-producing cells in human fat: evidence of differences between visceral and subcutaneous deposits. Arterioscler Thromb Vasc Biol 2002; 22:173-178.
[114] Alessi MC, Bastelica D, Mavri A, Morange P, Berthet B, Grino M, et al. Plasma PAI-1 levels are more strongly related to liver steatosis than to adipose tissue accumulation. Arterioscler Thromb Vasc Biol 2003; 23:1262-1268.
[115] Esmon CT. The interactions between inflammation and coagulation. Br J Haematol 2005;131:417-430.
[116] Devaraj S, Xu DY, Jialal I. C-reactive protein increases plasminogen activator inhibitor-1 expression and activity in human aortic endothelial cells: implication for the metabolic syndrome and atherothrombosis. Circulation 2003;107:398-404.

[117] Targher G. Non-alcoholic Fatty Liver Disease and Cardiovascular Disease. Curr Cardio Risk Rep 2010;4:32–39.
[118] Kantartzis K, Thamer C, Peter A, Machann J, Schick F, Schrami C, et al. High cardiorespiratory fitness is a an independent predictor of the reduction in liver fat during a lifestyle intervention in non-alcoholic fatty liver disease. Gut 2009; 58:1281-1288.
[119] Promrat K, Kleiner DE, Niemeier HM, Jackvony E, Kearns M, Wands JR, et al. Randomized controlled trial testing the effects of weight loss on nonalcoholic steatohepatitis. Hepatology 2010; 51:121-129.
[120] Assy N, Nassar F, Nasser G, Grosovski M. Olive oil consumption and non-alcoholic fatty liver disease. World J Gastroenterol 2009;15:1809-1815.
[121] Estruch R, Martinez- Gonzalez MA, Corella D, Salas- Salvado J, Ruiz- Gutierrez V, Covas MI, et al; PREDIMED study Investigators. Effect of a Mediterranean diet supplemented with nuts on metabolic syndrome status: one-year results of the PREDIMED randomized trial. Arch Intern Med 2008;22:2449-2458.
[122] Nseir W, Nassar F, Assy N. Soft drinks consumption and nonalcoholic fatty liver disease. World J Gastroenterol 2010;16: 2579-2588.
[123] Dunn W, Xu R, Schwimmer JB. Modest wine drinking and decreased prevalence of suspected nonalcoholic fatty liver disease. Hepatology 2008; 47:1947-1954.
[124] Harrison SA, Oliver D, Arnold HL, Gogia S, Neuschwander-Teri BA. Development and validation of a simple NAFLD clinical scoring system for identifying patients without advanced disease. Gut 2008; 57:1441-1447.
[125] Angulo P, Hui JM, Marchesini G, Bugianesi E, George J, Farrell GC, et al. Hepatology 2007; 45:846-854.
[126] Hwang ST, Cho YK, Yun JW, Park JH, Kim HJ, Park DI, et al. Impact of NAFLD on microalbuminuria in patients with prediabetes and diabetes. Intern Med J 2009; May 8. [Epub ahead of print]
[127] Smith RA, Cokkinides V, Brooks D, Saslow D, Brawley OW. Cancer screening in the United States, 2010: a review of current American Cancer Society guidelines and issues in cancer screening. CA Cancer J Clin 2010; 60:99-119.
[128] Marchesini G, Brizi M, Bianchi G, Tomassetti S, Zoli M, Melchionda N. Metformin in non-alcoholic steatohepatitis. Lancet 2001; 9285:893-894.
[129] Promrat K, Lutchman G, Uwaifo GI, Freedman RJ, Soza A, Heller T, et al. A pilot study of pioglitazone treatment for nonalcoholic steatohepatitis. Hepatology 2004; 1:188-196.
[130] Paradis V, Perlemuter G, Bonvoust F, Dargere D, Parfait B, Vidaud M, et al. High glucose and hyperinsulinemia stimulate connective tissue growth factor expression: a potential mechanism involved in progression to fibrosis in nonalcoholic steatohepatitis. Hepatology 2001; 34:73-44.
[131] Klonoff DC, Buse JB, Nielsen LL, Guan X, Bowlus CL, Holcombe JH, et al. Exenatide effects on diabetes, obesity, cardiovascular risk factors and hepatic biomarkers in patients with type 2 diabetes treated for at least 3 years. Curr Med Res Opin 2008;1:275-286.
[132] Balaban YH, Korkusuz P, Simsek H, Gokcan H, Gedikoglu G, Pinar A, et al. Dipeptidyl peptidase IV (DDP IV) in NASH patients. Ann Hepatol 2007; 4:242-250.

[133] Antonopoulos S, Mikros S, Mylonopoulou M, Kokkoris S, Giannoulis G. Rosuvastatin as a novel treatment of non-alcoholic fatty liver disease in hyperlipidemic patients. Atherosclerosis 2006;1:233-234.

[134] Gomez-Dominguez E, Gisbert JP, Moreno-Monteagudo JA, García-Buey L, Moreno-Otero R. A pilot study of atorvastatin treatment in dyslipemid, non-alcoholic fatty liver patients. Aliment Pharmacol Ther 2006;11:1643-1647.

[135] Browning JD. Stains and hepatic steatosis: perspectives from the Dallas Heart Study. Hepatology 2006; 44:466-471.

[136] Yoshiji H, Kuriyama S, Yoshii J, Ikenaka Y, Nakatani T, Tsujinoue H, et al. Angiotensin-II type 1 receptor interaction is a major regulator for liver fibrosis development in rats. Hepatology 2001; 34:745-750.

[137] Georgescu EF, Ionescu R, Niculescu M, Mogoanta L, Vancica L. Angiotensin-receptor blockers as therapy for mild-to-moderate hypertension-associated non-alcoholic steatohepatitis. World J Gastroenterol 2009;8:942-954.

[138] Sanyal AJ, Mofrad PS, Contos MJ, Sargeant C, Luketic VA, Sterling RK, et al. A pilot study of vitamin E versus vitamin E and pioglitazone for the treatment of nonalcoholic steatohepatitis. Clin Gastroenterol Hepatol 2004;12:1107-1115.

[139] Masterton GS, Plevris JN, Hayes PC. Review article: omega-3 fatty acids- a promising novel therapy for non-alcoholic fatty liver disease. Aliment Pharmacol Ther 2010;7:679-692.

[140] Miller ER 3rd, Pastor-Barriuso R, Dalal D, Riemersma RA, Appel LJ, Guallar E. Meta-analysis: high-dosage vitamin E supplementation may increase all-cause mortality. Ann Intern Med. 2005 ;142:37-46.

[141] Leuschner UF, Lindenthal B, Herrmann G, Arnold JC, Rössle M, Cordes HJ, Zeuzem S, Hein J, Berg T; NASH Study Group. High-dose ursodeoxycholic acid therapy for nonalcoholic steatohepatitis: a double-blind, randomized, placebo-controlled trial. Hepatology. 2010;52:472-9.

[142] Targher G, Day CP, Bonora E. Risk of cardiovascular disease in patients with nonalcoholic fatty liver disease. N Engl J Med. 2010 30;363:1341-50.